RESPIRATION in HEALTH and DISEASE

Third Edition

REUBEN M. CHERNIACK, M.D.

D.Sc. (Man.), F.R.C.P.(C), F.R.C.P., F.A.C.P., F.C.C.P.

Cetalie and Marcel Weiss Chairman, Department of Medicine,
National Jewish Hospital and Research Center;
Professor and Vice Chairman, Department of Medicine,
University of Colorado

LOUIS CHERNIACK, M.D.

F.R.C.P., F.R.C.P.(C), F.A.C.P., F.C.C.P.

Associate Professor of Medicine, Emeritus,
University of Manitoba

W. B. SAUNDERS COMPANY • 1983

- *Philadelphia*
- *London*
- *Toronto*
- *Mexico City*
- *Rio de Janeiro*
- *Sydney*
- *Tokyo*

W. B. Saunders Company: West Washington Square
Philadelphia, PA 19105

1 St. Anne's Road
Eastbourne, East Sussex BN21 3UN, England

1 Goldthorne Avenue
Toronto, Ontario M8Z 5T9, Canada

Apartado 26370—Cedro 512
Mexico 4, D.F., Mexico

Rua Coronel Cabrita, 8
Sao Cristovao Caixa Postal 21176
Rio de Janeiro, Brazil

9 Waltham Street
Artarmon, N.S.W. 2064, Australia

Ichibancho, Central Bldg., 22-1 Ichibancho
Chiyoda-Ku, Tokyo 102, Japan

Library of Congress Cataloging in Publication Data

Cherniack, Reuben M.

Respiration in health and disease.

Bibliography: p.

Includes index.

1. Respiratory organs—Diseases.   2. Respiration.
I. Cherniack, Louis.   II. Title. [DNLM: 1. Respiration.
2. Respiratory tract diseases. WF 140 C521r]

RC731.C45 1983   616.2   83–14300

ISBN 0–7216–2527–4

Respiration in Health and Disease   ISBN   0-7216-2527-4

Last digit is the print number: 9   8   7   6   5   4   3   2   1

PREFACE

This book is once again directed at the student. The mechanism of development of symptoms and signs, and the correlation of clinical, radiologic, morphologic and functional disturbances are again emphasized. We have attempted to summarize current knowledge in pulmonary physiology and the role of effector cells and the immune system in defending the lungs against foreign agents. In addition, current concepts of the development of chronic respiratory disease and the principles of therapy have been updated.

The first edition of this text was dedicated to Dr. Joseph Doupe, and the foreword was written by Dr. Lennox Bell. Both were friends and mentors of my brother and me, and we benefited extensively from their counsel and frequent constructive criticism. When we began to write this third edition, we again wanted to dedicate it to these two men. Although this remains very appropriate, I especially want this third edition to be devoted to my brother, Dr. Louis Cherniack, who passed away while this edition was being written. Louis was a scholar and a gentleman. He was an exceptional clinician and teacher who continually stressed the importance of a thorough history and had the uncanny ability to demonstrate pathology in the lung by physical examination. Rounds with Louis were always stimulating and challenging at the same time. I hope the book will live up to all his expectations.

We wish to thank the many additional students and confreres who have provided helpful suggestions and criticisms along with their encouragement. We especially wish to thank Drs. Arnold Naimark and Vic Chernick, who contributed to the second edition of the book and whose contributions have influenced significantly certain areas in this edition. Special acknowledgment is once again given to Nancy Joy, whose excellent illustrations in the first edition have stood the test of time and form the basis of most of the figures in this edition, and to Peggy Hammond, whose outstanding secretarial assistance and enthusiasm were immeasurably valuable and without whom this book would likely never have been completed. The additional secretarial assistance of Susan Krois, Billie Wilson, Lydia Titus and Sandy Sarris is also gratefully acknowledged.

REUBEN M. CHERNIACK

CONTENTS

Section II   MANIFESTATIONS OF RESPIRATORY DISEASE

9
PRIMARY MANIFESTATIONS OF PULMONARY DISEASE 163

10
SECONDARY MANIFESTATIONS OF PULMONARY DISEASE 183

Section III   ASSESSMENT OF RESPIRATORY DISEASE

11
CLINICAL ASSESSMENT.. 195

12
RADIOLOGIC ASSESSMENT... 231

13
LABORATORY ASSESSMENT 243

Section IV THE PATTERNS OF RESPIRATORY DISEASE

14
AIRWAY DISEASE

15
LUNG PARENCHYMAL DISEASE

16
PULMONARY VASCULAR DISEASE

17
PLEURAL DISEASE

18
CHEST WALL AND DIAPHRAGMATIC DISEASE

Section V RESPIRATORY FAILURE

19
PATHOPHYSIOLOGY OF RESPIRATORY FAILURE....................... 365

20
MANAGEMENT OF CHRONIC RESPIRATORY FAILURE 374

21
MANAGEMENT OF ACUTE RESPIRATORY FAILURE 389

SUGGESTED ADDITIONAL READING

INDEX

INTRODUCTION

The main functions of the respiratory system are to supply oxygen to the cells of the body and to remove carbon dioxide from them. The oxygen is transported into the lungs during inspiration, and carbon dioxide is eliminated in the expired air. The oxygen is carried from the lungs to the tissues, and the carbon dioxide from the tissues to the lungs, via the circulation. To generate the mechanical energy needed for ventilation between the atmosphere and lungs and circulation between the lungs and the tissues, active work must be performed by the respiratory muscles and the heart. As we shall see, it is possible to regulate the bulk transport of gases between the environment and the lungs, or their convective transport between the lungs and the tissues, by influencing the activity of respiratory and cardiac muscles.

To understand how gas exchange takes place in either the lungs or the tissues, one must understand certain physical properties of gases as well as their behavior. For instance, if a volume of gas is placed in a container, it expands until it fills the container, because the gas molecules diffuse very rapidly throughout it. The gas exerts a pressure that is related to the amount of bombardment of the walls of the containing vessel by the molecules of the gas. If a mixture of two or more gases is confined within the same space, each gas behaves independently, as if it alone were in that space. In other words, the molecules of each gas are uniformly distributed throughout the space, and the pressure that each gas exerts depends on its own concentration, regardless of the concentration of the other gases.

The pressure that a gas exerts, whether alone or mixed with other gases, is called the *partial pressure,* or the *tension,* of that gas, and is expressed in mm. Hg, or *torr.* It is indicated by the letter *P* preceding the symbol for the gas; e.g., P_{O_2} is the partial pressure of oxygen, and P_{CO_2} that of carbon dioxide. The total pressure exerted by a mixture of gases is the arithmetic sum of the partial pressures of all the gases that make up the mixture. For instance, the total pressure of air at sea level is 760 mm. Hg, and this is the sum of the partial pressures of the oxygen, carbon dioxide, nitrogen and the inert gases (such as argon and neon) that it contains. Since ambient air contains 20.94 per cent oxygen, 0.04 per cent carbon dioxide and 79 per cent nitrogen, their partial pressures are 159, 0.3 and 600 mm. Hg, respectively.

According to *Boyle's law,* the pressure of a gas will rise when the volume of the container is reduced, because the molecules of gas are then closer together and they increase their bombardment of the walls of the container. Similarly, according to *Gay-Lussac's law,* the pressure of a gas will rise when its temperature is raised, provided the volume is kept constant, because the speed of molecular movement increases, and as a result, there is greater bombardment of the gas molecules on the boundaries of the confining space.

When the partial pressure of a gas is different in two parts of a system, there will be a concentration gradient between the two parts. The gas will diffuse readily between the two parts of the system, and because its pressure is higher in one part, it will diffuse from the region with a high concentration to the region of low concentration. If the system is left undisturbed, the gas will continue to diffuse until its partial pressure is the same in both parts of the system. The rate at which it diffuses depends on its diffusing properties and the steepness of the concentration gradient.

Similarly, if one exposes a liquid free of gas to air, gases will diffuse from the air phase to the liquid phase until the partial pressure of each of the gases is the same in the two phases. The volume of gas transferred from the air phase to the liquid phase before the partial pressure comes to equilibrium is ordinarily related to the solubility of the gases in the liquid phase. For example, if 1 liter of blood plasma is exposed to a continuous stream of water-saturated gas with a P_{O_2} of 100 mm. Hg, oxygen will be taken up by the plasma until its P_{O_2} is also 100 mm. Hg. Since the solubility of O_2 in plasma is 0.003 ml./mm. Hg/100 ml. plasma, the total amount of oxygen transferred will be approximately 3 ml.

When the respiratory muscles contract during inspiration, ambient air enters the alveoli and, as a result, the alveolar P_{O_2} is raised and the P_{CO_2} is lowered. The blood that enters the lungs (mixed venous) comes from the tissues, where oxygen has been extracted and carbon dioxide has been added; i.e., the P_{O_2} in the blood is low and the P_{CO_2} is high. Because of the difference in partial pressures between the alveoli and the mixed venous blood (for oxygen 100 versus 40 mm. Hg, and for carbon dioxide 40 versus 46 mm. Hg), oxygen moves into the pulmonary capillary blood and some of the carbon dioxide moves from the blood into the alveoli. As the diffusion of oxygen and carbon dioxide proceeds, the alveolar P_{O_2} falls and the alveolar P_{CO_2} rises. When the respiratory muscles relax, expiration occurs, and the oxygen-depleted and carbon dioxide–enriched alveolar gas leaves through the airway. With each succeeding inspiration, the alveolar gas is once again refreshed. Depending on the state of activity of the body, this cycle is repeated 10 to 50 times a minute.

The expired P_{O_2} will be higher than that in the alveoli, because this gas is diluted by inspired air that has filled the dead space and thus has not taken part in gas exchange. In addition, the average P_{O_2} in the pulmonary capillary blood leaving the lungs is normally slightly less than 100 mm. Hg, because the gas exchange in the lung is not perfect. The P_{O_2} may be even lower in the systemic circulation, because blood that is coming from poorly ventilated alveoli, or that has not been exposed to alveoli at all, is admixed with the arterialized blood leaving well-ventilated alveoli.

After the blood leaves the lungs and then the left ventricle, it is distributed to the tissues by the arteries and arterioles so that the metabolic processes of life, which require oxygen and produce carbon dioxide, are supported. Because oxygen is taken up from the blood by the tissue cells, the P_{O_2} falls to approximately 40 mm. Hg at the level of the tissue capillaries. In the tissues, the oxygen diffuses from the blood to its intracellular binding site, and the carbon dioxide diffuses from the cells to the blood. The tissue P_{O_2} is not known, so the gradient between the capillary P_{O_2} and that in the intracellular sites of oxygen utilization cannot be determined.

In the pages that follow, the processes involved in the events that occur during respiration will be described in some detail in order to set the stage for both a discussion of the disturbances in function produced by disease and the functional interventions that constitute therapy.

BASIC CONSIDERATIONS

- MECHANICS OF BREATHING
- PULMONARY VENTILATION, BLOOD FLOW AND GAS EXCHANGE
- GAS TRANSPORT AND ACID-BASE BALANCE
- CONTROL OF BREATHING
- RESPIRATION UNDER STRESS
- SPECIAL ASPECTS RELATED TO THE NEWBORN INFANT
- APPLICATION OF PULMONARY PHYSIOLOGY TO PULMONARY FUNCTION TESTING
- DEFENSES OF THE RESPIRATORY SYSTEM

1

MECHANICS OF BREATHING

The lungs can be viewed as an inverted tree, with the trachea its trunk and the bronchi the branches that lead to the gas-exchanging alveoli. The trachea and the cartilaginous bronchi divide dichotomously and asymmetrically into successively smaller branches, down to the terminal bronchioles. There are from 20 to 22 bronchial subdivisions, which give rise to more than a million tubes. Cartilaginous rings and plates extend in the tracheobronchial tree as far as the bronchioles, which are 1.0 to 2.0 cm. in diameter. There is an abrupt transition from the terminal bronchioles to the respiratory bronchioles, which radiate into the alveolar ducts, and these, in turn, give rise to the alveolar sacs. These sacs consist of groups of alveoli that have a radius of approximately 55 to 65 microns. It has been estimated that there are about 15 million alveolar ducts and about three hundred million alveoli in the human lungs and that they occupy an area of 40 to 100 square meters, depending on body size.

Expansion of the chest occurs when the inspiratory muscles contract and air enters the lungs and distends the tracheobronchial tree (Fig. 1). All portions of the tracheobronchial tree become enlarged. The trachea elongates and dilates, as do all of the bronchi, which lengthen and widen, the greatest increase in cross-sectional area taking place in the distal portions of the bronchial tree. The alveolar ducts also elongate and widen, and the openings into the alveolar sacs increase in size. There is smooth muscle in the bronchi and bronchioles and contractile tissue in the alveolar ducts, and it is thought that in certain disorders the alveolar ducts and small airways may be constricted. As a result, the lung volume and distensibility of the lungs are reduced, and gas distribution is impaired in these conditions.

The expansion of the chest normally takes place in three dimensions: anteroposterior, transverse and longitudinal. This three-dimensional increase in volume during inspiration occurs because contraction of the scalene and intercostal muscles elevates the ribs and because the diaphragm descends.

The volume of air that is breathed in during inspiration or out during expiration is called the *tidal volume* (V_T). Although usually stated to be

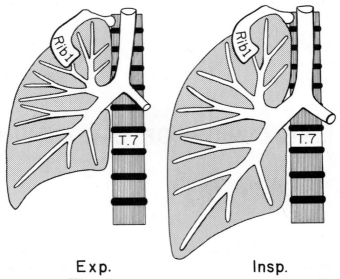

Figure 1. The change in size of the tracheobronchial tree during respiration.

about 500 ml. under resting conditions in healthy individuals, its absolute amount varies from one person to another as well as with the activity of each person. By multiplying the tidal volume by the respiratory rate, the ***minute ventilation*** ($\dot{V}_E$) can be determined.

THE SUPPORTING STRUCTURES—THE THORACIC CAGE

The human thorax is constructed in such a manner that it is sufficiently rigid to protect the vital organs it contains and yet is pliable enough to function as a bellows during the ventilatory cycle. The rigidity is provided by the bony ribs, and the pliability by the movable joints of the ribs at their vertebral and sternal ends. The sternum is held in position by its connection with the ventral ends of the ribs, which are under continuous elastic tension, even when the respiratory muscles are relaxed. The elastic thoracic cage always returns to its original position when it is compressed in any direction.

The first seven ribs are attached to the sternum, and the cartilages of the next three ribs are attached to the cartilage of the seventh rib. The remaining two ribs, the "floating ribs," do not connect with either the sternum or other ribs.

THE FORCE GENERATORS—THE RESPIRATORY MUSCLES

THE SCALENE MUSCLES

During inspiration, contraction of the scalene muscles, which arise from the transverse processes of the cervical vertebrae, raises the anterior end of the first rib, together with the manubrium sternum. This increases the anteroposterior diameter of the upper outlet of the thorax and helps to stabilize the upper chest cage so that contraction of the intercostal muscles results in elevation of the remaining ribs.

THE INTERCOSTAL MUSCLES

The first to the sixth ribs are connected with one another by the intercostal muscles, whose fibers run downward and forward. Contraction of these intercostal muscles results in an upward and forward movement of this part of the thorax. There is very little lateral movement of the first four ribs, which overlie the upper lobes of the lungs, and the increase in size of this portion of the chest cage is predominantly in an anteroposterior direction (Fig. 2, third rib). The fifth and sixth ribs, which are situated approximately over the middle lobe of the right lung and the lingular segment of the left lung, have a greater radius of curvature than the upper four ribs. As a result, inspiratory elevation of these two ribs increases both the anteroposterior and the transverse diameter of that portion of the thoracic cage.

The seventh to the tenth ribs, which overlie the lower lobes of the lungs, differ from the other ribs in that their anterior ends are situated at almost the same level as their posterior ends. In addition, they are more sharply curved. Inspiratory movement of these ribs primarily increases the transverse diameter of this portion of the thoracic cage while the anteroposterior diameter decreases slightly (Fig. 2, ninth rib).

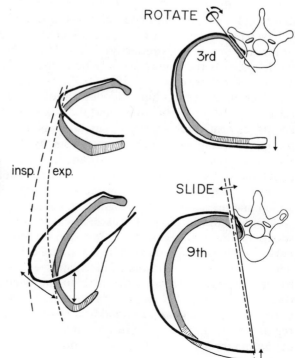

Figure 2. Anteroposterior and superior views of an upper and lower rib during inspiration and expiration.

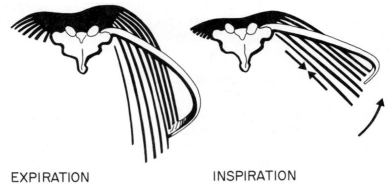

EXPIRATION   INSPIRATION

Figure 3. Because of its dome shape, contraction of the diaphragm during inspiration results in elevation of the ribs, with a consequent increase of the transverse diameter of the chest.

THE DIAPHRAGM

The diaphragm is the principal muscle of inspiration; its contraction increases the volume of the thoracic cage in a vertical direction, and tends to increase the transverse diameter of the lower thoracic cage as well. The transverse diameter increases because the muscular fibers of the diaphragm run in a vertical direction from their attachment at the costal margins. Since the diaphragm is normally dome-shaped, contraction of its fibers moves the lower ribs in an upward and lateral direction (Fig. 3). However, when the diaphragm becomes flattened and loses its dome shape, as in emphysema, it behaves like a flat sheet of muscles. Under such circumstances, contraction of the diaphragm is less effective in increasing the longitudinal dimension of the lungs, and there may actually be narrowing of the transverse diameter of the lower thorax.

During quiet breathing, the descent of the diaphragm during inspiration raises the abdominal pressure, and the pressure falls during expiration. This results in protrusion of the upper abdominal wall during inspiration, and recession during expiration. Apart from its function in normal breathing, the diaphragm also plays an important role in other respiratory acts such as coughing, sniffing and sneezing. In addition, in conjunction with contraction of the abdominal muscles, contraction of the diaphragm raises the intra-abdominal pressure, so that it assists in defecation, vomiting and parturition.

Unlike the intercostal muscles, which are innervated from the corresponding thoracic segments of the spinal cord, the diaphragm derives its nerve supply from the third, fourth and fifth cervical segments via the phrenic nerves. The lateral portions of the diaphragm and the crura are innervated by nerves arising between the sixth to the twelfth thoracic segments. It is thus possible for the diaphragm to continue to function even when the intercostal muscles are paralyzed as a result of a lesion in the upper thoracic region or the administration of a spinal anesthetic. Paralysis of both leaves of the diaphragm apparently need not cause significant disability, provided that the intercostal muscles are functioning normally and that the lungs are healthy.

THE MUSCLES OF THE ABDOMINAL WALL

The muscles of the abdominal wall (the external oblique, the internal oblique, the transversus abdominis, and the rectus abdominis muscles), which arise from the superficial surfaces of portions of the lower eight ribs or their cartilages, do not normally participate in the breathing act. However, during a maximum expiration, they do contract and cause depression of the lower ribs of the chest cage. As indicated above, the abdominal muscles are also important during coughing, sneezing and defecation because they increase the rigidity of the abdominal wall, so that the intrathoracic pressure can be raised to high levels.

SECONDARY RESPIRATORY MUSCLES

The secondary respiratory muscles are also attached to the ribs, but they do not ordinarily take an active part in breathing. However, they do come into play if one hyperventilates markedly, as may occur during severe exertion in healthy individuals, as well as in the dyspneic patient.

THE DIMENSIONS—LUNG VOLUMES

Breathing takes place within the boundaries of the maximal excursions of the respiratory apparatus. These maximum excursions in both an inspiratory and an expiratory direction are determined by a balance of forces— the elastic forces of the respiratory apparatus and the muscle forces that are applied to the chest cage.

The maximum volume of air that can be contained in the lungs is called the *total lung capacity* (TLC). At TLC, the elastic forces of the lungs and chest wall tending to deflate the lungs are balanced by the inspiratory muscle forces. The *residual volume* (RV) is the amount of air that is still in the lungs at the end of a maximal expiration. At RV, the elastic forces (mainly the chest wall) tending to expand the lungs are balanced by the maximum expiratory muscle forces and the extent of elevation of the diaphragm.

The TLC is comprised of a group of subdivisions. The primary subdivisions do not overlap and are called "volumes," whereas secondary divisions, termed "capacities," do overlap. The *vital capacity* (VC) is the maximal amount of air that a subject is able to expire after a maximal inspiration (i.e., from TLC). The *functional residual capacity* (FRC) is the amount of air in the lungs at the end of a normal expiration. It can be subdivided into two components: the *expiratory reserve volume* (ERV) and the *residual volume* (RV). The ERV is the maximal volume of air that can be expired beyond the FRC or the resting level. The *inspiratory capacity* (IC) is the maximum volume of air that can be inspired from the FRC. Clearly, the tidal volume is included in this subdivision, and the *inspiratory*

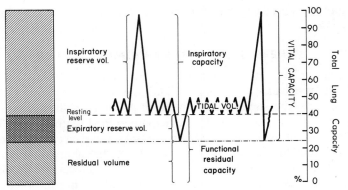

Figure 4. The subdivisions of lung volume shown as a proportion of total lung capacity. The block diagram on the left is included for future reference in other figures.

reserve volume (IRV) is the maximal volume of air that can be inspired, over and above the tidal volume, from the FRC.

Figure 4 illustrates these subdivisions as approximate proportions of the TLC, because although their absolute values vary considerably, even in normal persons, and are related to the age, sex and size of the person, the proportion of the TLC that each of the lung volume subdivisions occupies is remarkably similar. The FRC is normally about 40 per cent, the IC about 60 per cent, VC about 70 to 75 per cent and RV about 25 to 30 per cent of the TLC. This principle is also illustrated in Table 1, where the values obtained in two males of the same age but of different size are shown.

Except for the vital capacity, almost all of the lung volume compartments are estimated with reference to the normal end-expiratory position of the chest, i.e., the FRC. The FRC can be determined by measuring the dilution of an inert gas, but a physical method, which is based on Boyle's law and employs a body plethysmograph, is now the most common method used. Here the amount of air in the lungs is determined while the subject is sitting in the body plethysmograph and breathing through a mouthpiece-shutter system (Fig. 5). The shutter is closed at the end of a normal expiration (i.e., FRC), thus trapping the gas within the chest at that lung volume. When the subject makes gentle inspiratory and expiratory efforts against the closed shutter, the air in the chest is alternately compressed and decompressed,

TABLE 1. Lung Volumes in Two Males of Equal Age But Different Size

Lung Volume	Height, ml.	180 cm. % TCL	Height, ml.	150 cm. % TLC
Total lung capacity	8000	100	4800	100
Vital capacity	6000	75	3500	73
Inspiratory capacity	4300	54	2500	52
Functional residual capacity	3700	46	2300	48
Residual volume	2000	25	1300	27
Expiratory reserve volume	2300	21	1000	21

Figure 5. This model illustrates the physical method of calculating lung volume (V_{TG}). The relationship (K) between volume change (ΔV) and pressure change in the box (ΔP_p) is determined so that pressure changes can be used to determine volume changes. When the shutter (S) is closed at FRC, the subject tries to inspire and expire so that the air in the chest is decompressed and compressed. As the chest volume increases the box volume decreases, and vice versa. The relationship between the mouth pressure (P_{aw}) and the pressure in the box (P_p) is plotted on an oscilloscope. Since the pressure in the lungs at end-expiration was 970 cm. H_2O,

$$V_{TG} = 970 \times \frac{\Delta P_P \times K}{\Delta P_{aw}}.$$

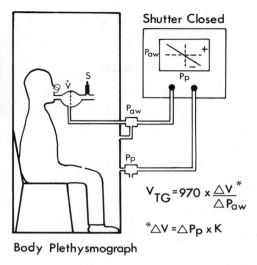

Shutter Closed

$$V_{TG} = 970 \times \frac{\Delta V}{\Delta P_{aw}} \ ^*$$

$$^*\Delta V = \Delta P_p \times K$$

Body Plethysmograph

thus creating a positive and negative pressure in the lungs and the opposite changes in the plethysmograph. By relating the changes in mouth pressure (which are equal to alveolar pressure, or P_{aw}) and the changes in thoracic gas volume (as reflected by changes in box pressure, or P_P), the amount of gas in the lungs at the point of shutter closure, which is called the **thoracic gas volume** (V_{TG}), can be calculated:

$$V_{TG} = 970 \times P_{aw}/P_P$$

where 970 is the barometric pressure, minus water vapor pressure, in cm. H_2O at sea level.

The remaining lung volume compartments are estimated with reference to the FRC, using an ordinary recording spirometer. The TLC is calculated by having the subject inspire maximally from FRC (i.e., IC) and adding the IC to FRC. As we have seen, the RV cannot be measured with the spirometer; it is calculated by determining the maximal amount of air that can be expired from the FRC (i.e., the ERV) and subtracting that from the FRC.

RESPIRATORY PRESSURES

The lung is invested with a serous membrane called the **visceral pleura,** and its reflection onto the chest wall is called the **parietal pleura.** A thin film of fluid separates the two pleural surfaces, and the pressure in this potential space, which is variously called the intrapleural, pleural or intrathoracic pressure, reflects the forces exerted by the lungs or chest wall on the pleural space. The retractive elastic force of the lungs that tends to pull them away from the chest wall is registered as a negative pleural pressure, because it is opposed by the tendency of the chest wall to pull further away

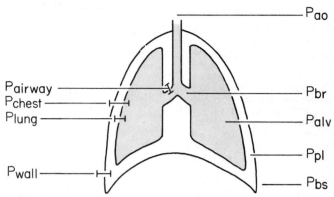

Figure 6.   Respiratory pressures:

P_{ao} = pressure at airway opening (usually atmospheric pressure)
P_{br} = pressure in the bronchi
P_{alv} = pressure in terminal air spaces (syn.: intrapulmonary pressure)
P_{pl} = pressure in pleural space (syn.: intrapleural pressure, intrathoracic pressure)
P_{bs} = pressure at body surface (usually atmospheric pressure)

Transmural pressures in the chest:

$P_{airway} = P_{br} - P_{pl}$ = pressure tending to widen or narrow the airways
$P_{chest} = P_{alv} - P_{bs}$ = pressure tending to inflate or deflate lungs and chest wall together (transthoracic pressure)
$P_{lung} = P_{alv} - P_{pl}$ = pressure tending to inflate or deflate the lungs, depending on sign (transpulmonary pressure)
$P_{wall} = P_{pl} - P_{bs}$ = pressure tending to expand or collapse chest wall, depending on sign

from the lungs. In a healthy person the mean pleural pressure at the end of a normal expiration is about 5 cm. H_2O below atmospheric pressure (i.e., 965 cm. H_2O).

The balance of elastic forces acting in the chest at the end of a normal expiration, i.e., at FRC, is indicated in Figure 6. Since there is no air moving and the gas inside the lung is in continuity with the atmosphere through the airways, the pressures at the airway opening, in the bronchi, in the alveoli and at the body surface are all equal to atmospheric pressure (970 cm. H_2O). The pressure difference between the inner and outer surfaces of the lungs (P_{lung}), which is often referred to as the ***transpulmonary pressure,*** is a measure of the net force acting on the lungs, and is represented in Figure 6 as $P_{alv} - P_{pl}$. The difference between the pleural pressure and that acting at the body surface (P_{wall}) is a measure of the net force acting on the chest wall, and is represented as $P_{pl} - P_{bs}$.

BALANCE OF ELASTIC FORCES

The position of the chest cage when the muscles are relaxed (i.e., at the end of a normal expiration, or at FRC) is determined by the balance between the elastic forces of the lungs, which tend to reduce their volume, and the elastic forces of the chest wall, which tend to increase it:

$$P_{lung} = P_{wall}$$

or

$$P_{alv} - P_{pl} = P_{pl} - P_{bs}$$

This is illustrated in Figure 7, where a model of the lung–chest wall system, in the form of a two-plate piston within a container, is depicted. Note that each of the plates is attached to a set of springs, that the two sets of springs are pulling in opposite directions, and that a rubber balloon, representing the pleural cavity, separates the two plates. The springs attached to the left plate represent the elastic resistance of the lungs, and those attached to the right plate represent that of the chest wall. In this illustration, the piston is at its "resting position," where the forces that are being exerted by the two sets of springs are equal. Clearly this is analogous to the equilibrium situation that exists in the human thorax at the resting level, or FRC.

In Figure 8 the mechanical analogue is used to illustrate the relationship between the elastic forces of the lung and chest wall at different lung volumes. When the piston is pulled out as far as possible (*A*), a situation analogous to that at TLC, the springs representing the elastic forces of the lung are stretched, while those representing the elastic forces of the chest wall are compressed and actually attempting to re-expand. As a result, both

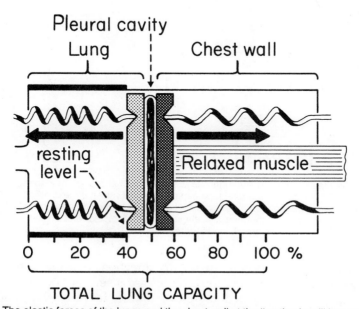

Figure 7. The elastic forces of the lungs and the chest wall at the "resting level" in a mechanical analogue. The springs on the left represent the force of lung elasticity, and those on the right represent the elastic forces of the chest wall. The forces being exerted by the two springs are equal, so the piston is stationary. This is analogous to the situation in the human at functional residual capacity.

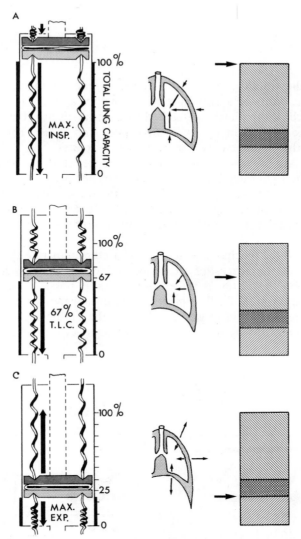

Figure 8. The elastic forces of the lung and the chest wall at maximum inspiration (TLC), at approximately 67 per cent of the total lung capacity, and at maximum expiration (RV). On the left, the stretch on the springs of the mechanical analogue is shown. In the center, the relative propensities of the forces of the lung and chest wall are depicted, and on the right, the lung volume at which these forces are acting is represented.

elastic forces are exerted in an expiratory direction, i.e., the piston (or the lung) has a marked propensity to recoil toward a smaller volume.

As the piston is allowed to return toward its original position, the stretch on both springs diminishes. At a particular point, thought to be about 65 to 70 per cent of TLC (Fig. 8B), the "chest wall" spring is completely relaxed and does not exert a force in any direction whereas the "lung" spring continues to exert a force in an expiratory direction. Near this volume, then, the piston (and the lungs) will tend to move in an expiratory direction until the pull of the "chest wall" spring is equal to the pull of the "lung" (i.e., until FRC is reached).

If the piston is pushed past its resting position, as occurs when one expires to a volume less than FRC (Fig. 8C), there is less stretch of the "lung" spring, so that its retractile force is small; however, the "chest wall" spring is stretched more, so that its tendency to recoil is increased. In this situation, then, the net force is in an inspiratory direction; i.e., there is a propensity for the volume to increase until, once again, the pull of the two sets of springs in opposite directions is equal.

The relationship between the elastic forces of the lungs and chest wall at different lung volumes is analogous to the situation in the human (Fig. 9). The net balance between the two elastic forces (termed **relaxation pressure**) is determined by having the subject relax against a complete obstruction at the different lung volumes. In this figure, pressures tending to increase lung volume are negative, and those tending to decrease lung volume are positive. Again, the forces exerted by the lung and chest wall at FRC are equal and pulling in opposite directions, so that the relaxation pressure is equal to atmospheric pressure, or zero. At lung volumes above FRC, the elastic force of the lung, which is tending to empty it, is greater than that of the chest wall tending to fill it, so that the relaxation pressure is positive. At very high lung volumes, the relaxation pressure is more positive, because the lung and chest wall forces both act in an expiratory direction. At lung volumes below FRC, the inspiratory pull of the chest wall is greater than the expiratory pull of the lungs, so that the relaxation pressure is negative. Clearly then, as in the mechanical analogue, there is a propensity

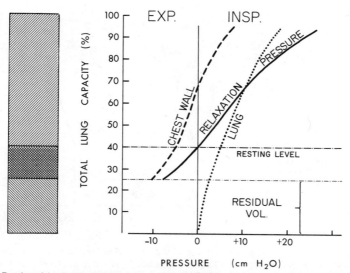

Figure 9. Depicted is the pressure derived at different lung volumes when a subject relaxes against a complete obstruction (relaxation pressure). This pressure is the resultant net balance between the elastic forces of the lung and the chest wall at all levels of lung volume.

for the lung volume to return to the "resting level" at any volume above or below FRC.

ELASTIC BEHAVIOR OF THE LUNG

The elastic behavior of the springs in the mechanical analogue can be described by the force necessary to stretch and hold them at a certain length. The elastic behavior of the lung can also be described by its force-displacement characteristics, and in a three-dimensional apparatus such as the respiratory system, it is considered conveniently in terms of pressure and volume. By changing the volume in the lungs and noting the change in pressure required to maintain the new volume, or by changing the pressure and noting the change in volume that results, one can derive information about the elastic properties of the lung. In either case, one can describe the elastic behavior accurately only if the values of pressure and volume are recorded under static conditions, i.e., when there is no airflow.

Since one cannot empty the lungs completely, it is not possible to describe the total pressure-volume behavior of the lungs in intact man. Nevertheless, much important information has been gained by studying the elastic behavior of excised lungs, as is shown in Figure 10. If the excised lung is made completely airless, and increments of pressure are then applied, the lung does not begin to inflate until the applied pressure reaches 15 to 20 cm. H_2O. With further increases in pressure, the lung inflates further but in

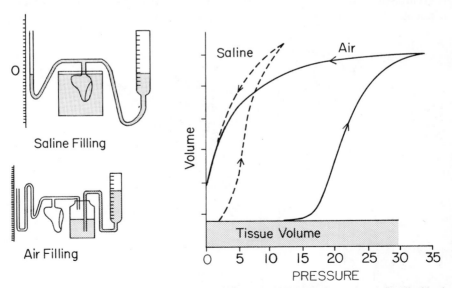

Figure 10. The pressure-volume relationship of the excised airless lung when inflated with air and with saline. With saline filling, the lung is immersed in saline to counterbalance the effects of hydrostatic pressure. The "deflation limbs" of the air and saline curves diverge at high lung volumes as a result of surface tension at the air tissue interface.

an uneven manner. Areas of the lung are seen to pop open here and there until, finally, at a pressure of about 40 cm. H_2O, the lung is completely inflated. When the pressure around the lung is reduced again, the lung deflates along a pressure-volume curve that differs from that inscribed during the application of pressure. The lung deflates uniformly, and even when the inflation pressure has fallen to zero, it remains slightly inflated. The difference between the inflation and deflation curves and the failure of the lung to return to its original state after deformation is called *hysteresis.* Subsequent inflations and deflations result in pressure-volume curves that exhibit much less hysteresis and follow more closely the deflation limb of the initial pressure-volume curve.

When the lungs are inflated with saline instead of air, they begin to expand at a much lower pressure, fill uniformly and require less pressure to fill them completely. When the lungs empty little hysteresis is noted. The difference between air and saline filling is attributed to the fact that the surface tension that exists at the air-tissue interface during inflation with air is much greater than the negligible amount of surface tension existing at the liquid-tissue interface during saline filling.

These pressure-volume characteristics that are demonstrated with air and saline filling indicate that the retractive force of the lung has two components: that due to surface tension and that due to the elastic elements in the tissue.

SURFACE FORCES

Examination of the deflation limb of the air and saline pressure-volume curves in Figure 10 indicates that, at high lung volumes, almost half of the retractive force of the lung is due to *surface tension,* whereas the effect of surface tension is negligible at low lung volumes. The surface tension is minimal at low lung volumes because of the presence in the lung of surface-active material (*surfactant*) that has special physical and chemical characteristics. Surfactant is formed in the terminal units of the lung, and is generally believed to be a product of a large granular epithelial cell, the alveolar type II cell. The surface of the terminal lung units (i.e., the alveoli, alveolar ducts and respiratory bronchioles) is lined with this material, which is rich in disaturated lecithins. These phospholipids account for the surface tension–lowering effects of the lining material.

The surface tension exerted by a liquid may be measured in an apparatus such as that shown in Figure 11, in which the pull of the liquid surface on a platinum strip is registered. Saline exerts a surface tension of about 70 dynes/cm., and this value does not vary with expansion or contraction of the surface. When surfactant is added to the saline the surface tension falls. Compression of the surface film by movement of the barrier results in an even further fall in tension to as low as 1 to 2 dynes/cm., probably because surfactant molecules become concentrated in the surface. Such behavior may explain why there is a greater difference between air and saline pressure-volume curves at high lung volumes than at low lung volumes. When the

Plan View

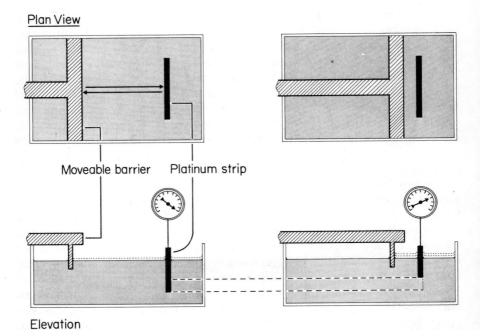

Elevation

Figure 11. Measurement of surface tension. The apparatus consists of a trough containing an aqueous solution, which is shown in two views. On the surface, lung washings form a film; a barrier moves horizontally to increase or decrease the area of the surface film. Surface tension pulls down the platinum strip. As the barrier compresses the surface film, the tension drops *(right)* and rises again when the barrier is moved back *(left)*.

surface area (volume) is great, the surface tension is high, and when the surface area (volume) is small, the surface tension is low.

The physiologic importance of surfactant may be appreciated by considering the factors that affect the pressure inside an alveolus. The *law of LaPlace* states that the pressure (P) inside a spherical structure is directly proportional to the tension (T) in the wall and inversely related to the radius of curvature (r).

$$P = 2T/r$$

Thus, for a given tension in the wall of a sphere, the pressure necessary to keep the structure from collapsing will become greater as its radius of curvature becomes smaller. Assuming that this is true of the lung alveoli, then surfactant, by decreasing the tension, contributes to the stability of the lung by allowing small air spaces to remain open at relatively low transpulmonary pressures. Furthermore, the fact that surfactant lowers the surface tension when the surface area is small means that the ratio 2T/r may be the same in alveoli of different sizes, and as a result, they can be stable at the same transpulmonary pressure.

Clearly then, a deficiency of surfactant would be expected to render the lung unstable and to promote collapse (atelectasis). Indeed, impaired surface activity has been found in lungs of children dying of hyaline membrane disease, in patients suffering from the adult respiratory distress syndrome, and in a wide variety of experimental conditions, including exposure to high concentrations of oxygen. In all of these situations, atelectasis is a prominent feature. Figure 12 illustrates measurements of the surface tension of extracts of lung tissue obtained from a normal and an atelectatic lung. Since many substances can interfere with pulmonary surfactant, notably certain factors in the fibrinolytic system, it is still not possible to be certain whether abnormal surface activity is due to a primary effect on surfactant production or is secondary to inhibition of surfactant by interfering substances.

TISSUE ELASTICITY

The air and saline pressure-volume curves indicate that, over the tidal breathing range, most of the retractive force of the lung is due to the elastic tissue elements in the lung. From the histology of the respiratory system we know that the structures in the lung that resist deformation (i.e., stretch) are collagen and elastin. The net elastic retraction of the lung is influenced by nutritional factors, at least in young growing animals, and changes in collagen and elastin content of the lung have been demonstrated in disease in both animals and man. In the context of this discussion, an increased resistance to deformation means that the structure is stiffer and that there is an increase in elasticity.

Tissue retractive forces are increased in pulmonary fibrosis and decreased in emphysema. In fibrosis the greater elastic force is apparently due

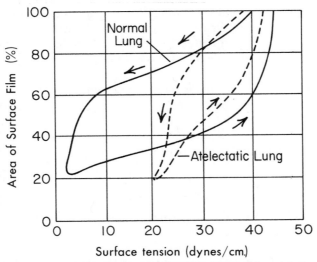

Figure 12. Surface area tension diagrams obtained on compression and decompression of the surface of a saline extract of the lungs of a normal infant and of lungs from an infant with hyaline membrane disease.

to an increase in fibrous connective tissue in the lung; in emphysema the decrease in elastic forces is due to destruction of alveolar walls and a loss of elastic elements. The stiffness or retractive force of the lung is also increased when the pulmonary vessels are engorged with blood or when the interstitial spaces are filled with fluid. In addition, contraction of muscle or contractile elements that are present even in the small alveolar ducts can increase the elastic retractive force. The alveolar ducts contract when histamine is injected into the pulmonary circulation or when blood clots lodge in the pulmonary vascular bed. They are also thought to be constricted in active cigarette smokers. Like the smooth muscle in large airways, the alveolar duct smooth muscle is relaxed by beta-2-adrenergic agents.

ESTIMATION OF ELASTIC RESISTANCE

The elastic resistance, or *elastance,* of the total respiratory apparatus, the chest wall or the lungs, is expressed as the change in pressure per unit change in volume:

$$\text{Elastance} = \Delta \text{ pressure}/\Delta \text{ volume}$$

In practice, however, the elastic property of each part of the system is generally expressed in terms of its *compliance,* which expresses the dimensions of change in volume per unit change in pressure:

$$\text{Compliance} = \Delta \text{ volume}/\Delta \text{ pressure}$$

Thus the compliance of the respiratory apparatus is $\Delta V/\Delta P_{chest}$; the compliance of the lungs is $\Delta V/\Delta P_{lung}$; and the compliance of the chest wall is $\Delta V/\Delta P_{wall}$. Clearly, the values obtained are the reciprocal of their elastance.

The concept of compliance of the lungs is depicted in the mechanical analogue and in the lung in Figure 13. It can be seen that, in "healthy lungs" (*A*), the application of a distending pressure of 5 cm. H_2O results in an "inspiration" of 1 liter of air. Thus, the compliance of these "lungs" is 1.0/5, or 0.20 l./cm. H_2O. The application of the same pressure to "lungs" that have lost elasticity (as in emphysema) results in an "inspiration" of 2 liters of air (*B*). In this case, the compliance is 2.0/5, or 0.40 l./cm. H_2O. When the lungs are stiff (as in pulmonary fibrosis) the same pressure induces a volume change of only 0.5 liter (*C*). Here, the compliance is 0.5/5 or 0.10 l./cm. H_2O.

LUNG COMPLIANCE

The compliance of the lung may be assessed in the spontaneously breathing subject by measuring the change in pressure across the lungs (transpulmonary) from end-expiration to end-inspiration (i.e., at points of zero flow), along with the change in volume. Although either pleural or esophageal pressure may be measured, it is usually the esophageal pressure that is determined.

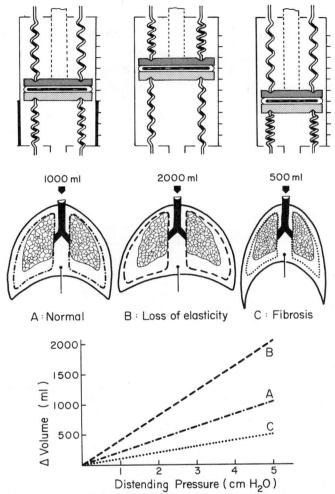

Figure 13. The stretch on the springs represents the distention of the lungs produced by a change in applied or distending pressure of 5 cm. H_2O in normal lungs **(A)**, lungs that have lost elasticity **(B)**, and lungs that are fibrotic **(C)**. The change in volume induced by the change in pressure is also plotted.

Dynamic Compliance

When the compliance of the lungs is determined during spontaneous breathing (i.e., the tidal volume is divided by the change in transpulmonary pressure from end-expiration to end-inspiration), it is called **dynamic compliance** (C_{dyn}). However, as we shall see below, the calculated compliance of the lungs is very dependent on the lung volume. To overcome this problem, lung compliance measured during spontaneous breathing is corrected for the lung volume at which it was measured. "Compliance per unit lung volume" is termed **specific compliance**.

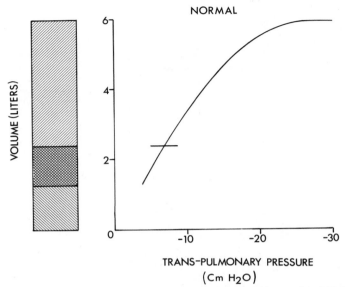

Figure 14. The relationship between transpulmonary pressure and lung volume (static pressure volume curve of the lung) in a healthy individual is shown. As is seen on the lung volume graph, the horizontal line on the pressure curve represents the resting level or functional residual capacity.

The **dynamic compliance** is also significantly influenced by alterations of flow resistance in the lung. This will be considered in more detail when the factors determining flow resistance are discussed.

Pressure/Volume Relationship of the Lungs

In practice, the elastic properties of the lung are assessed by measuring the transpulmonary pressure at different lung volumes under static conditions (i.e., when there is no airflow) over the entire range of the inspiratory and expiratory vital capacity. When the static pressures during expiration are plotted against the lung volume at which they were determined, a pressure-volume curve is derived (Fig. 14). Clearly, the expiratory static pressure-volume curve of the lung is the same as the curve depicting the lung elastic recoil in Figure 9.

It is apparent that the slope of the pressure-volume curve between two particular volumes is the compliance of the lung over that volume. However, since the pressure-volume curve of the lung is alinear, the "compliance" value will vary and depend on the portion of the curve over which it is determined. The lungs of a person breathing near total lung capacity will appear to be stiffer than those of another person breathing near functional residual capacity, even though the intrinsic elastic properties of the lungs of the two individuals may be identical. In practice then, it is important to derive the complete static pressure-volume relationship of the lungs over the entire expiratory vital capacity whenever possible.

Examples of the static pressure-volume relationship of the lungs that are found in three pulmonary disorders are compared with that found in healthy individuals in Figure 15. Shown are the relationships found in a patient who has lost lung elastic recoil (i.e., emphysema), one whose lungs have an increased elastic recoil (i.e., lung fibrosis) and one whose lungs are overdistended because of asthma. It can be seen that the curve is shifted upward (lung volume is greater) and to the left (pressure is lower) in the patient with emphysema, and downward (lung volume is less) and to the right (pressure is greater) in the patient with pulmonary fibrosis. Note that the curve is also shifted upward and to the left in asthma, but the slope of the curve is unaltered.

TOTAL COMPLIANCE

The compliance of the chest or the total respiratory apparatus can be determined by measuring the change in FRC or resting level that results when a positive pressure is applied to the airways or when a negative pressure is applied to the external surface of the chest. As we have seen in Figure 9, it can also be determined from the *relaxation pressure* curve. The compliance of the respiratory system has been shown to be approximately 0.12 l./cm. H_2O in healthy subjects. The compliance of the respiratory apparatus is low when the compliance of the lungs or the chest wall is reduced.

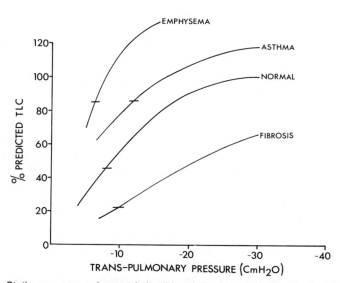

Figure 15. Static pressure–volume relationship of the lung in a healthy individual and in patients suffering from pulmonary fibrosis, asthma, and emphysema is shown. Note that the curve is shifted down and to the right (a given lung volume is associated with a higher pressure) in the patient with fibrosis, and up and to the left (a given lung volume is associated with a lower pressure) in asthma and emphysema. In asthma the slope of the curve is unchanged, whereas in emphysema the slope is increased.

Although it would appear to be comparatively simple to determine the compliance of the respiratory apparatus, it must be pointed out that the respiratory muscles must be in a state of either complete relaxation or paralysis in order to obtain an accurate assessment. Complete relaxation of the respiratory muscles is extremely difficult to attain except in a well-trained subject; therefore, this method is not always practical. Similarly, although the compliance of the lungs and chest wall (either together or separately) can be measured when the respiratory muscles are paralyzed, one is never certain that the values are similar to those that occur during spontaneous breathing.

CHEST WALL COMPLIANCE

To measure the compliance of the chest wall, it is necessary to determine the total compliance and the lung compliance simultaneously. As we have seen previously, this entails measurement of the change in transpulmonary (esophageal-mouth differential) pressure and FRC before and after either a positive pressure is applied to the upper airway, a negative pressure is applied to the external surface of the chest, or the relaxation pressure is determined. By using these techniques, the compliance of the chest wall has been estimated to be approximately 0.20 l./cm. H_2O in healthy subjects. In obese individuals, on the other hand, the compliance of the chest wall has been found to be greatly reduced, averaging about 0.08 l./cm. H_2O.

FLOW RESISTANCE

During breathing, contraction of the respiratory muscles must apply sufficient force to overcome the resistance to airflow in the tracheobronchial tree, the frictional resistance of tissues sliding over one another in the lung parenchyma (tissue viscous resistance) and the chest wall, and the elastic resistance (Fig. 16). Inertia, which must also be overcome during acceleration and deceleration of gas or tissues, is also present, but is generally considered to be negligible. The flow resistance of the airways and the frictional resistance of lung tissue are encountered only when the volume of the lung is changing (i.e., there is airflow). Unlike the force required to overcome the elastic resistance, which is stored during expansion of the lung, the energy expended in overcoming these resistances is dissipated as heat because of friction. Conversely, like the elastic resistance, which is proportional to lung volume, flow resistance is also influenced by the lung volume.

In Figure 16, a nozzle or airway, which has a flow resistance, as well as the frictiional resistance developed by the plates sliding along the walls of the container have been added to the mechanical analogue. Clearly, the flow resistance of the multibranched tracheobronchial tree and tissues of the human lung is distributed in a much more complex fashion, but the model allows demonstration of how the elastic and flow-resistive properties of the lung can be separated during breathing.

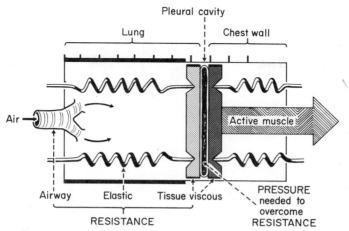

Figure 16. The resistances that must be overcome in order to move air into the lungs during breathing are illustrated. In addition to the elastic resistance offered by the two sets of springs, there is resistance to movement when the muscle contracts because of flow resistance in the airways and the sliding of tissues over one another. Thus the pressure in the pleural space that the muscles must develop is the sum of that required to overcome the elastic resistance of the lung to distention and the flow resistance.

TOTAL FLOW RESISTANCE

To calculate total flow resistance (R), one uses an equation that is similar to **Ohm's law** for electrical circuits, which relates flow of the current to the electromotive force. In the case of airflow resistance, one relates the pressure (P_R) required to produce a given rate of airflow ($\dot{V}$):

$$R = P_R/\dot{V} \quad \text{in cm. } H_2O/l./sec.$$

During inspiration and expiration, the pressure difference (P_T) between the pleural space (or esophagus) and the airway opening is made up of two components: the pressure necessary to overcome the lung elastic resistance (P_{el}), and that necessary to overcome the resistance to the flow of gas (P_R) through the airways and the tissue viscous resistance:

$$P_T = P_{el} + P_R$$

In practice, one can determine the pressure required to overcome flow resistance from simultaneous recordings of changes in lung volume, airflow and pleural (or esophageal) pressure during breathing (Fig. 17). When one plots the simultaneous changes of volume and pleural pressure during inspiration and expiration against one another, a **pressure-volume loop** is formed, the boundaries of the loop being derived from the pleural pressure changes at different degrees of lung inflation during the respiratory cycle. Since at the extremes of the volume cycle (i.e., at the ends of expiration and inspiration) there is no airflow, then P_R = zero, so that all of the pressure is being applied to the elastic resistance:

$$P_T = P_{el}$$

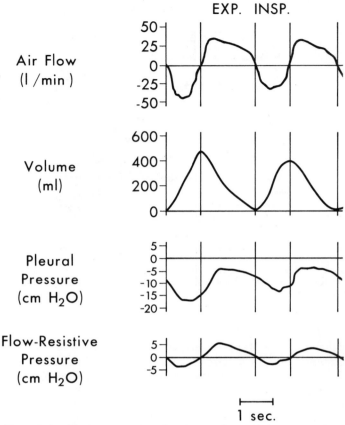

Figure 17. The relationship between pleural pressure, flow-resistive pressure, airflow, and volume is shown in the model. Note that the flow-resistive pressure is atmospheric at end expiration and end inspiration when there is no airflow. The compliance can be determined by dividing the volume change between these points by the change in pleural pressure.

Since the elastic resistance of the lungs is linearly related to the state of lung distension over the tidal volume range, one can calculate the elastic component of the total pressure at any instant during the breath.

$$Compliance = \frac{Volume}{P_{el}}$$

and

$$P_{el} = \frac{Volume}{Compliance}$$

Now, since at any instant in the respiratory cycle:

$$P_R = P_T - P_{el}$$

the pressure necessary to overcome the total flow resistance (P_R) at any moment during the respiratory cycle is:

$$P_R = P_T - (\text{Volume/Compliance})$$

A pressure volume loop and total flow resistance in a healthy subject is illustrated in Figure 18. A straight line joining the points of end-expiration and end-inspiration represents the pressure required to overcome the elastic resistance at any given instant during the breathing cycle. At any given moment during the breathing cycle, then, the pressure necessary to overcome the flow resistance (P_R) is the difference between the total pressure and that required to overcome the elastic resistance. If the rate of airflow at the same instant is known, one can derive a pressure-flow plot (Figure 18B), and flow resistance can be calculated. Here, inspiration is shown in the upper right quadrant and expiration in the lower left. It can be seen that the pressure change is linearly related to the airflow up to a certain point, after which there is a disproportionate increase in the pressure required to produce a further increase in airflow. The linear portion of the curve is primarily due to laminar resistance, and the deviation from the linear relationship is due to turbulent resistance. In healthy individuals, the flow resistance ranges between 1.0 and 2.0 cm. $H_2O/l./sec.$ of airflow, and about one-tenth of the resistance at a flow rate of 1 l./sec. is due to turbulence.

When there is airway obstruction, there is a marked increase in the pressure required to overcome flow resistance during both inspiration and expiration, so that the pressure-volume loop is considerably widened. This

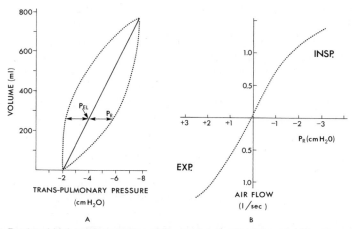

Figure 18. Depicted is the determination of flow resistance from the simultaneous relationship between volume and transpulmonary pressure (P_T) during a breath **(A)**. The elastic component of the transpulmonary pressure (P_{EL}) is derived by a line joining the points of end expiration and end inspiration. The pressure necessary to overcome flow resistance (P_R) at any particular instant is the difference between P_T and P_{EL}. When P_R is plotted against the simultaneously measured rate of air flow **(B)**, flow resistance can be derived from the slope of the linear portion of the curve ($\Delta P_R/\Delta \dot{V}$).

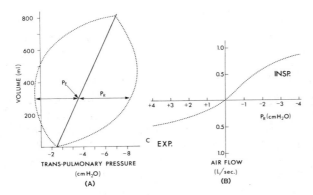

Figure 19. Pressure-volume (A) and pressure-flow (B) relationships during a breath in a patient with asthma. The pressure (P_R) required to overcome flow (V) is markedly increased. Note that the pressure becomes positive during expiration, indicating that extra work is performed during this phase.

is demonstrated in Figure 19, which illustrates a pressure-volume loop and pressure-flow plot during a breath; these were derived in a patient suffering from increased resistance to airflow. In patients suffering from bronchitis, or during acute asthmatic attacks, flow resistance may be 10 to 15 times that observed in healthy individuals.

TISSUE VISCOUS RESISTANCE

Using techniques that measure flow resistance during the inhalation of gases that have a greater or lesser viscosity than that of air, it is possible to calculate by extrapolation the resistance that would be present if a gas possessing no viscosity whatsoever were being inhaled. The pressure required to overcome the tissue viscous resistance can then be derived. This pressure has also been determined by the simultaneous estimation of the pressure required to overcome total flow resistance and that necessary to overcome airway resistance. The tissue viscous resistance has been found to form only a small part of the total flow resistance; the major resistance is that which occurs in the airways. Therefore, it is the airway resistance or total flow resistance that is usually determined.

AIRWAY RESISTANCE

The airway resistance (R_{aw}) component of the total flow resistance is given by the formula:

$$R_{aw} = P_{aw}/\dot{V}$$

In practice, the airway resistance is usually determined in a body plethysmograph by measuring the relationship between airflow and the plethysmograph pressure (V/P_P) while the subject pants through an unobstructed flow meter (Fig. 20). The airway pressure during the panting maneuver is then derived from the ratio of airway and plethysmograph pressure (P_{aw}/P_P), which is obtained when the airway is occluded (i.e., in determining lung volume). Then:

$$R_{aw} = P_{aw}/P_P/\dot{V}/P_P \quad \text{in cm. } H_2O/l./sec.$$

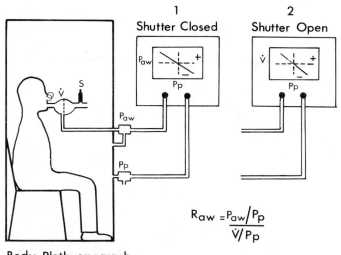

Body Plethysmograph

Figure 20. Measurement of airway resistance (R_{aw}) in the body plethysmograph is shown. With the shutter closed, the ratio between mouth pressure (P_{aw}) and box pressure (P_p) is determined. The relationship between P_p and airflow ($\dot{V}$) is then estimated while the subject pants through the unobstructed pneumotachograph. Now $R_{aw} = P_{aw}/\dot{V}$.

Factors Affecting Airway Resistance

Under normal circumstances, flow resistance is determined by the velocity of airflow, the physical properties of the gas being breathed, the lung volume and the factors determining the cross-sectional area of the airways available for flow.

Velocity of Flow. As indicated previously, the relationship between airflow and driving pressure is not a simple one. At low levels of airflow, gas moves in a streamline or laminar fashion, and flow and pressure are linearly related. At higher levels of airflow, the pressure-flow relationship departs from linearity (see Figs. 18*B* and 19*B*), because turbulence is created and this increases the resistance. The laminar component of airflow is proportional to the velocity of airflow, and the turbulent component is related to the square of the airflow velocity. Both laminar and turbulent resistance are affected by the physical characteristics of the respired gas.

Physical Characteristics of the Respired Gas. Since airway resistance is the result of friction between the flowing gas and the walls of the airways, as well as friction within the air stream itself, it is evident that any property of the gas tending to affect friction will affect the airway resistance. Thus, as originally proposed by Rohrer, the drop between the pressure in the alveolus (P_{alv}) and that of the mouth (P_{ao}) can be represented by the following equation:

$$P_{alv} - P_{ao} = K_1\dot{V} + K_2\dot{V}^2$$

Where $\dot{V}$ is flow, K_1 is a constant reflecting gas viscosity and K_2 is another constant reflecting gas density.

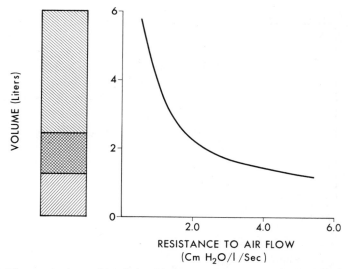

Figure 21. The graph shows the relationship between resistance to airflow and lung volume in a normal individual. The airways are more distended at higher lung volumes because the transpulmonary pressure is more negative, so that the flow resistance is lower at high lung volumes.

Gases with low density, such as helium, reduce the airway resistance, whereas gases with high density, such as sulfur hexafluoride, increase airway resistance. The barometric pressure will also affect the flow resistance, because the density of the gas is altered. In deep-sea divers, the increased density of the gas may raise the airway resistance sufficiently to interfere with breathing, whereas at higher altitudes, the airway resistance is decreased.

Lung Volume. The flow resistance varies with lung volume; it is less at high lung volumes than at lower lung volumes (Fig. 21), because, as lung volume increases and pleural pressure becomes more subatmospheric, those parts of the tracheobronchial tree that are exposed to the pleural pressure increase in size. Conversely, at lower lung volumes, the airways decrease in size as the pleural pressure rises. Clearly then, interpretation of measurements of airflow resistance requires knowledge of the absolute lung volume at which the measurements were made. The relationship between the inverse of the flow resistance, which is called *airway conductance* (G_{aw}), and lung volume, is essentially linear. For that reason, one generally expresses flow resistance as conductance per unit volume, or *specific conductance* (SG_{aw}), which is virtually independent of body size or the lung volume at which the subject was breathing.

Cross-Sectional Area of Airways. The cross-sectional area of the airways is determined by the lung volume and the balance between those forces tending to narrow the airways and those tending to widen them. Those tending to narrow the airways include the pressure surrounding the airways (peribronchial pressure) and the force exerted by contraction of bronchial smooth muscle. The forces tending to keep the airways open include the pressure inside the bronchi at any moment (intraluminal pressure) and the tethering action of the surrounding connective tissue. As we have seen, as lung volume increases and pleural pressure becomes more subatmospheric, those parts of the tracheobronchial tree that are exposed to the pleural pressure will increase in size because of the increase in transbronchial pressure. During passive expiration the airways decrease in size again as the transbronchial pressure falls.

The influence of peribronchial and intraluminal pressures on airway caliber is particularly important during a forced expiration. This is illustrated by assessing the rate of airflow during expirations of increasing force at different lung volumes (Fig. 22). If one plots the airflow rates at a particular

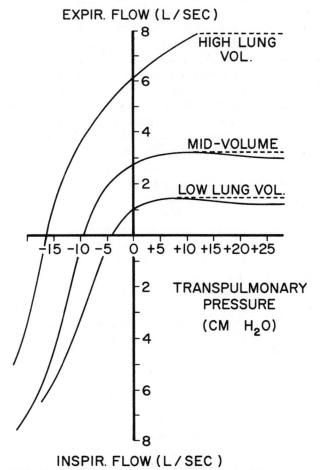

Figure 22. Isovolume pressure-flow curves obtained in a normal subject at three levels of lung inflation are illustrated. At high lung volume, maximum expiratory flow increases with increasing effort. At lower lung volumes increasing pressure raises the airflow rate up to a maximum, and further effort produces no further increase in flow, presumably because of airways compression (see Figure 23).

lung volume against the corresponding effort or transpulmonary pressure, an *isovolume pressure-flow curve* is obtained. Notice that with forced inspirations, the maximal airflow rate ($\dot{V}_{max}$) achieved at each lung volume essentially depends on the amount of effort that is developed. On the other hand, with forced expirations, $\dot{V}_{max}$ at a particular lung volume is not as directly related to the degree of effort. At high lung volumes, the airways are wide open, so that very high expiratory flow rates can be achieved. Just as in a forced inspiration, $\dot{V}_{max}$ appears to be related to the amount of effort exerted at high lung volumes. At lung volumes below about 75 per cent of the vital capacity, the flow rate also increases with effort, but only up to a certain point. Beyond this point, the flow rate does not increase with further effort or greater driving pressure, and it may even fall slightly. Since the resistance to airflow is represented by the ratio of pressure to flow, it is clear that once the maximal expiratory flow rate has been achieved at any particular lung volume, the resistance to airflow rises in direct proportion to the driving pressure. This rise in flow resistance with increasing effort is due to dynamic compression of the airways.

The concept of dynamic compression is very important and may be better understood with the aid of another model, such as that shown in Figure 23. In this model, the respiratory system is depicted at a particular moment during the forced expiratory effort. The pleural pressure (P_{pl}), which reflects the amount of expiratory effort being exerted, is assumed to be 20 cm. H_2O, and the elastic recoil pressure of the lung (P_{el}) is assumed to be 10 cm. H_2O. At this moment, then, the pressure in the alveoli (P_{alv}) is 30 cm. H_2O (i.e., the sum of the lung elastic recoil pressure and the pleural pressure). Clearly the intrabronchial pressure must vary along the airways and diminish from the alveolus (30 cm. H_2O) to the airway opening (0 cm. H_2O). It is also apparent that there is a point in the airways at which the intrabronchial pressure is equal to the pressure surrounding it (i.e., 20 cm. H_2O, or the pleural pressure). This point in the airway has been called the *equal pressure point* (EPP).

In the *downstream airways* (i.e., between the EPP and the mouth), then, the intrabronchial pressure is less than the peribronchial (pleural) pressure, so that there is a net force tending to compress these airways. The greater the amount of effort that is generated, the higher will be the pleural pressure and the more the downstream airways will be compressed; they may even close.

Partitioning of Airway Resistance

A substantial proportion of the total airway resistance is present in the upper respiratory tract. The nasal passages, the nasopharynx, the larynx and the trachea have been shown to contribute about 20 per cent of the flow resistance at low rates of airflow and as much as 45 per cent at higher rates of flow. Most of the remainder of the resistance to airflow resides in airways greater than 2 mm. in diameter. Peripheral airways that are smaller than 2 mm. in diameter, which are far more numerous than large airways, provide

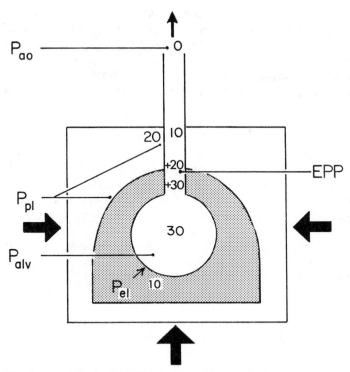

Figure 23. The forces acting in the chest during a forced expiratory effort are depicted. The heavy arrows indicate compression of the thorax by contraction of the expiratory muscles. P_{pl} equals the pleural pressure, in this case 20 cm. H_2O. P_{el} equals elastic recoil pressure of the lung, in this case 10 cm. H_2O. P_{alv} equals pressure in the alveolus = P_{pl} (20) + P_{el} (10) = 30 cm. H_2O. Note that the pressure in the airways drops from the alveolar pressure (30 cm. H_2O) to the mouth or P_{ao} (or atmospheric pressure). EPP indicates the "equal pressure point," i.e., the point in the airway at which the intramural and extramural pressures are equal, in this case 20 cm. H_2O. Farther downstream from the equal pressure point, toward the airway opening, there is a transmural pressure tending to narrow or close the airway.

a total cross-sectional area for airflow that is many times that of the central airways, and therefore constitute only 10 to 15 per cent of the total airway resistance. The flow through each individual peripheral airway is slight, and there is very little pressure drop across them. For this reason, the total airway resistance may be little altered, even when there is significant disease of the small peripheral airways and the ventilation of the air spaces distal to them is seriously impaired. Fortunately, there are now a number of determinations that are thought to reflect alterations in the peripheral airways. In general, these are based on the interrelationship between lung elastic recoil and the flow resistance in the airways that subtend them.

Upstream Resistance. As we have seen in Figure 23, the airways that are downstream from the EPP are subject to compression during a forced expiration, because the pressure surrounding the airways is greater than the pressure inside the airways. Figure 23 also indicates that the pressure responsible for airflow in the **upstream airways** (i.e., between the EPP and the alveoli) is the difference between the pressure in the alveoli and the intrabronchial pressure at the EPP. Since the pressure in the airways at the EPP is equal to the pleural pressure, the driving pressure in the upstream segment of the airways is $P_{alv} - P_{pl}$, or the elastic recoil pressure of the lungs (P_{el}). Thus, the **upstream resistance** (R_{us}) at any volume can be calculated:

$$R_{us} = P_{el}/\dot{V}_{max}$$

Since, as we have seen, it is possible to determine the relationship between the static lung elastic recoil pressure and lung volume, a plot of the relationship between lung elastic recoil pressure and maximal expiratory flow ($\dot{V}_{max}$) at equivalent lung volumes allows visualization of the pressure-flow relationships (i.e., the flow resistance) of the upstream segment of the airways.

Maximal Expiratory Flow Rate. From the foregoing, it is apparent that the $\dot{V}_{max}$ at any lung volume is related to the lung elastic recoil (P_{el}) and the resistance to airflow in the airways that are upstream from the EPP (R_{us}):

$$\dot{V}_{max} = P_{el}/R_{us}$$

Clearly then, a lower than expected $\dot{V}_{max}$ may be due to an increased upstream resistance (i.e., airway narrowing), a reduced driving pressure (i.e., loss of elastic recoil) or both disturbances. Figure 24 indicates examples of a lower-than-expected $\dot{V}_{max}$ in two patients. In one case, the flow rate is low because the upstream resistance is elevated. In the other case, the upstream resistance is normal, but the driving pressure is reduced (i.e., the patient has emphysema). As a corollary, it should be clear that if the lung elastic recoil pressure at a particular lung volume is greater than expected (such as in pulmonary fibrosis), then the $\dot{V}_{max}$ at any lung volume should be greater than expected, unless the upstream resistance is proportionately elevated. In other words, in patients with pulmonary fibrosis, a "normal" $\dot{V}_{max}$ is indicative of an increase in upstream resistance.

Frequency Dependence of Compliance. As has been discussed, it is possible to recognize disease of the peripheral lung units when the upstream resistance is increased. However, in early disease of the peripheral units, the disturbances are frequently spotty and the upstream resistance may not be sufficiently elevated to be recognized as abnormal. The nonuniformly distributed disturbances of the peripheral lung units may be recognized by measurement of parameters that are affected by the rate at which these parts of the lung can fill or empty, and that depends on their respective flow resistances and compliances, i.e., the distribution of time constants in the lung.

This concept of time constants in the lung is best illustrated by reference to an electrical analogue. The emptying of an elastic reservoir, such as the lung, through a resistive conduit, such as the airways, resembles the discharging of a capacitor through a resistor. If the charge (I) on the capacitor

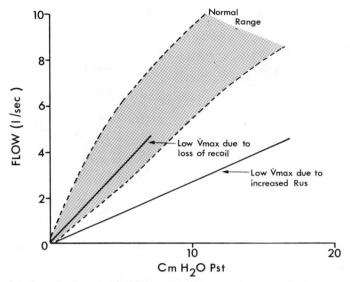

Figure 24. The graph shows the relationship between the static elastic recoil pressure of the lung (P_{st}) and air flow ($\dot{V}_{max}$ determined during an FVC). The stippled area represents the range in healthy individuals. Note that the $\dot{V}_{max}$ is lower than normal when there is a loss of lung elastic recoil (the pressure-flow relationships are normal, but the driving pressure is reduced), or when there is an increased upstream resistance (R_{us}); i.e., a given flow rate is associated with a greater-than-normal pressure.

is plotted as a fraction of the initial charge (I_o) against time, then an exponential curve is obtained whose equation is;

$$I/I_o = e^{-Kt}$$

The constant K is equal to 1/RC, where R is the resistance and C the capacitance. When the exponent has a value of unity (i.e., $K_t = 1$) the equation becomes

$$I/I_o = e^{-1} = 1/e = 0.37$$

and

$$t = 1/k = 1/1/RC = RC$$

In this capacitance-resistance system, the time it takes the charge to fall to 37 per cent of its initial value is called the time constant, and this is equal to the product of the resistance and capacitance.

The same considerations apply to a lung unit; the time it takes a lung unit to fill or empty depends on its time constant or the product of its resistance and compliance:

$$R \text{ (cm. } H_2O/l./sec.) \times C \text{ (l./cm. } H_2O) = sec.$$

When two or more parallel units in the lung are subjected to the same inflation or deflation pressure, they will each fill or empty at a rate that is

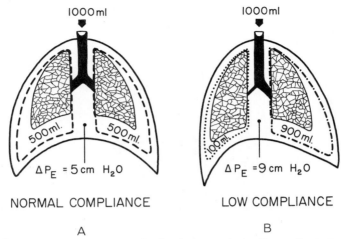

Figure 25. Represented is the effect of a local airway obstruction on the pressure-volume relationship of two lungs that have the same elastic properties when 1000 ml. of air is inhaled during breathing. When there is no difference in flow resistance, the major impedance to lung distention is the elastic resistance, and both lungs share the inspired volume equally. When there is local obstruction, particularly at rapid respiratory rates (high flow rates), the major impedance will be flow resistive, the inspired volume will be distributed unequally, and the calculated compliance of the lungs will be lower.

determined by their individual time constants. If the time constants of the units are the same, the units will fill or empty uniformly. Conversely, if the time constants of the lung units are not equal, they will fill or empty nonuniformly. Thus, when there are local alterations in the mechanical properties of the lungs, such as may occur when the airway resistance or the compliance of the alveoli varies throughout the lung, then the distribution of gas in the lung will be altered. Thus alterations in the periphery of the lung will be indicated by tests that reflect the distribution of gas (such as the single-breath nitrogen test).

By influencing the distribution of gas in the lung, inequality of the time constants throughout the lung also affects the measurement of dynamic lung compliance, particularly at rapid breathing rates. The mechanism of this phenomenon is shown in Figure 25, where, for simplicity, two lungs are depicted. In the normal situation *(A)* the complicance of each lung and the flow resistance of each airway are the same. A change in pressure of 5 cm. H_2O across the lungs between end-expiration and end-inspiration brings 500 ml. into each lung. In this case, then, the compliance of each lung is 500/5, or 0.100 l./cm. H_2O, and the compliance of both lungs is 1.0/5, or 0.200 l./cm. H_2O. It is interesting that, in healthy lungs, the dynamic compliance of the lungs does not change even when the respiratory rate is increased to about 60/min. This is remarkable, since it means that the distribution of elastic and flow-resistive properties of the lung units is such that the time constants, and therefore the distribution of inspired gas, remain the same over this range of respiratory rates.

When there is localized airway obstruction, the dynamic compliance is frequently reduced. This is illustrated in Figure 25B, where the compliance of each lung is unchanged and is the same as in A, but where flow resistance is increased in one of the airways. If the tidal volume is inhaled exceedingly slowly, the resistance to airflow is minimal, the major impedance to the change in volume is the elastic recoil of each lung, and the calculated dynamic lung compliance is virtually unaltered. On the other hand, if the tidal volume is inhaled rapidly, the principal impedance to the volume change is the flow resistance, and, since those of the two lungs (and therefore the time constants) are markedly dissimilar, the lungs do not share equally in the volume change. The majority of the flow will take place through the airway with the lower resistance, and this lung will undergo greater inflation. If the same total volume of air is to be inspired into the lungs under these circumstances, then a greater pressure change will be necessary across the more inflated lung. As a result, the calculated dynamic compliance of the lungs will be reduced. The faster the breathing rate, the lower will be the measured compliance. At extremely high frequencies, virtually all of the volume change could take place in and out of one unit, and when this occurs, the calculated dynamic compliance will be approximately one-half of that obtained during exceedingly slow breathing. In the example shown in Figure 25B, the pressure must change by 9 cm. H_2O in order to bring 900 ml. into the unobstructed lung; so the calculated dynamic compliance is 1.0/9, or 0.111 l./cm. H_2O. The compliance would fall an equal amount if the flow resistance were the same in two units, but their compliance was different. A fall in lung compliance with increasing respiratory rate is called *frequency dependence of compliance*. The presence of *frequency dependence of compliance* in a patient whose static pressure-volume characteristics of the lung and airway resistance are normal is thought to reflect an alteration in the peripheral lung units.

WORK OF BREATHING

To overcome the impedances to breathing offered by the mechanical properties of the lung and the chest wall, work must be performed by the respiratory muscles. Work is usually defined as a force acting through a distance, and is expressed in dynes/cm.^{2} × cm.^{3}. Conventionally, the work of the respiratory muscles is determined from the product of the change in the pressure, which is the force developed divided by the surface area over which it acts; and the volume, which is used as an index of the change in length or distance.

Four aspects of the work of breathing are of particular importance in understanding pulmonary disability: (1) the total amount of mechanical work that is performed during breathing; (2) the relationship between the amount of work performed and that portion of the total ventilation which actually takes part in gas exchange, i.e., the alveolar ventilation; (3) the amount of oxygen consumed by the respiratory muscles while they are performing this work; and (4) the relationship between the amount of work necessary and the development of muscle fatigue.

TOTAL MECHANICAL WORK OF BREATHING

The total amount of work performed during breathing is the sum of the amount performed to overcome elastic resistance and that necessary to overcome flow resistance. The amount performed to overcome the elastic resistance of the total respiratory system may be estimated from the *relaxation pressure curve*. However, there is no direct method available for measuring the total amount of work being done on the lung, the respired gases, the chest wall, the diaphragm and the abdominal contents while a subject is breathing, because no technique has been devised to determine the frictional resistance of the chest wall. Two indirect methods of estimating total mechanical work of breathing have been described. In the first method, a ventilator is substituted for the respiratory muscles of a paralyzed or "completely relaxed" subject, and it is presumed that the force exerted and the resultant movements of the chest are similar to those resulting from the action of the respiratory muscles during breathing. In the second method, the total mechanical work is calculated indirectly from the change in oxygen consumption brought about by an increase in ventilation, and the efficiency with which added respiratory work loads are handled. Because the efficiency of the respiratory muscles appears to be constant over a wide range of added work loads, it is possible to calculate the total work of breathing.

MECHANICAL WORK DONE ON THE LUNGS

The amount of mechanical work performed solely on the lungs during a breathing cycle can be estimated by measuring the simultaneous changes in intrathoracic pressure and volume. Figure 26 demonstrates the information that can be derived from a plot of the pressure and volume measurements (i.e., a pressure-volume loop) over the period of a complete breathing cycle. The area of the trapezoid *(OACD)* represents the amount of work necessary to overcome the elastic resistance during inspiration, whereas the work required to overcome flow resistance during both inspiration and expiration is calculated from the area of the loop (AB^1CB^2). The portion of the loop that falls to the right of the line ABC represents the work necessary to overcome inspiratory flow resistance, and the portion of the loop that falls to the left of the line ABC represents the mechanical work required to overcome expiratory flow resistance.

During quiet breathing in healthy individuals, virtually all of the work is carried out during inspiration, because the elastic recoil of the lungs is sufficient to overcome the frictional resistance of both airflow and the tissues during expiration. Indeed, the expiratory work loop does not usually fill the entire trapezoid, and some of the elastic energy built up during inspiration is dissipated in the form of heat. When a portion of the expiratory work loop falls outside the trapezoid, it means that the intrathoracic pressure

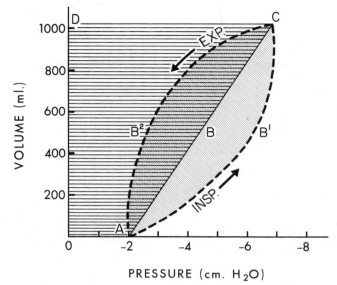

Figure 26. The mechanical work done on the lungs during a breathing cycle. The work necessary to overcome elastic resistance equals the area of trapezoid OACD. Mechanical work necessary to overcome inspiratory flow resistance equals area AB¹CB. Mechanical work necessary to overcome expiratory flow resistance equals ABCB².

became positive during expiration, and this signifies that expiratory muscular work was required for that part of the expiration.

The amount of mechanical work carried out on the lungs during a breath is calculated from the sum of the work necessary to overcome elastic resistance, the resistance to airflow during inspiration, and, when applicable, the work necessary to overcome that portion of the expiratory flow resistance work loop which falls outside of the elastic work trapezoid. The amount of work performed may vary from breath to breath, and one generally determines the mechanical work carried out on the lungs over a minute by multiplying the average amount of work done during a breath by the respiratory rate.

In normal subjects the amount of mechanical work performed on the lungs has been estimated to be approximately 0.3 to 0.7 kg.m./min. In patients suffering from chronic airflow limitation, such as bronchial asthma or emphysema, the mechanical work necessary to overcome flow resistance is markedly increased, so that the pressure-volume loop is widened (Fig. 27A); whereas, in pulmonary fibrosis, much more work must be performed to overcome the increased elastic resistance of the "stiff lungs" (Fig. 27B), but the work required to overcome flow resistance is often little altered. In patients suffering from respiratory disease, the work of breathing frequently increases disproportionately when the ventilation increases, and it is likely that an increase in mechanical work plays a role in limiting a patient's activity.

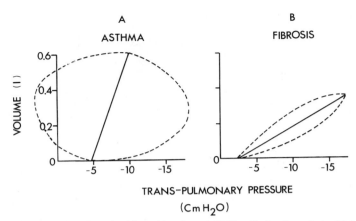

Figure 27. The mechanical work of breathing in a patient suffering from bronchial asthma is shown in **A,** and that in a patient suffering from pulmonary fibrosis is shown in **B.** Note that the flow resistance loop falls outside of the elastic work area in the patient with asthma. Thus additional work was necessary to overcome flow resistance during expiration in this patient.

MECHANICAL WORK AND ALVEOLAR VENTILATION

There appears to be a relationship between the mechanical work of breathing and the rate and depth at which a person breathes. It can be shown mathematically that for any given alveolar ventilation there is an optimum respiratory rate at which the work is minimal. As is illustrated in Figure 28A, at a respiratory rate that is less than the optimum, the flow-resistive work is low, but because larger tidal volumes are necessary to achieve the required alveolar ventilation, the amount of work required to overcome the elastic resistance is increased. At a respiratory rate that is greater than the optimum, the tidal volume is smaller, so that less work is required to overcome elastic resistance. However, the flow-resistive work will be increased, roughly in proportion to the increase in respiratory rate.

Patients with respiratory disease also appear to breathe at a rate and depth at which the work of breathing is minimal. When the elastic resistance is increased, as in disorders of the lung, such as fibrosis, or of the chest wall, such as kyphoscoliosis, the respirations tend to become rapid and shallow (Fig. 28B), probably because even small increases in tidal volume increase the amount of work required to overcome the elastic resistance. Because the elastic resistance is increased, the curve representing elastic work is shifted upward; i.e., the amount of work performed is greater at any respiratory rate, and the rate at which the total work is minimal is increased. Conversely, if the flow resistance is increased, as in bronchial obstruction, the respirations tend to become slower and deeper (Fig. 28C). This is because the curve representing the work to overcome flow resistance is shifted upward, and a fast respiratory rate entails an increased amount of work to overcome flow resistance.

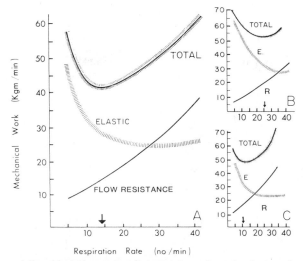

Respiration Rate (no./min)

Figure 28. The relationship between respiratory rate and mechanical work of breathing at a given alveolar ventilation. In the healthy individual **(A)** an increase in respiratory rate is associated with a fall in tidal volume, so that elastic work (E) is reduced, but the increase in rate and therefore airflow resistance results in a rise in the work required to overcome flow resistance (R). As a result of these divergent effects, there is a respiratory rate at which the total work of breathing is minimal.

In a patient with a restrictive disorder **(B)**, the elastic work is greater at any respiratory rate, and as a result the total work of breathing is minimal at a higher respiratory rate than in the healthy individual. In a patient with an obstructive disorder **(C)**, the flow-resistive work is greater at any respiratory rate, so that the total work is least at a lower respiratory frequency than in the healthy individual.

OXYGEN COST OF BREATHING

To perform the mechanical work of breathing, the respiratory muscles require oxygen. The oxygen consumption of the respiratory apparatus has been estimated by determining the difference between the oxygen consumption during resting breathing and that during an increased ventilation. Figure 29 illustrates the change in oxygen consumption associated with increases in ventilation in a healthy subject and in patients with respiratory insufficiency. A healthy person is able to increase ventilation considerably without much rise in oxygen consumption, the oxygen cost of breathing ranging between 0.3 and 1.8 ml./l. of ventilation at ventilations up to about 50 l./min., clearly a very small proportion of the total oxygen consumption. At ventilations above 50 l./min. the ventilatory apparatus uses a greater proportion of the total oxygen consumption; at still higher ventilations, the oxygen cost per unit of ventilation becomes progressively greater and may constitute a significant proportion of the total oxygen consumption. In the example shown, the oxygen requirement of the respiratory apparatus in the healthy individual is about 30 per cent of the total oxygen consumption when the ventilation is 70 l./min.

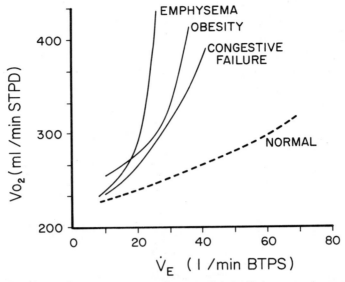

Figure 29. The change in oxygen consumption associated with increases in ventilation in a normal subject and in patients with respiratory insufficiency is shown. In the patients, small increases in ventilation are associated with marked increases in oxygen consumption; i.e., the oxygen cost of breathing is higher.

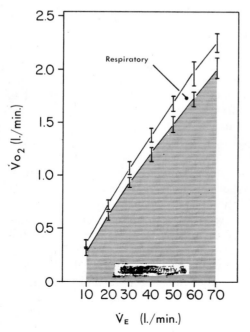

Figure 30. The relationship between ventilation and oxygen consumption during increasing exercise in normal subjects. The oxygen consumption at each ventilation is subdivided into a respiratory and a nonrespiratory component.

Figure 29 also shows that in patients suffering from chronic airflow limitation (such as emphysema), obesity or congestive heart failure, the oxygen cost of breathing, even at a low ventilation, may be four to ten times that of healthy individuals and may amount to as much as 25 per cent of the total oxygen consumption. In addition, it can be seen that the ventilation at which the oxygen consumption increases disproportionately is very much lower in the patients with respiratory insufficiency. In such patients, then, any activity that necessitates an increased ventilation may be associated with a greater energy requirement of the respiratory muscles, and this may play a major role in the respiratory insufficiency.

Oxygen Cost of Breathing and Exercise

It has been suggested that exercise tolerance may depend on the relationship between the total oxygen uptake and the oxygen consumption of the respiratory muscles during the exercise. The relationship between ventilation and oxygen consumption during increasing exercise in healthy subjects and patients with emphysema are shown in Figures 30 and 31, respectively. The total oxygen consumption during exercise is divided into the portion required by the respiratory apparatus and that consumed by the nonrespiratory tissues. In healthy subjects, the proportion of the exercise oxygen consumption being used by the respiratory apparatus at low ventilations (i.e., low exercise loads) is very small (roughly 2 per cent of the total) so that 98 per cent of the oxygen is available for the rest of the body. As the severity of the exercise increases, the greater ventilation is associated with an increased oxygen cost of breathing, so that the respiratory apparatus takes a larger proportion of the total oxygen uptake. In the patients with emphysema, the amount of oxygen consumed by the respiratory muscles is greater at each level of ventilation, so that the oxygen available for nonrespiratory work is reduced. In such situations, a stage may be reached at which the oxygen consumption is insufficient to meet the needs of both the respiratory muscles and the other exercising muscles. As a result, either the exercising muscles, the respiratory muscles or both must go into more oxygen debt, and exercise tolerance may be limited.

Figure 31. The relationship between ventilation and oxygen consumption during increasing exercise in patients with emphysema. The oxygen consumption at each ventilation is subdivided into a respiratory and a nonrespiratory component.

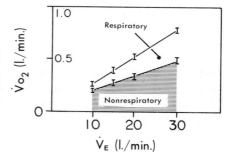

Efficiency of the Respiratory Muscles

The efficiency of a system is represented by the relationship between mechanical work and the energy consumption. In the case of the respiratory muscles

Efficiency (%) = 100 × (mechanical work (kg.m.) / oxygen cost (kg.m.)

As described earlier, the mechanical work performed on the lungs can be determined approximately by using the esophageal pressure as an index of the intrathoracic pressure, but the total work performed in moving the lung, chest wall and abdominal contents cannot be measured directly in the spontaneously breathing subject. Nevertheless, the efficiency with which an added respiratory work load is handled has been used to calculate the efficiency of the respiratory muscles. Using this technique, the efficiency of the respiratory muscles has been found to vary between 5 and 10 per cent in healthy subjects, and it is apparently even lower in patients with cardiorespiratory disease. The mechanism of the reduced efficiency of the respiratory muscles in cardiorespiratory disease has not been elucidated, but a similar reduction in efficiency can be induced in healthy subjects if they breathe against added resistive loads or inhale hypoxic gas mixtures.

MECHANICAL WORK AND RESPIRATORY MUSCLE FATIGUE

Recently, it has been suggested that respiratory muscle fatique may play an important role in respiratory insufficiency. Like any muscle, respiratory muscles will continue to work indefinitely without becoming fatigued so long as the product of its efficiency and the rate of energy that is being supplied to the muscle is greater than or equal to its muscle power and energy consumption (oxygen cost). However, all muscles have a finite endurance time, and they will fail as a force generator if the product of the energy supply and the efficiency is less than the muscle power. Clearly then, there may be a predisposition to the development of fatigue if the efficiency of the respiratory muscles is reduced, or the oxygen supply to the muscles is diminished (as would occur with a low O_2 content or cardiac output) or there is a marked increase in the amount of mechanical work required to overcome an increased impedance to breathing, as occurs with airflow limitation or stiff lungs. Thus it is not unreasonable to presume that if the mechanical work of breathing is increased and the oxygen cost of the respiratory muscles exceeds the rate of oxygen supplied to them, fatigue will develop.

It has been demonstrated that inspiratory muscle fatigue will develop even in healthy individuals at transdiaphragmatic pressures that are greater than 40 per cent of the maximum achievable when such individuals breathe through an external resistance. The muscle fatigue comes on sooner if the individual is inhaling a hypoxic gas mixture or is breathing at an increased lung volume. It has also been shown that the respiratory muscles are weaker in undernourished individuals, so these individuals might be expected to demonstrate respiratory muscle fatigue earlier. Similarly, one might expect that all muscles, including the respiratory muscles, will be prone to become fatigued when neurologic disease, myopathy or muscular atrophy develop.

Several studies have suggested that the respiratory muscles are fatigued in patients with respiratory failure and that this may be important during the process of weaning from a ventilator. There seems to be an inherent attempt to overcome fatigue of the respiratory muscles when it develops, and it appears that patients tend to alternate their breathing pattern, using either the diaphragm predominantly or the intercostal/accessory muscles. This results in asynchronous movements of the abdomen as the rib cage expands, and indeed this has been described in patients with severe cardiorespiratory disease or acute respiratory failure.

Thus fatigue of the respiratory muscles may be a very important clinical event that must be recognized. Clearly, if respiratory muscle fatigue is an important factor in pulmonary disability and in respiratory failure, then it is possible that respiratory muscle training will improve endurance and that this is an essential aspect of the management of patients with cardiorespiratory insufficiency. Although the clinical relevance has not been fully elucidated, it has been demonstrated that respiratory muscle training increases strength and endurance in patients with chronic airflow limitation or cystic fibrosis and in quadraplegic individuals.

PULMONARY VENTILATION, BLOOD FLOW AND GAS EXCHANGE

As we have seen in Chapter 1, the respiratory pump provides the pulmonary ventilation by moving gas into and out of the lungs, and this provides oxygen to the pulmonary capillary blood and removes carbon dioxide from the blood. The transport of oxygen from the lungs to the tissue cells and of carbon dioxide from the tissues to the lungs depends on the convective movement of blood in the circulatory system. In this chapter, the special features of the ventilation and the circulation of the lung will be discussed.

PULMONARY VENTILATION

Normally, we breathe about 6 to 7 liters of air per minute. Practically speaking, however, it is not the amount of air we breathe that is all-important; rather, it is the amount that is concerned in the exchanges of gases with the blood, a process that takes place only in the alveoli. About 20 to 30 per cent of the inspired air is normally wasted, because it fills the parts of the respiratory system that serve as the conducting airway, i.e., the dead space, and is eliminated during the next exhalation.

DEAD SPACE

The mouth, nose, pharynx, larynx, trachea, bronchi and bronchioles are the conducting system for air and are collectively called the *anatomic dead space*. Actually the division between the ventilation of dead space and that of the alveoli is not that sharp, for areas of lung that are overventilated relative to their perfusion also may contribute to the dead space. Thus, functionally, the dead space is really a physiologic not an anatomic concept;

it may be defined as the volume of the inspired gas that does not take part in gas exchange. The *physiologic dead space* therefore includes the volume of the anatomic dead space and the volume of the inspired gas that ventilates alveoli that are not perfused by capillary blood flow.

In healthy young persons the physiologic dead space is equal to the anatomic dead space and is approximately 150 ml. at rest, or about 20 to 30 per cent of the tidal volume. In patients suffering from pulmonary disease, there is considerable ventilation of alveoli whose perfusion is inadequate or even absent as well as overventilation of other alveoli that are normally perfused, so that the physiologic dead space is increased.

Measurement of Physiologic Dead Space

Calculation of the physiologic dead space is based on Bohr's formula, which states that the expired air consists of a mixture of two components, one from the physiologic dead space, which has the same composition as the inspired air, and an alveolar component, which has given up oxygen and received carbon dioxide.

Thus, for any gas,

$$V_T \times F_T = (V_D \times F_D) + (V_A \times F_A)$$

where V represents a gas volume and F a fractional gas concentration; the subscripts signify the specific gas volume referred to, T being tidal gas, D dead space gas and A alveolar gas.

In most cases, physiologic dead space is calculated using carbon dioxide as the reference gas. Since $V_A = V_T - V_D$, and the concentration of CO_2 in the dead space is the same as that of the inspired air (i.e., virtually zero), the equation becomes

$$V_T \times F_E CO_2 = (V_T - V_D) \times F_A CO_2$$

and

$$V_D/V_T = \frac{F_A CO_2 - F_E CO_2}{F_A CO_2}$$

or, when expressed in terms of the partial pressures,

$$V_D/V_T = \frac{P_A CO_2 - P_E CO_2}{P_A CO_2}$$

For instance, if the tidal volume were 500 ml., the respiratory rate 12/minute, and the concentrations of carbon dioxide in the expired and alveolar gases 4 and 6 per cent, respectively, then

$$V_D = 500 \times \frac{6-4}{6} = 167 \text{ ml. and } V_D/V_T = 1/3$$

As long as the lungs are healthy, the end-tidal $P CO_2$ is a fairly accurate reflection of the mean $P_A CO_2$. However, in patients with cardiorespiratory disease, it is difficult to obtain a representative alveolar sample, so that, in practice, arterial P_{CO_2} is substituted for the alveolar P_{CO_2} when one calculates the physiologic dead space.

ALVEOLAR VENTILATION

As air is inspired into the lungs and carried toward the alveolar spaces, it becomes saturated with water, which evaporates from the surfaces of the airways. Water vapor is similar to any other gas in that it exerts a partial pressure and behaves independently from the other gases in a mixture. On the other hand, since it is in equilibrium with the liquid phase, it behaves differently from other gases in one respect: its partial pressure depends almost completely on the temperature and is almost independent of the barometric pressure. At normal body temperature (37°C) the partial pressure of water vapor is 47 mm. Hg.

The total pressure of gases in the alveolar air corresponds to that of the ambient barometric pressure. Since water vapor is present, the total pressure of dry alveolar gas is equal to the barometric pressure minus 47 mm. Hg. Analyses of the concentrations of gases in alveolar air or expired air are reported in terms of the dry gas, so that to determine its partial pressure,

$$P_A = F_A \times (P_B - 47)$$

where P_B is barometric pressure, P the partial pressure and F the fractional concentration of the alveolar gas, A.

Since the concentrations of oxygen, carbon dioxide and nitrogen in the alveolar air are approximately 14, 6 and 80 per cent, respectively, their partial pressures at sea level are approximately 100, 40 and 570 mm. Hg, respectively. However, the gas concentrations in the alveoli are not constant and are changing from moment to moment during inspiration and expiration. In addition, the concentrations are not the same in different parts of the lung, because the distribution of air and blood is not uniform. Each individual alveolus can be viewed as an equilibration chamber, the composition of its gas representing a balance between the fresh air entering the alveoli, which raises the P_{O_2} and lowers the P_{CO_2}, and the gas entering from the mixed venous blood, which lowers the P_{O_2} and raises the P_{CO_2}. Clearly then, any stated value for an alveolar gas concentration or partial pressure is some sort of average figure and does not describe the actual situation in all parts of the lung.

Measurement of Alveolar Ventilation

From knowledge of the tidal volume (V_T), and the frequency of breathing (f), the minute ventilation (V_E) can be calculated.

$$\dot{V}_E = V_T \times f$$

Since $V_T = V_D + V_A$, the alveolar ventilation per minute $(\dot{V}_A)$ can be calculated if one knows the size of the physiologic dead space.

$$\dot{V}_A = (V_T - V_D) \times f$$

The alveolar ventilation may also be calculated directly from the Bohr equation. Since the concentration of carbon dioxide in the dead space is virtually zero, then

$$\dot{V}_E F_E = \dot{V}_A F_A \quad \text{and} \quad \dot{V}_A = \dot{V}_E \times F_E/F_A$$

where $\dot{V}$ is the ventilation/minute and F the fractional gas concentration of E, the expired, and A, the alveolar, ventilation, respectively.

In the example used for calculation of the dead space, the alveolar ventilation is

$$\dot{V}_A = 6.0 \times 0.4/0.6 = 4 \text{ l./min.}$$

Clearly, for a given-sized dead space, a reduction or an increase in minute ventilation per se will result in a similar rise or fall in alveolar ventilation. Even if the minute ventilation were to remain constant, however, a change in the size of the dead space or in tidal volume or respiratory frequency would affect the alveolar ventilation (Table 2). The alveolar ventilation falls despite a constant minute ventilation if the dead space increases *(a)*. This situation arises particularly in patients with emphysema, in whom the physiologic dead space is increased. If the minute ventilation and the dead space are constant, the alveolar ventilation also falls when the tidal volume falls *(b)* or when the respiratory rate increases *(c)*. Such a reduction in alveolar ventilation because of rapid shallow breathing may be encountered in patients who are suffering from kyphoscoliosis or severe obesity. For any given minute ventilation, then, an increase in the dead space or a decrease in the tidal volume has the same net effect, namely, a reduction in the alveolar ventilation, with consequent effects on the arterial blood gas tensions. If an increase in dead space and a decrease in the tidal volume should occur simultaneously, the situation would, of course, be severely aggravated.

Alveolar Ventilation and Carbon Dioxide Production

The absolute level of the alveolar ventilation does not determine the effectiveness of gas exchange; rather the adequacy of the alveolar ventilation must be judged in relation to the body's metabolic consumption of oxygen or carbon dioxide production. In practice, one generally relates it to the metabolic carbon dioxide production, which, in a steady state, is equal to the amount of carbon dioxide being eliminated by the alveoli. This, in turn, is the difference between the amounts of carbon dioxide entering and leaving the alveoli per unit time. Since there is virtually no CO_2 in the inspired air, then

$$\dot{V}CO_2 = \dot{V}_A \times F_A CO_2$$

where $\dot{V}CO_2$ is the amount of CO_2 eliminated from the lungs, $\dot{V}_A$ the alveolar ventilation and $F_A CO_2$ the concentration of CO_2 in the alveoli,

and

$$F_A CO_2 = \dot{V}CO_2/\dot{V}_A$$

TABLE 2. Effect on Alveolar Ventilation of Change in (a) Dead Space, (b) Minute Ventilation and (c) Respiratory Pattern

$\dot{V}_E$ (l./min.)	V_T (l.)	f (No./min.)	V_D (l.)	$\dot{V}_A$ (l./min.)
a. 8.0	0.50	16	0.15	5.6
8.0	0.50	16	0.25	4.0
8.0	0.50	16	0.35	2.4
b. 8.0	0.50	16	0.15	5.6
6.4	0.40	16	0.15	4.0
4.8	0.30	16	0.15	2.4
c. 8.0	0.80	10	0.15	6.5
8.0	0.50	16	0.15	5.6
8.0	0.25	32	0.15	3.2

Or, when expressed in terms of the partial pressure of CO_2,

$$P_ACO_2 \text{ (mm. Hg)} = 0.863 \times \dot{V}CO_2 / \dot{V}_A$$

The factor 0.863 corrects for the fact that the CO_2 production is expressed as a dry gas volume at a standard temperature and pressure (STPD), whereas the alveolar ventilation is expressed as a wet gas volume at body temperature and pressure (BTPS). An analogous relationship can be derived between alveolar ventilation and the alveolar PO_2.

In practice, it is difficult to obtain a valid sample of the mixed alveolar gas, since, as we have seen, the alveolar gas is different in various parts of the lung, even in healthy individuals. However, there is usually very little difference between the arterial PCO_2 and that of the mixed alveolar gas; so the arterial PCO_2 provides an excellent measure of the "effective" alveolar PCO_2 and the ability of the alveolar ventilation to cope with the metabolic production of carbon dioxide. On the other hand, the arterial PO_2 is usually very different from the alveolar PO_2, because it is influenced by many other factors besides the alveolar ventilation.

When the alveolar ventilation is insufficient to cope with a given CO_2 production, *alveolar hypoventilation* is present, and the alveolar (and arterial) PCO_2 is higher than normal (i.e., greater than 45 mm. Hg at sea level). Conversely, *alveolar hyperventilation* is present when the alveolar ventilation is greater than is necessary to cope with the CO_2 production; so the alveolar (and arterial) PCO_2 is lower than normal (i.e., less than 35 mm. Hg at sea level).

DISTRIBUTION OF PULMONARY VENTILATION

Ventilation of the alveoli is not enough to ensure an adequate exchange of oxygen; the incoming air must be distributed uniformly so that each alveolus receives its share. However, even in young healthy persons, and particularly in older persons, the inspired air is not distributed uniformly throughout the lungs. This is because the pleural pressure is different at various levels in the chest.

At the top of the pleural space, i.e., at the apex of the lung when one is standing or seated or at the sternal margin if one is supine, the tendency for the lung to retract away from the chest wall is added to by the force of gravity (weight of the lung), and the lung is pulled further away from the chest wall. At the bottom of the pleural space, the weight of the lung counteracts the tendency of the lung to pull away from the chest wall so that the pleural surface of the lung is pushed against the chest wall. As a result, the pleural pressure is more negative at the top of the lung than it is at the bottom. The pleural pressure increases by about 0.25 cm. H_2O/cm. of distance from the top to the bottom of the lungs. Because of this regional difference in pleural pressure, the lung units are at different portions of their individual pressure-volume relationships, and the air spaces near the top of the lung are more expanded than are those near the bottom.

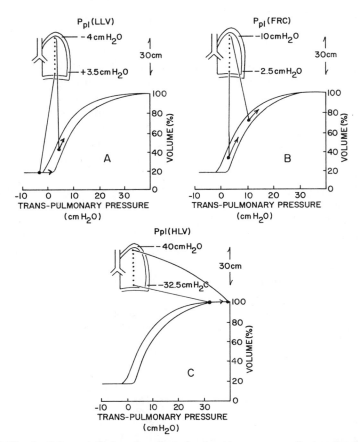

Figure 32. Graphs **A** through **C** show the effect of a pleural pressure gradient on the distribution of ventilation (the pressure is assumed to fall at a rate of 0.25 cm. of water per cm. of vertical distance). At low lung volumes **(A)** the pleural pressure at the base may exceed airway pressure so that this region is not ventilated and the initial part of inspiration is delivered to the apex of the lung. During an inspiration from FRC **(B)** air is distributed to the upper and lower parts of the lung. Because the pressures at the apex and base are taken to be −10 and −2.5 cm. of H_2O, respectively, the two regions are on different parts of the pressure-volume curve, and the lung units at the base are smaller than those at the apex. On inspiration the lung units at the base have a greater change in volume than do those at the apex. At FRC, therefore, ventilation decreases with vertical distance up the lung. At high lung volumes **(C)** both upper and lower lung regions are on the flat part of the pressure-volume curve and exhibit changes in volume that correspond to changes in transpulmonary pressure.

The distribution of inspired air to the different lung regions will depend upon the lung volume at which one is breathing (Fig. 32). At very low lung volumes, the airways in the dependent portions of the lung tend to be closed, because the pleural pressure is greater than the airway pressure. Thus, if one were breathing at a very low lung volume, the upper part of the lung would be ventilated more than the lower part *(A)*, which would receive little, if any, ventilation. During normal breathing, i.e., at FRC *(B),* both the upper and lower parts of the lung are ventilated, but the air spaces in the upper zone are on the less steep portion of the pressure-volume curve, so they tend to fill somewhat less than those at the base. If one were to breathe at lung volumes close to TLC, the changes in volume at the top and bottom, though minimal, would tend to be smaller *(C)*, since both the upper and lower regions are on the flat part of the pressure-volume curve.

As we have seen in Chapter 1, the distribution of the inspired gas will also be affected by regional differences in time constants of the peripheral lung units, which may result from patchy alterations of the mechanical resistances offered by the lung parenchyma, the airways or the extrapulmonary structures. Figure 33 illustrates the effect of a localized obstruction on the distribution of gas, as exemplified by the moment-to-moment nitrogen concentration in the expired air following a maximum inspiration of pure oxygen. When both airways are widely patent, the inspired gas enters both lungs almost synchronously and equally, and expiration takes place in the same fashion *(A)*. There is no nitrogen in the first part of the expired gas, because pure oxygen is being exhaled from the dead space. After this, the nitrogen concentration rises in a curvilinear fashion, because gas containing nitrogen from the alveolar spaces mixes with the oxygen from the dead

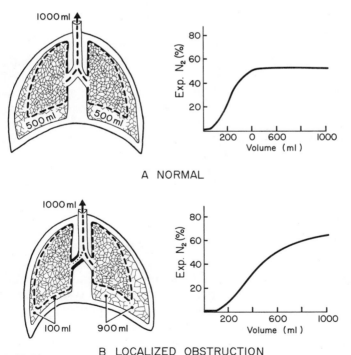

Figure 33. The effect of a localized airway obstruction on the distribution of air is depicted. Normally **(A)**, air is distributed synchronously and equally, and expiration takes place in the same manner. As a result, the nitrogen concentration reaches a virtual plateau. With localized airway obstruction **(B)**, inspired oxygen moves predominantly into areas of lung that offer least resistance. During expiration, air moves out of the unobstructed lung first, and the asynchronous delivery of air results in a rising nitrogen concentration curve.

space. The last portion of the expired nitrogen concentration curve is almost a plateau, indicating that the nitrogen concentration of the gas coming from each lung is virtually the same. The very slight rise in the plateau is probably due to sequential emptying of different areas of the lungs.

When there is a localized alteration in flow resistance (Fig. 33B), the inspired oxygen is not distributed equally between the two areas. Instead, it moves into and distends the area offering the least resistance before it enters the other. As a result, the nitrogen in the unobstructed area will be diluted more, and hence its concentration will be lower, than in the obstructed area. During the ensuing expiration, one again sees pure oxygen initially, and then the curvilinear rise in nitrogen concentration, but this time air moves out of the unobstructed lung first, and the air leaving the obstructed lung is delayed. The asynchronous delivery of air from the two lungs (and hence differing nitrogen concentrations) results in a rising nitrogen concentration curve.

Clearly then, assessment of the distribution of a gas such as oxygen or a relatively insoluble reference gas such as helium or hydrogen provides information about the uniformity of the distribution of time constants in the lung. The rate at which nitrogen in the lung is diluted when pure oxygen is inhaled, or the time taken for the lungs and a spirometer to reach equilibrium with respect to a foreign gas, such as helium or hydrogen, is used clinically to assess the distribution of time constants in the lung, and like the frequency dependence of compliance, an abnormal gas distribution implies a non-uniform distribution of time constants in the lung. An abnormal distribution of inspired gas is encountered clinically in a variety of disorders characterized by regional variations in flow resistance (as in bronchial asthma, chronic bronchitis, bronchiectasis and emphysema), regional areas of reduced lung compliance (as in emphysema) or increased lung compliance (as in pulmonary congestion and interstitial fibrosis), alterations in chest wall compliance (as in kyphoscoliosis) and non-uniform application of forces to the chest wall by the respiratory muscles (as in muscular dystrophy, local muscular weakness or paralysis).

PULMONARY CIRCULATION

The pulmonary circulation resembles the systemic circulation in that it has a pump (the right ventricle), a distributing system (the pulmonary arteries and arterioles), an exchange system (the pulmonary capillaries), and a collecting system (the pulmonary venules and veins). However, the pulmonary circulation is characterized by a low pressure and a relatively low resistance to flow, and its vessels have much thinner walls and are more easily distensible. As a result, the pulmonary vessels are more susceptible to relatively small changes in extravascular pressure than are the systemic vessels. Furthermore, whereas systemic capillaries are surrounded by tissue and tissue fluid, the pulmonary capillaries are surrounded by a fluid of much lower density—the air in the alveoli. Because of these two factors, pulmonary blood flow is markedly affected by gravity and any changes in transpulmonary pressure associated with spontaneous or artificial ventilation.

FUNCTIONS OF THE PULMONARY CIRCULATION

Gas Exchange. The main function of the pulmonary circulation is to conduct mixed venous blood through the alveolar capillaries so that sufficient oxygen can be added and a proper amount of carbon dioxide can be removed.

Reservoir for Left Ventricle. The pulmonary vessels contain about 900 ml. of blood, of which more than half is in readily distensible veins. These veins, in essence, constitute a blood reservoir, which supplies blood to fill the left ventricle and maintains its output, even when the right ventricular pump falls behind for a few beats. Thus, the left ventricular stroke volume (output per beat) has been shown to remain unchanged for several beats, even when the pulmonary artery is completely blocked by a balloon. The larger the left atrium and the more distended the pulmonary veins, the more capacious will be the reservoir.

Protective Function. The pulmonary vessels act as a filter to trap and prevent small blood clots from reaching and blocking systemic arteries, arterioles or capillaries. Because the lungs can perform their gas exchange function with fewer than half of their conducting and exchange vessels, the body can tolerate block of some pulmonary vessels far better than it can tolerate block of coronary or cerebral vessels. The pulmonary vascular bed is the site of the rapid inactivation of certain endogenous substances, such as the prostaglandins, as well as the rapid activation of angiotensin.

Nutrition. The nutrition of the alveoli and alveolar ducts is provided by the pulmonary capillary blood flow. In the absence of a pulmonary circulation, the bronchial arteries can provide an adequate blood supply through new or expanded channels, but this requires several weeks to develop.

PULMONARY VASCULAR DISTENSIBILITY AND COLLAPSIBILITY

The compliance (capacitance or volume distensibility) of the pulmonary vascular bed is far greater than that of the systemic vascular bed. Unlike analogous systemic vessels, the pulmonary arteries are more distensible than the pulmonary veins, and the large arteries are more compliant than the small ones. The pulmonary capillary bed as a whole exhibits a good deal of overall volume distensibility, and individual capillaries vary widely in the amount of blood they contain. For instance, there is more blood in the capillaries at the bottom of the lung than at the top. The resistance to flow through the capillary bed can fall if previously closed capillary channels open, such as when the intracapillary pressure rises above the extravascular pressure. Presumably, capillaries do not dilate actively, but disease or change in their chemical environment may stimulate their dilation. For instance, whereas red blood cells file through one by one or may even have to squeeze through normal capillaries, the capillaries may be so wide in mitral stenosis that three or four red blood cells can flow through abreast.

The high compliance of pulmonary vessels allows the volume of blood in the lungs to change over fairly wide limits with relatively little change in pressure. This is advantageous because any transient discrepancies in the volume output of the right and left ventricles can be accommodated by the pulmonary blood reservoir. Normally about 10 per cent of the total circulating blood volume is in the lungs. The distribution of blood between the pulmonary and systemic vascular beds varies with posture and the state of contraction of pulmonary in relation to systemic vascular smooth muscle, as well as with any factor that tends to influence the difference between intra-abdominal and intrathoracic pressures.

About 30 per cent of the total pulmonary blood volume is in the arteries, about 10 per cent is in the capillaries, and about 60 per cent is in the veins. Normally the pulmonary capillary bed contains only about 75 ml. of blood, with more at the bottom of the lung than at the top, and this volume is contained in a multitude of capillaries whose surface area has been estimated at 70 m.^{2} and whose capacity is about 200 ml.

During a normal inspiration, the fall in pleural pressure distends the intrathoracic portions of the venae cavae and right atrium. As a result, blood flow into the heart increases and the right ventricular stroke volume rises. The left ventricular stroke volume also increases, but to a smaller extent, and as a result, the pulmonary blood volume increases during inspiration. By contrast, during artificial ventilation, the application of intermittent positive pressure at the airway raises the mean intrathoracic pressure, and this impedes the venous return to the heart, thereby resulting in a decrease in pulmonary blood volume. The amount of blood in the pulmonary capillaries increases as much as threefold during exercise. There is also an increase in pulmonary capillary blood volume when pulmonary congestion is present, as a result of an increased pulmonary venous pressure.

PULMONARY VASCULAR PRESSURE

Table 3 indicates the normal range of pulmonary vascular pressures and other hemodynamic values. The pressures in the pulmonary circulation must be considered in light of the surrounding environment, and there are three types of pressures used in studies of pulmonary hemodynamics.

Intravascular Pressure

The *intravascular pressure* in the pulmonary vessels, when expressed in relation to atmospheric pressure, is not the same even in similar vessels in all parts of the pulmonary circulation, because it is influenced by gravity. In a man of ordinary height, the distance between the top (apex) and bottom (base) of the lung is about 30 cm. If the main pulmonary trunk is considered to be midway between the apex and base when one is in the upright position, then the column of blood between the pulmonary trunk and the arterioles in the apex of the lung will be 15 cm. high (equivalent to 11 mm. Hg), and there will be a similar column of blood between it and the arterioles in the base.

TABLE 3. Normal Range of Hemodynamic Values

Pressures		Normal Range
Mean right atrial (P_{RA})		2–10 mm. Hg
Right ventricle (P_{RV})	systolic:	15–30 mm. Hg
	diastolic:	0– 5 mm. Hg
Pulmonary artery (P_{PA})	systolic:	15–30 mm. Hg
	diastolic:	5–12 mm. Hg
	mean:	11–18 mm. Hg
Pulmonary capillary wedge (P_{CWP}):		5–12 mm. Hg
Hemodynamics		
Cardiac output (C.O.)		4.4–8.9 l./min.
Cardiac index (C.O./BSA)		3.5 ± 0.7 l./min./m.²
Stroke volume (SV)		60–129 ml. beat
Stroke volume index (SV/BSA)		46 ± 3/beat/m.²
Pulmonary vascular resistance (PVR)		70 ± 20 dyne/sec./cm.$_{-5}$
Arteriovenous O_2 difference ($C_{(a-v)}O_2$)		4.0 ± 0.6 ml./100 ml.

Thus, if the pressure in the main pulmonary artery is 22/9 mm. Hg, there will be a differential pressure of 11 mm. Hg ($22-11$) during systole in the upper part of the lung, so that there will be blood flow. However, during diastole (when the differential pressure is $9 - 11$, or -2, mm. Hg), blood flow will stop briefly in this uppermost part of the lung. At the base of the lung the pressure will be $(22 + 11)/(9 + 11)$, or 33/20, mm. Hg. This increase in absolute pressure in the dependent vessels will distend them and therefore diminish their resistance to blood flow. The effect of gravity on the intravascular pressures will be less when one lies on one's side, since the lungs are not as wide as they are long, and will be still less when one lies prone or supine.

Transmural Pressure

The *transmural pressure* is the difference between the intravascular pressure and that of the tissue surrounding it. A greater pressure in the vessel tends to distend it, just as the transpulmonary pressure distends the lungs. A greater pressure in the tissue surrounding the vessel tends to compress or collapse the vessel. The pressure around the pulmonary arteries and veins is the intrathoracic pressure. The pressure around the smaller intrapulmonary vessels (arterioles, capillaries and venules) is difficult to measure, because it is neither the air pressure in the alveoli nor the intrapleural pressure, but some pressure in between. For some purposes the pulmonary circulation can be divided into two functional groups: those that behave as if they are exposed to the pleural pressure (extra-alveolar vessels) and those that behave as if they were exposed to the alveolar pressure (alveolar vessels). However, the pressure at the immediate outer surface of these vessels may differ in absolute value from the pleural or alveolar pressure. For example, it is thought by some that the alveolar pressure is not transmitted in full to the capillary surface because some of it is dissipated across the air-liquid interface.

Driving Pressure

The ***driving pressure*** is the difference in pressure between two points in a vessel. This difference in pressure is what overcomes frictional resistance and is responsible for the blood flow between these two points. The driving pressure for the total pulmonary circulation is the difference between the pressure at the beginning of the pulmonary circulation (the pulmonary artery) and that at the other end (the left atrium). The mean pulmonary artery pressure, the pulmonary capillary pressure and the left atrial pressure are approximately 14, 6 and 5 mm. Hg, respectively, in a healthy individual. In this case, then, the total driving pressure is 14 − 5, or 9 mm. Hg. In a patient with mitral stenosis, the left atrial pressure may rise to 21 mm. Hg, the pulmonary capillary pressure to 23 mm. Hg and the mean pulmonary artery pressure to 30 mm. Hg. In this situation, the total driving pressure remains the same (30 − 21, or 9, mm. Hg), but the capillary pressure is considerably elevated (23 instead of 6 mm. Hg), and this is close to the colloidal osmotic pressure of the plasma proteins.

It must be emphasized that the pressure may be extremely high in the pulmonary artery and normal in the pulmonary capillaries. For example, in a patient with primary pulmonary hypertension due to arteriosclerosis of the pulmonary vessels, the mean pulmonary artery pressure may be 90 mm. Hg (nearly equal to the mean systemic arterial pressure), but the pulmonary capillary pressure and left atrial pressure may be normal. The total driving pressure is very high (90 − 5, or 85, mm. Hg) because of an increased resistance to flow through the arterioles, and this imposes a very heavy work load on the right ventricle and may lead to right ventricular strain, hypertrophy and possibly failure. However, there is no danger of pulmonary edema, because the pulmonary capillary pressure is normal. Conversely, an elevation of the capillary pressure to only about 25 mm. Hg, which would not usually impose a severe strain on the right ventricle, may lead to fulminating pulmonary edema and death.

PULMONARY BLOOD FLOW

Pulmonary blood flow may be measured by many techniques. One method is the direct Fick method, which requires measurements of the O_2 uptake/min. and the O_2 concentration in the arterial (a) and mixed venous blood ($\bar{v}$):

$$\text{Blood flow (l./min.)} = \text{oxygen uptake (ml./min.)}/\text{a} - \bar{v}$$
$$\text{difference for } O_2 \text{ (ml.)}$$

Other methods of measuring pulmonary blood flow use dye or thermal dilution techniques or a body plethysmograph. The plethysmograph method is of special interest because it measures instantaneous flow through the pulmonary capillaries. With this method it has been shown that pulmonary capillary blood flow is pulsatile. This is because the arteriolar resistance is normally low in the pulmonary circulation, and the pulmonary arterial pulse is transmitted to the capillary blood.

PULMONARY VASCULAR RESISTANCE

Just as with airway resistance, the pulmonary vascular resistance is calculated by an equation similar to Ohm's law for electrical circuits. Again, one must determine the driving pressure (P_R) and the flow ($\dot{Q}$):

$$R = P_R/\dot{Q}$$

where P_R is measured in dynes/cm.^{2} (force/unit area), $\dot{Q}$ is measured as cm.^{3}/sec. and R becomes (dynes $\times$ sec.)/cm.^{5}.

In practice, the driving pressure is usually expressed in mm. Hg and flow in liters/minute, so that the resistance unit is mm. Hg/l./min. Thus, in the normal circulation, with a driving pressure of 9 mm. Hg. and a blood flow of 6 l./min., the resistance is 9/6, or 1.5, mm. Hg/l./min, i.e., almost 10 per cent of the resistance in the systemic circulation. Most of this resistance to flow occurs in the arterioles and the capillaries; there is little resistance to flow in the venous system, the pressure difference between the end of the pulmonary capillaries and the left atrium being less than 1 mm. Hg.

Factors Affecting Pulmonary Vascular Resistance

Neural Influences. The pulmonary vessels are well supplied with both sympathetic and parasympathetic nerve fibers, but under normal conditions, pulmonary vasomotor tone appears to contribute little to the total resistance of the pulmonary vessels. However, the pulmonary vascular resistance can be altered as a result of neural influences, and in animals, the pulmonary vascular resistance decreases following stimulation of systemic baroreceptors and increases following stimulation of the aortic body chemoreceptors.

Chemical Influences. The pulmonary vascular resistance is also affected by chemical influences. Hypoxia causes constriction of the pulmonary blood vessels and probably affects both the precapillary and postcapillary vessels. This vasoconstriction is likely not mediated by neural reflex mechanisms, since it also occurs in the isolated lung. On the other hand, isolated pulmonary vascular smooth muscle does not appear to contract in response to hypoxia unless remnants of lung parenchyma are attached to it. Although this suggests that hypoxia acts by causing the lung parenchyma to release a substance that induces vasoconstriction, none has been identified.

The pulmonary blood vessels exhibit a variable response to hypercapnia. When vasoconstriction occurs it is probably due to an increased H^+ concentration, since vasoconstriction does not result when hypercapnia is associated with a normal pH. Indeed, acidemia, per se, results in pulmonary vasoconstriction, and the presence of acidemia of either respiratory or metabolic origin potentiates the vasoconstrictor response to hypoxia.

Pharmacologic Influences. Certain agents, such as histamine, epinephrine, norepinephrine, angiotensin, serotonin, *E. coli* endotoxin and alloxan, also cause constriction of the pulmonary vessels. The direct effects of these vasoactive substances may be masked by passive changes in transmural pressure that develop because of the effect of these agents on the heart and systemic vessels. Furthermore, the vasoconstriction induced by agents such as epinephrine may be offset by their effects on airway smooth muscle. For example, bronchodilation may increase the ventilation of a portion of lung, and the resultant rise in partial pressure of oxygen and fall in the partial pressure of carbon dioxide may offset the increase in vascular resistance produced by epinephrine. Other agents, such as isoproterenol, acetylcholine and oxygen and vasodilating agents, dilate constricted pulmonary arterioles, and recently it has been suggested that calcium blocking agents may reduce pulmonary hypertension.

Pathologic Disturbances. The pulmonary vascular resistance is elevated in a variety of conditions. Intraluminal obstruction caused by thrombi or emboli (blood clots, parasites, fat cells, air, or tumor cells); diseases of the vascular wall, such as sclerosis, endarteritis, polyarteritis, or scleroderma; destructive or obliterative diseases, such as emphysema and interstitial pulmonary fibrosis; or compression of vessels by a mass may elevate the pulmonary vascular resistance. The increased resistance may be in the artery, arterioles, capillaries, venules or veins. If the increased resistance is in the venules or veins, then the transmural pulmonary capillary pressure rises, and pulmonary edema may result. As we have seen earlier, if the resistance is in the arteries or arterioles, the pulmonary artery pressure will be elevated, but the pulmonary capillary pressure will be normal. In any location, an increase in pulmonary vascular resistance is followed by an increased right ventricular pressure and right ventricular strain.

DISTRIBUTION OF PULMONARY BLOOD FLOW

Like the distribution of gas, the distribution of blood flow in the lungs is profoundly influenced by gravity, the intraluminal pressures in the pulmonary blood vessels and the pressures surrounding them. This interrelationship between pressures within and around the pulmonary vessels is best demonstrated in a simple mechanical model (Fig. 34), where a collapsible tube representing a pulmonary capillary is surrounded by the alveolar pressure (P_{alv}). For flow to occur through this "capillary," the perfusing pressure, i.e., pulmonary artery pressure (P_{PA}), must exceed all of the pressures downstream. For a given pulmonary artery pressure, the capillary is narrowed, its resistance increased and its flow decreased, if the alveolar pressure is elevated. The venous pressure (P_V) has no influence on blood flow as long as it is lower than the alveolar pressure. However, if the venous pressure exceeds the alveolar pressure, it will constitute an effective "back pressure" and interfere with blood flow. Under these circumstances, the amount of flow will depend on the difference between P_{PA} and P_V. This arrangement has been likened to a waterfall, where the flow over the fall is independent of the height of the fall.

Since, as we have seen, the lung has an appreciable height between apex and base, the model is expanded in Figure 35 to include a series of parallel collapsible "capillaries" that are surrounded by the same P_{alv} everywhere (2 cm. H_2O), and the effect of gravity on the pulmonary artery pressure and blood flow distribution has been introduced. P_{PA} is represented by the inflow reservoir, which is kept filled to a height of 23 cm. H_2O above the "artery" at the lowest part of the lung. The height of the fluid in the outflow reservoir, which overflows when its fluid level is more than 11 cm. above the "vein" in the lowest part of the lung, is analogous to the left atrial pressure (P_{LA}). In this model, the amount of blood flow through each "capillary" depends on the perfusing pressure, i.e., the height of the channel.

In the upper part of the model (which in the lung has been called zone 1) the P_{alv} of 2 cm. H_2O exceeds P_{PA}, which is zero. Thus, the vessels are compressed and there is no blood flow.

In the middle part of the model (called zone 2 in the lung), P_{PA} exceeds both P_{alv} and P_{LA}. In this zone, therefore, blood flow occurs, but the amount of flow in each "capillary" depends on the gradient between the inflow pressure and the alveolar pressure ($P_{PA} - P_{alv}$). This, in turn, will vary with the height of the vessel, and will be less at the top of this zone than at the bottom.

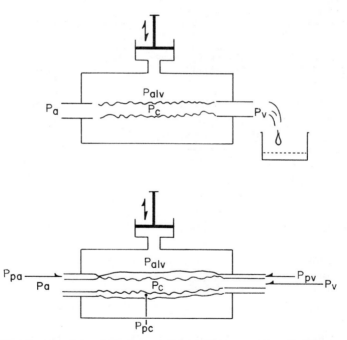

Figure 34. The upper model represents a small pulmonary vessel ("capillary") as a collapsible tube that is exposed to a variable extramural pressure analogous to alveolar pressure (P_{alv}). When the outflow pressure, or "venous" pressure (P_v), is lower than P_{alv}, it does not influence flow through the vessel. Flow will be determined by the dimension of the collapsible vessel and the inflow, or "arterial", pressure (P_a). The dimension of the vessel is determined by its transmural pressure, i.e., the difference between its intraluminal and extraluminal pressures ($P_{alv} - P_c$). Only when P_v exceeds P_{alv} is it reflected "back," hence constituting an effective "back pressure" that influences flow.

The lower model has additional elements representing extramural forces acting on the "extra-alveolar" and "intra-alveolar" portions of the vessel. These include periarterial (P_{pa}) and perivenous (P_{pv}) forces such as interstitial pressure and smooth muscle tone. Pericapillary forces (P_{pc}) may include those related to the surface tension of the alveolar lining layer.

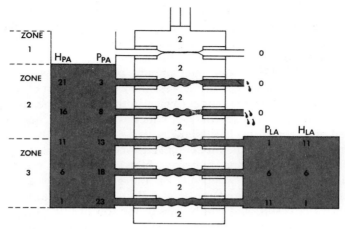

Figure 35. This model represents the pulmonary vascular bed. H_{PA} is height of inflow reservoir. P_{PA} represents pulmonary artery pressure. H_{LA} represents height of outflow reservoir. P_{LA} is left atrial pressure. Alveolar pressure (P_{alv}) equals 2 cm. of water throughout the system. In zone 1, P_{alv} exceeds P_{PA} so that there is no flow. In zone 2, P_{PA} exceeds P_{alv} so that flow varies with height, being greater near the bottom than at the top of the zone. In zone 3, P_{PA} exceeds P_{alv}, but P_{alv} is less than P_{LA}. Since P_{PA} and P_{LA} increase by equal amounts throughout this zone, flow through each channel in this zone is the same and does not vary with height.

In the lower part of the model (zone 3), P_{PA} exceeds P_{alv} in every channel, but the alveolar pressure is less than the outflow pressure (P_{LA}). The amount of flow through each capillary in this zone will depend on the difference between pulmonary artery pressure and the corresponding venous pressure ($P_{PA} - P_{LA}$). In this zone, the pulmonary artery pressure and venous pressure increase equally with distance down the lung, so that the driving pressure, and therefore the flow in each channel, is approximately the same and is not affected by the height, as it was in zone 2.

In the lungs, the same principles apply, but the inflow and outflow tubes are distensible rather than rigid, and they are affected by the transmural pressure acting on them. In addition, unlike the model, there is usually blood flow during systole in zone 1, and the blood flow in zone 3 of the lung varies with height. Blood flow is influenced by the resistance in the capillaries, which, in turn, is determined by their distensibility and the local transmural pressure.

In the human lung, then, the blood flow is less at the apex than at the base of the upright lung (sitting or standing), owing to the effect of gravity. When one lies down, the apical-basal blood flow difference is largely abolished, because the two parts of the lung are nearly at the same hydrostatic level, but there is still a gradient in flow between the upper and lower parts of the lung. If one lies on one side, there is more of a hydrostatic gradient and the dependent lung is better perfused than the contralateral lung. During exercise, blood flow at the top of the lung increases relatively more than it does at the base, although a perfusion gradient remains down the lung.

The distribution of blood flow in the lung will be altered when the pulmonary artery pressure and circulating blood volume are elevated (as might occur in heart failure) or when the pulmonary artery pressure and circulating blood volume are low (as occurs in severe hypotension and shock). Like the distribution of ventilation, the distribution of perfusion is altered by changes in flow resistance and distensibility (compliance) of the pulmonary vessels in different regions in the lung. It will also be affected by pulmonary vascular occlusion, embolization or thrombosis in pulmonary blood vessels, or by obliteration of part of the pulmonary vasculature caused by emphysema or fibrosis.

GAS EXCHANGE

Ideal gas exchange requires that there be good matching of the distribution of the incoming air and the capillary blood flow of a given alveolus and that the partial pressures of oxygen and carbon dioxide in the pulmonary capillaries come into equilibrium with those in the alveoli. One generally assesses the status of gas exchange by determining the partial pressures of oxygen and carbon dioxide in the arterial blood as well as the difference between the oxygen tensions in the alveolar gas and the arterial blood ($P_{(A-a)}O_2$). To determine this difference, the "ideal" alveolar P_{O_2} is calculated.

"IDEAL" ALVEOLAR P_{O_2}

Unlike the arterial P_{O_2}, which can be measured directly, it is not possible to measure the true alveolar P_{O_2}, which, as we have seen, is constantly changing. Instead, an "ideal" or "effective" value for the alveolar P_{O_2} is calculated, using the alveolar equation and the alveolar P_{CO_2}. This equation is based on the hypothesis that the arterial P_{CO_2} is representative of the P_{CO_2} of all of the perfused alveoli and that the gas exchange ratio of these alveoli is equal to that of the lungs as a whole:

$$P_AO_2(\text{ideal}) = F_IO_2(P_B - 47) - P_ACO_2(F_IO_2 + [1 - F_IO_2]/R)$$

Although this equation looks formidable, it really is quite simple to estimate the ideal P_AO_2. The first part of the equation is simply the calculation of the partial pressure of oxygen in moist inspired air (P_B being the barometric pressure and 47 the partial pressure of water). Instead of P_ACO_2, one uses the P_aCO_2, since it is representative of the mean P_{CO_2} in all of the perfused alveoli. The latter part in brackets will vary with the inspired oxygen concentration and the respiratory quotient (R). If 100% oxygen is inhaled, the value within the brackets becomes I and the equation is simply the difference between the inspired P_{O_2} and the P_ACO_2:

$$P_AO_2 = P_IO_2 - P_ACO_2/R$$

In the majority of clinical situations, one does not collect expired gas along with an arterial blood sample; so the respiratory quotient is not available. However, if room air is being breathed while the blood is drawn, an R of 0.8 is assumed; if an oxygen-enriched gas is being inhaled, one assumes an R of 1.0. A simplified version of the equation is generally used:

$$P_AO_2 = P_IO_2 - (P_aCO_2/0.8)$$

or

$$P_AO_2 = P_IO_2 - (P_aCO_2 \times 1.25)$$

ALVEOLO-ARTERIAL Po₂ GRADIENT

The effective alveolar oxygen tension is used to determine the gradient or difference between the mean alveolar and the mean arterial oxygen tensions $(P_{(A-a)}O_2)$:

$$P_{(A-a)}O_2 = P_IO_2 - (P_aCO_2 \times 1.25) - P_aO_2$$

In healthy young individuals, the $P_{(A-a)}O_2$ is between 5 and 10 mm. Hg while the individual is breathing room air; this value increases as one gets older. The $P_{(A-a)}O_2$ is also greater than expected when there is mismatching of the ventilation and perfusion in the lung, true venous admixture or a diffusion defect.

MATCHING OF VENTILATION AND PERFUSION

It is the relationship between the alveolar ventilation $(\dot{V}_A)$ and the pulmonary capillary blood flow $(\dot{Q})$ that determines the gas composition of the blood leaving the lung. The amount of oxygen taken up from the lungs $(\dot{V}O_2)$ over a given period of time is equal to the difference between the amount inspired and the amount expired from the alveolar gas in that time:

$$\dot{V}O_2 = \dot{V}_A(F_IO_2) - \dot{V}_A(F_AO_2)$$

Similarly, the oxygen taken up from the alveolar gas by the blood equals the difference between the amount leaving the lung in the systemic arterial blood and the amount delivered to the lung in the mixed venous blood:

$$\dot{V}O_2 = \dot{Q}(C_aO_2) - \dot{Q}(C_{\bar{v}}O_2)$$

The two equations representing oxygen uptake can then be combined as follows:

$$\dot{V}_A(F_IO_2 - F_AO_2) = \dot{Q}(C_aO_2 - C_{\bar{v}}O_2)$$

From this, the relationship between alveolar ventilation and perfusion $(\dot{V}_A/\dot{Q})$ can be derived:

$$\dot{V}_A/\dot{Q} = (C_aO_2 - C_{\bar{v}}O_2)/(F_IO_2 - F_AO_2)$$

Now one can see that at a fixed inspired oxygen concentration (F_IO_2) and a given level of mixed venous oxygen content $(C_{\bar{v}}O_2)$, the oxygen contents of the arterial blood and the alveolar gas are determined by the ratio of the alveolar ventilation to perfusion.

A similar expression can be derived for carbon dioxide exchange, namely

$$\dot{V}_A/\dot{Q} = (C_{\bar{v}}CO_2 - C_aCO_2)/F_ACO_2$$

Since in a steady state the $\dot{V}_A/\dot{Q}$ ratios for O_2 must be identical to the $\dot{V}_A/\dot{Q}$ ratios for CO_2, we may write

$$\dot{V}_A/\dot{Q} = (C_aO_2 - C_{\bar{v}}O_2)/(F_IO_2 - F_AO_2) = (C_{\bar{v}}CO_2 - C_aCO_2)/F_ACO_2$$

Clearly then, for given values of F_IO_2, $C_{\bar{v}}O_2$ and $C_{\bar{v}}CO_2$, the concentrations of oxygen and carbon dioxide in the alveolar air, and hence their partial pressures, will be determined by the ratio of ventilation to perfusion. By graphic analysis (as in an O_2-CO_2 diagram presented in Fig. 36) it is possible to determine, for given values of F_IO_2, $C_{\bar{v}}O_2$, and $C_{\bar{v}}CO_2$, the values of P_AO_2 and P_ACO_2 that would satisfy the equation at different degrees of $\dot{V}_A/\dot{Q}$ mismatching.

As we have seen, neither the distribution of the inspired gas nor that of the pulmonary blood flow is uniform throughout the lungs, even in healthy individuals. In Figure 37 we can see that the matching of the blood and gas distribution ($\dot{V}_A/\dot{Q}$ ratio) is also not uniform throughout the lung, and it is different at the top and bottom of the lung. It is also apparent that since the ventilation/perfusion ratios are high at the top of the lung and low at the bottom, the gas tensions in blood leaving alveoli are not the same in the different regions. Under normal circumstances, however, this amount of mismatching is not sufficient to materially interfere with gas exchange, and the partial pressures of oxygen and carbon dioxide in the mixed arterial blood are nearly the same as those in the mixed alveolar gas.

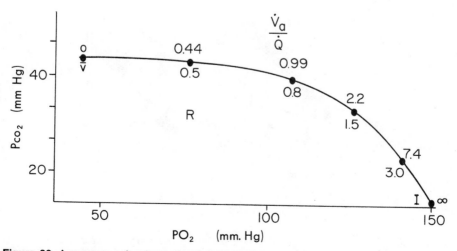

Figure 36. A curve may be drawn that joins the points (representing the values of P_{O_2} and P_{CO_2}) that are determined by given values for the respiratory exchange ratio (R), the ventilation/perfusion ratio ($\dot{V}_A/\dot{Q}$), the composition of mixed venous blood ($\bar{V}$) and inspired air (I).

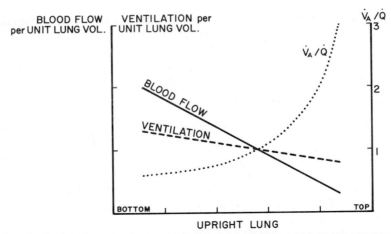

Figure 37. Regional blood flow and ventilation. Both ventilation and blood flow decrease from bottom to top, but the ratio between them changes so that the upper regions are overventilated in relation to their perfusion and the lower regions are relatively undervenilated.

Venous-Admixture–Like Perfusion

If inadequately ventilated alveoli are well perfused (Fig. 38A) or, in the extreme case, if there is continued perfusion of alveoli receiving no ventilation because they are full of exudate or because the airway leading to them is blocked (a low ventilation/perfusion ratio), the blood flowing past these alveoli will receive little, if any, oxygen and give up no carbon dioxide. This poorly aerated blood then mixes with fully "arterialized" blood coming from other pulmonary capillaries, i.e., it is a *venous-admixture–like perfusion,* and the mixed arterial blood will have a lower PO_2 and a slightly elevated

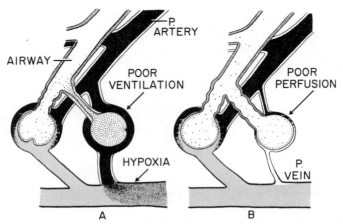

Figure 38. This figure shows the effect of alterations of ventilation/perfusion relationships on gas exchange. **A,** Low $\dot{V}_A/\dot{Q}$ areas contributing poorly oxygenated blood to the systemic circulation—an effect that is similar to that resulting from venous admixture (shunt). **B,** High $\dot{V}_A/\dot{Q}$ areas contribute gas to the mixed expired air, which is high in O_2 and low in CO_2 concentration—an effect similar to that resulting from an increase in dead space.

P_{CO_2}. Hypercapnia may not develop if there is sufficient hyperventilation of the rest of the perfused alveoli, but because of the shape of the oxyhemoglobin dissociation curve, this only adds a limited amount of oxygen to the blood and the arterial hypoxemia is not corrected to any significant degree.

Dead-Space–Like Ventilation

When the ventilation of alveoli is maintained but their perfusion is limited (Fig. 38B), or, in the extreme case, when there is no blood flow, such as occurs when an embolus or thrombus occludes a pulmonary artery, a high ventilation/perfusion ratio is present. This has been termed "alveolar dead-space" or **dead-space–like ventilation,** because the gas leaving such alveoli takes little, if any, part in gas exchange and its composition is much like the gas in the tracheobronchial tree. Adequate oxygenation and carbon dioxide elimination, as evidenced by the presence of normal arterial oxygen and carbon dioxide tensions, is frequent when there is excessive dead-space–like ventilation. However, the large amount of wasted ventilation means that the $P_{(A-a)}O_2$ will be elevated and the proportion of the ventilation that takes part in gas exchange, i.e., the alveolar ventilation, may be lower than required, unless the total ventilation is increased.

It is important to emphasize that hypoxemia can develop, even though the total alveolar ventilation and the total pulmonary blood flow are within normal limits, if the matching of ventilation and perfusion of alveoli is not uniform throughout the lungs. Conversely, even though blood or gas distribution in the lung is abnormal, the gas exchange can remain effective if the alterations in ventilation are matched by similar alterations of blood flow. For example, a decrease in ventilation of an area of the lung can lead to local constriction of the blood vessels so that blood flow is directed away to areas of lung that are better ventilated. Similarly, airways supplying alveoli whose blood flow becomes restricted may constrict and thereby divert more of the air to alveoli with a normal or better-than-normal blood supply. Nonuniform ventilation-perfusion ratios throughout the lung result in an elevated $P_{(A-a)}O_2$, but there may be no difference between the partial pressures of the gases in a particular alveolus and its capillary.

Mismatching between ventilation and perfusion, along with an elevated $P_{(A-a)}O_2$ and hypoxemia, is common in patients suffering from pulmonary disease, both abnormally high and low ventilation/perfusion ratios frequently coexisting. In the early stages of these conditions, compensatory hyperpnea may ensure an adequate effective alveolar ventilation, so that the P_aCO_2 may be normal, but the hypoxemia will persist. In the later stages, however, because of the mechanical disturbances in the lungs, the patient may be unable to increase ventilation sufficiently to provide an adequate alveolar ventilation, so that the low arterial P_{O_2} is associated with an elevated P_{CO_2} (i.e., alveolar hypoventilation).

TRUE VENOUS ADMIXTURE, OR SHUNT

The most gross example of blood and gas mismatching that may be imagined is one in which some pulmonary capillary blood does not come

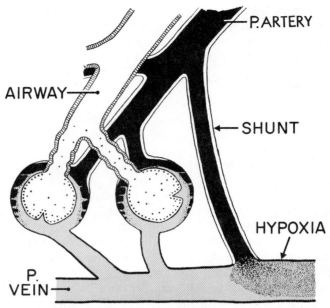

Figure 39. Poorly oxygenated blood, which does not come into contact with alveoli, is added to arterialized blood coming from ventilated alveoli. This is called true venous admixture or right-to-left shunt.

into contact with any alveoli at all, so that mixed venous blood is added to arterialized blood; i.e., ***true venous admixture,*** or a right-to-left shunt exists (Fig. 39).

Even in healthy individuals, approximately 2.5 per cent of the pulmonary blood flow enters the arterialized systemic circulation via the pulmonary veins and the thebesian and the bronchial veins, which empty into the left side of the heart. In some congenital heart lesions, where blood is shunted from the right to the left side, and in a pulmonary arteriovenous aneurysm, where blood is shunted from the pulmonary artery to the pulmonary veins, the amount of true venous admixture increases. In such conditions, the $P_{(A-a)}O_2$ is elevated and considerable arterial hypoxemia may be present. Because ventilation is generally increased as a result of the hypoxemic stimulus, hypocapnia is common.

In practice, a qualitative assessment of the amount of venous admixture present—i.e., the proportion of the cardiac output that is acting like a shunt $(\dot{Q}_S/\dot{Q}_T)$—can be derived from equations that use the calculated effective alveolar PO_2 and either the arterial oxygen content or saturation:

$$\dot{Q}_S/\dot{Q}_T = \frac{C_{(c'-a)}O_2}{C_{(c'-\bar{v})}O_2}$$

or

$$\dot{Q}_S/\dot{Q}_T = \frac{S_{(c'-a)}O_2}{S_{(c'-\bar{v})}O_2}$$

where C is the content and S the saturation of oxygen in the mean end-capillary (c'), arterial (a), and mixed venous ($\bar{v}$) blood. It is usually assumed that the mean end-capillary P_{O_2} is the same as the effective $P_{A}O_2$. The end-capillary and arterial oxygen contents and saturations are estimated from the respective partial pressures of oxygen, and the mixed venous content is usually estimated by assuming an a-$\bar{v}$ content difference of 5 vol. per cent and a saturation difference of 25 per cent.

Calculations are usually made by sampling the arterial P_{O_2} after the subject has been breathing 100% oxygen for 20 minutes. If the $P_{a}O_2$ is greater than 100 mm. Hg, then the hemoglobin in the pulmonary end-capillary and the arterial blood will be fully saturated, and any difference in oxygen content between the end-capillary and arterial blood resulting from a greater-than-normal amount of shunting will be reflected by the amount of oxygen in physical solution in the blood. For instance, we know that 1 gm. of hemoglobin will carry 1.34 ml. of oxygen and that 0.003 ml. of oxygen will be dissolved in the blood for every mm. Hg partial pressure. If while a person is breathing 100 per cent oxygen at sea level ($P_B = 760$), the $P_{a}O_2$ is 500 mm. Hg, the $P_{A}CO_2$ is 40 mm. Hg and the person's hemoglobin is 20 gm./100 ml., then

$$P_{A}O_2 = (760 - 47) - 40 = 673 \text{ torr}$$

and since $P_{A}O_2 = P_{c'}O_2$, then

$$C_{c'}O_2 = (20 \times 1.34) + (673 \times .003) = 28.82 \text{ ml./100 ml. of blood}$$

and

$$C_{a}O_2 = (20.0 \times 1.34) + (500 \times .003) = 28.30 \text{ ml./100 ml. of blood}$$

If the a-$\bar{v}$ oxygen content difference is 5 ml./100 ml., then

$$\dot{Q}_S/\dot{Q}_T \text{ (\% shunt)} = \frac{28.82 - 28.30}{28.82 - 23.30} \times 100 = 9.4\%$$

DIFFUSION OF GAS

The transfer of oxygen and carbon dioxide between the alveolar gas and the pulmonary capillary blood is entirely passive. It is brought about by diffusion across the blood-gas barrier, which consists of the alveolar epithelium, the basement membranes, the capillary endothelium, plasma, the intracellular fluid and the red blood cell. The rate of diffusion across the blood-gas barrier depends on the solubility of the particular gas in liquid, its density, the partial pressure difference between the alveolar air and the capillary blood, and the surface area that is available for diffusion. Even

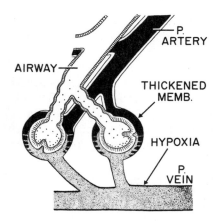

P.
ARTERY

AIRWAY

THICKENED
MEMB.

HYPOXIA

P.
VEIN

Figure 40. The effect of a diffusion defect on gas exchange. Note that the blood leaving the alveoli (the end-capillary blood) has not come into equilibrium with alveolar gas.

though it is a larger molecule than oxygen, the solubility of carbon dioxide is almost 25 times as great, and it diffuses about 20 times more rapidly between air and blood than does oxygen.

The difference in partial pressures across the alveolocapillary membrane depends on the slope of the dissociation curve for each gas; it is greatest at the point at which the venous blood enters the capillary and lowest at the point at which the blood leaves the capillary. The changes in the partial pressures of oxygen and carbon dioxide in the blood as it passes along the lung capillary have been estimated to take one cardiac cycle, i.e., approximately 0.75 second at rest.

Contrary to earlier beliefs, an impaired diffusion of oxygen from the alveolar air to the pulmonary capillary blood, as is shown in Figure 40, is seldom the primary cause of a low arterial oxygen tension. With the possible exception of a relatively rare group of cases that have a specific type of alveolar pathology, arterial hypoxemia in pulmonary disease, even when it is severe, usually results from mismatching of ventilation and perfusion, or alveolar hypoventilation. It is likely that no significant difference in partial pressure of carbon dioxide between gas and blood ever develops, because an overall resistance to diffusion that is great enough to cause a significant carbon dioxide gradient would be associated with such a fantastic partial pressure difference for oxygen that survival would be impossible.

Diffusing Capacity

A qualitative estimate of the diffusing capacity of the lungs can be obtained by using oxygen or carbon monoxide, either of which has a great affinity for hemoglobin. To calculate the diffusing capacity of the lungs for oxygen (D_LO_2) or carbon monoxide (D_LCO), one must know the amount of gas diffusing across the blood-gas barrier per minute ($\dot{V}O_2$ or $\dot{V}CO$) and the mean partial pressure gradient of the gas between the alveolus and the pulmonary capillary ($P_{\overline{A-c}}$):

$$D_LO_2 = \dot{V}O_2/P_{\overline{(A-c)}}O_2$$

and

$$D_LCO = \dot{V}CO/P_{\overline{(A-c)}}CO$$

Volume of Diffusing Gas. $\dot{V}O_2$ and $\dot{V}CO$ can be determined by estimating the difference between the amount of gas inhaled and the amount exhaled:

$$\dot{V}O_2 = \dot{V}_I(F_IO_2) - \dot{V}_E(F_EO_2)$$

and

$$\dot{V}CO = \dot{V}_I(F_ICO) - \dot{V}_E(F_ECO)$$

where V_I and V_E are the inspired and expired volume/min., respectively, and F the concentration of the particular gas in the inspired (I) and the expired (E) air.

Mean Alveolocapillary Partial Pressure Gradient. $P_{\overline{(A-c)}}O_2$ is a single figure that expresses the integral, with respect to time, of a changing gradient between the alveolus and the pulmonary capillary. As is shown in Figure 41, the gradient for oxygen varies along the course of the pulmonary capillary and diminishes from the point at which the venous blood arrives at the alveolus to that point along the course of the capillary at which the partial pressures of the gas phase and the blood phase approach equilibrium. Figure 41 also shows that the calculated mean pulmonary capillary oxygen tension, with respect to time, is determined by identifying the value of P_{O_2} at which the shaded areas designated X and Y are equal. It is this mean gradient that is used to calculate the diffusing capacity of the lungs for oxygen.

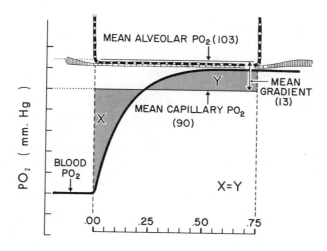

Figure 41. The change in the partial pressure of oxygen as blood passes along the pulmonary capillary. The mean alveolocapillary gradient is also shown.

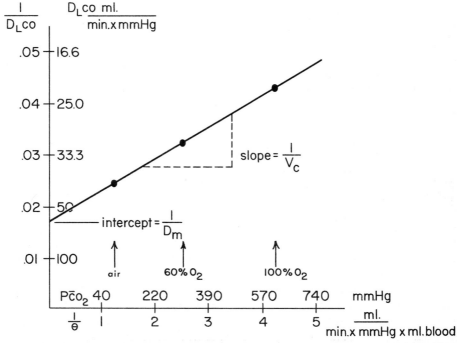

Figure 42. The diffusing capacity of the lungs for carbon monoxide ($D_L$co) measured at three levels of inspired oxygen concentration. A linear relationship is obtained when the reciprocal of the diffusing capacity is plotted against the mean capillary Po_2 ($P_{\bar{c}}O_2$) or the reciprocal of the reaction coefficient $\left(\dfrac{1}{\theta}\right)$.

The $P_{(\overline{A-c})}co$ is much easier to determine because of the remarkable affinity of CO for hemoglobin. Because measurable quantities of CO can diffuse into the pulmonary capillary blood without producing a significant partial pressure in the plasma, the partial pressure of carbon monoxide in the capillary is considered to be zero, and the $P_{(\overline{A-c})}co$ equal to the mean alveolar CO tension. This is not quite accurate, however, since it has been shown that the speed of the reaction between carbon monoxide and hemoglobin is slow, and therefore there is a significant resistance to the transfer of the gas from the alveolus to the hemoglobin molecule. Although there is little supportive evidence, the same may be true for oxygen. This suggests that measurements of the diffusing capacity of the lung are affected not only by the resistance of the blood-gas barrier but also by chemical reactions within the red blood cell.

If one uses carbon monoxide as the gas in question, one may express the resistance to the diffusion of carbon monoxide as the reciprocal of the diffusing capacity:

$$I/D_L co = \frac{\text{partial pressure gradient}}{\text{CO uptake}}$$

The resistance to diffusion is made up of a membrane component (I/D_M) and a blood component (I/D_B):

$$I/D_L\text{CO} = I/D_M + I/D_B$$

D_B represents the volume of CO taken up by the blood in the pulmonary capillaries for each mm. Hg partial pressure. It is often expressed as $V_c \times \Theta$, where V_c is the volume of blood in the pulmonary capillaries and Θ is the amount of CO that one ml. of blood will take up for each mm. Hg partial pressure. Thus,

$$I/D_L\text{CO} = I/D_M + I/(V_c \times \Theta)$$

The amount of CO taken up by the blood, i.e., the value of Θ, falls in the presence of increased oxygen levels, because oxygen and carbon monoxide compete for Hb. This explains why the $D_L\text{CO}$ falls when the concentration of inspired oxygen is increased. Indeed, by determining the relationship of $D_L\text{CO}$ to inspired P_{O_2} (Fig. 42), it is possible to estimate the volume of blood in the pulmonary capillaries as well as the size of the membrane component of the resistance to diffusion.

GAS TRANSPORT AND ACID-BASE BALANCE

The uptake of oxygen from the alveoli and its distribution to the various organs and tissues of the body, as well as the transport of carbon dioxide from the tissues and its subsequent elimination from the lungs, are functions of the blood, particularly of hemoglobin. If the plasma consisted only of plasma and no red cells, the adult human heart would have to pump more than 100 l./min. through the pulmonary capillaries to meet the oxygen requirements of a man at rest, and about 800 l./min. during exercise. On the other hand, blood containing red cells picks up 60 to 70 times more oxygen than plasma alone, thus enabling the resting cardiac output to be only 5 to 6 l./min.

A number of complex reactions are involved in the transport of both oxygen and carbon dioxide in the blood, and these are illustrated in Figures 43 and 44. Of the total amount of oxygen and carbon dioxide in the blood, less than 5 per cent is present in simple solution. Reversible chemical reactions are responsible for the transport of the remainder of the two gases, and in both cases hemoglobin plays a major role.

OXYGEN IN THE BLOOD

The oxygen that diffuses from the alveoli into the pulmonary capillary blood is carried in the blood in two ways: as dissolved oxygen in physical solution in the plasma, and combined with the hemoglobin in the erythrocytes. Both of these amounts depend upon the partial pressure of oxygen in the arterial blood.

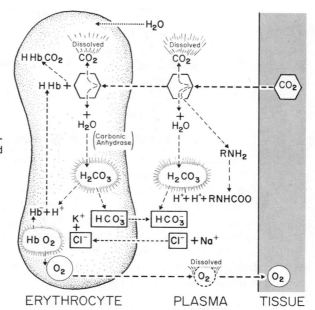

Figure 43. Gas exchange between systemic capillaries and the tissues.

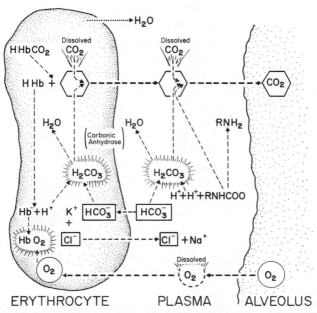

Figure 44. Gas exchange between the pulmonary alveoli and the capillaries.

OXYGEN IN PHYSICAL SOLUTION

The amount of oxygen that dissolves in a given volume of plasma is directly proportional to its partial pressure (0.03 ml./mm. Hg/l. plasma). Since the P_{O_2} in the arterial blood in healthy individuals is approximately 100 mm. Hg, the amount of oxygen in physical solution in the plasma is about 3.0 ml./l. plasma. In the venous blood, where the P_{O_2} is about 40 mm. Hg, there is 1.2 ml./l. plasma.

OXYGEN COMBINED WITH HEMOGLOBIN

Most of the oxygen in the blood is carried in the erythrocytes in combination with hemoglobin as oxyhemoglobin (HbO_2). One gram of hemoglobin is capable of combining chemically with 1.34 ml. of oxygen. Thus, in a healthy individual who has a hemoblogin content of 15 gm./100 ml., the blood is capable of carrying 20.10 vol. per cent of oxygen as oxyhemoglobin in addition to the comparatively small amount dissolved in the plasma. The hemoglobin does not usually combine with this amount of oxygen, however. The extent to which hemoglobin is actually combined with oxygen is usually expressed as the percentage saturation:

% saturation = 100 × oxygen content (HbO_2)/oxygen capacity (HbO_2 + Hb)

In a healthy individual breathing room air, the oxygen saturation of the arterial blood is about 97 per cent. The saturation of hemoglobin depends upon the partial pressure of the oxygen in the plasma. This relationship is illustrated in the *oxyhemoglobin dissociation curve,* which is shown in Figure 45. The characteristic S shape of this curve indicates that, unlike the dissolved oxygen, the amount of oxyhemoglobin formed in the red blood cell is not linearly related to the partial pressure. It means that the hemoglobin clings to oxygen over a fairly wide range of oxygen tension at the upper end of the scale and gives up oxygen readily at the lower oxygen tensions. The converse is also true, in that hemoglobin takes up oxygen very readily at the lower oxygen tensions but not at the higher ones. It should be noted that in a healthy individual breathing room air, the oxygen saturation will fall only slightly, even when there is a considerable fall in oxygen tension. In the hypoxic individual, on the other hand, even small changes in tension may be associated with a considerable reduction in oxygen saturation.

Figure 45 also shows that the amount of oxygen that is taken up or given off by hemoglobin depends not only on the partial pressure of oxygen in that tissue, but also on the partial pressure of carbon dioxide, the pH and the temperature of the blood. At a given partial pressure of oxygen, oxyhemoglobin will give up more oxygen when the carbon dioxide tension is high, the pH low (hydrogen ion concentration increased) or the temperature elevated. Conversely, less oxygen will be given up if the P_{CO_2} is low, the pH high (hydrogen ion concentration reduced) or the temperature lowered. The effect of these variables on the saturation of hemoglobin and the transport of oxygen is extremely important, because it acts as a safeguard for the welfare of the tissues. If the partial pressure of oxygen falls in the

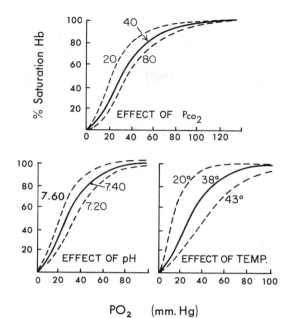

Figure 45. The effect of changes in P_{CO_2}, pH and temperature on the oxyhemoglobin dissociation curve.

tissues, such as occurs when the tissue activity is increased or when the blood supply is reduced, the carbon dioxide tension and hydrogen ion concentration both rise. As a result, the oxygen dissociation curve is shifted to the right and, therefore, the unloading of oxygen from the blood to the tissues is facilitated. Conversely, the fall in partial pressure of carbon dioxide tension as the blood passes through the lungs causes the dissociation curve to shift to the left, and this increases the capability of hemoglobin to take on an additional quantity of oxygen.

The oxyhemoglobin dissociation curve of fetal blood lies to the left of the adult curve, but the shape of the curve is similar to that of adult hemoglobin. Minor abnormalities in oxyhemoglobin dissociation have been found in a variety of metabolic or endocrine disorders in adult animals and in humans; these seem to be related to changes in the intracellular environment of hemoglobin rather than to changes in the hemoglobin itself. Recently, considerable attention has been directed at the possible role of 2,3-diphosphoglycerate (DPG), which is nearly equimolar with hemoglobin in human red blood cells, in accounting for the shift in the oxyhemoglobin dissociation curve seen in disease, because it lowers the affinity of hemoglobin for oxygen.

TISSUE OXYGEN

When oxygenated blood reaches the tissues, the oxygen diffuses rapidly from the blood into the tissue cells, because the oxygen tension of the tissue cells is low (probably less than 10 mm. Hg). As a result, the partial pressure of oxygen in the plasma falls to a very low level. As is indicated in the oxyhemoglobin dissociation curve, hemoglobin will relinquish oxygen readily when the Po_2 drops below 60 mm. Hg, so that oxygen is liberated from the red blood cells into the plasma, where it is then made available to the tissues. On the average, approximately 45 ml. of oxygen/l. of blood is given up by the blood to the tissues of the body. Even after all of the requirements of the tissues have been met, the oxygen saturation of the venous blood is still 70 to 75 per cent, under ordinary circumstances. Part of this remainder represents a reserve that can be drawn on by the tissues with only a slight further reduction in the partial pressure of oxygen.

HYPOXIA

At this point, it is appropriate to distinguish between *hypoxemia* and *hypoxia.* The term *hypoxemia* means that the oxygen content of the arterial blood is diminished, but it does not differentiate between a diminution caused by a reduced partial pressure of oxygen, a diminution caused by a lowered oxygen carrying capacity of the hemoglobin, or one caused by both mechanisms. The term *hypoxia* means that there is a decreased amount of oxygen available to the tissues, regardless of the cause or the location. Hypoxia may be present even though both the arterial oxygen tension and content are normal. It can be classified into four main types: hypoxic, anemic, circulatory and histotoxic.

HYPOXIC HYPOXIA

In *hypoxic hypoxia,* the oxygen tension in the blood that is being delivered to the tissues is lower than normal, so that the hemoglobin is incompletely saturated with oxygen; i.e., *hypoxemia* is present. Hypoxic hypoxia may be present in patients who are suffering from respiratory or cardiac disease, where the abnormality may be due to altered ventilation-perfusion ratios, true venous admixture, a diffusion defect, alveolar hypoventilation or a combination of these disturbances. This is also the type of hypoxia that occurs when the concentration of oxygen in the inspired air is low, e.g., at a high altitude.

ANEMIC HYPOXIA

In *anemic hypoxia,* the oxygen tension in the arterial blood is normal and the available hemoglobin is almost completely saturated with oxygen. However, because the hemoglobin content is lower than normal, both the oxygen content and the oxygen capacity of the blood are reduced. As a result, the tissues may not receive sufficient oxygen. This variety of hypoxia may be encountered in all of the anemic states, as well as in situations in which toxic substances combine with hemoglobin and prevent the uptake of oxygen, such as occurs in carbon monoxide poisoning or methemoglobinemia. In carbon monoxide poisoning, hypoxia develops because the affinity of carbon monoxide for hemoglobin is about 250 times greater than that of oxygen and the affinity of unbound iron atoms for oxygen is increased. Thus, the capacity of the hemoglobin to combine with oxygen is reduced, and that oxygen which is carried by the hemoglobin is firmly bound and not given up readily to the tissues. In methemoglobinemia, where the iron atoms are oxidized to the ferric state, the oxygen content and capacity of the blood are reduced similarly.

CIRCULATORY HYPOXIA

In *circulatory hypoxia,* the blood that arrives at the tissues may have a normal oxygen tension and content, but the quantity of blood, and therefore the oxygen supply to a particular organ, is not sufficient to meet its metabolic demands. It may develop when there is generalized circulatory insufficiency, such as congestive heart failure or shock, or when there is a localized obstruction of the blood flow to an organ. Similarly, a localized venous occlusion may produce local hypoxia because the flow of blood out of the capillaries is impeded. This form of hypoxia may also occur if the tissue requirements for oxygen exceed the available supply from the blood.

HISTOTOXIC HYPOXIA

There are a number of toxic substances, such as cyanide, that interfere with the ability of the tissues to use oxygen. Under such circumstances, the tissues may become exceedingly hypoxic, even though both the partial pressure and content of oxygen in the arterial blood are normal.

CARBON DIOXIDE IN THE BLOOD

The carbon dioxide that is produced in the tissues diffuses into the systemic capillaries and then is transported in the blood in several forms: in the dissolved state, as bicarbonate, and in combination with hemoglobin.

DISSOLVED CARBON DIOXIDE

Some of the carbon dioxide in the blood is transported in a physically dissolved form in both plasma and erythrocytes. The amount of carbon dioxide that is dissolved depends on its solubility coefficient, its partial pressure and the temperature. At body temperature, 0.067 vol. per cent, or 0.0301 mM./l., of carbon dioxide is dissolved in plasma for each mm. Hg partial pressure of carbon dioxide. In the arterial blood (P_{CO_2} approximately 40 mm. Hg), there is approximately 1.2 mM./l. of dissolved carbon dioxide, and in the venous blood (P_{CO_2} approximately 46 mm. Hg), there is 1.38 mM/l. of dissolved carbon dioxide.

Some of the dissolved carbon dioxide in the plasma reacts with water to produce carbonic acid (a process called **hydration**), which, in turn, dissociates into bicarbonate and hydrogen ions:

$$CO_2 + H_2O \rightleftharpoons H_2CO_3 \rightleftharpoons HCO_3^- + H^+$$

The hydration of CO_2 in the plasma is a very slow chemical reaction, and the concentration of dissolved carbon dioxide is about 1000 times greater than the concentration of carbonic acid. Consequently, there is only a small amount of bicarbonate actually formed in the plasma.

BOUND CARBON DIOXIDE

Even though there is only a small amount of bicarbonate formed in the plasma, the plasma bicarbonate content increases considerably when the blood traverses the tissue capillaries. This is because the red blood cells are capable of promoting the formation of bicarbonate from CO_2. They are able to do so for three reasons.

First, they contain an enzyme called **carbonic anhydrase,** which catalyzes the hydration of the CO_2 diffusing from the tissues through the plasma into the red blood cells to form carbonic acid at a rapid rate.

$$CO_2 + H_2O \underset{\text{carbonic anhydrase}}{\rightleftharpoons} H_2CO_3 \rightleftharpoons HCO_3^- + H^+$$

Second, the hemoglobin in the red blood cell provides basic groups that neutralize the H^+ ions formed by the dissociation of H_2CO_3, thereby promoting the formation of HCO_3^-:

$$Hb^- + H^+ + HCO_3^- \rightleftharpoons HHb + HCO_3^-$$

The formation of HCO_3^- in the red blood cells results in a concentration gradient between the cells and the plasma, so that the HCO_3^- diffuses quickly out of the cells. The red blood cell membrane is relatively impermeable to cations, and the exit of HCO_3^- creates an electrical imbalance. However, electrical neutrality is preserved by an influx of Cl^- ions into the red blood cells that is equivalent to the efflux of HCO_3^- ions. This phenomenon is called the **chloride shift.** In addition, the hydration of CO_2 and the dissociation of carbonic acid cause the osmolarity of the red blood cell to increase, and, as a result, water enters the cells and their volume increases.

Finally, red blood cells promote carbon dioxide transport because hemoglobin provides many more amino groups for the formation of carbamino compounds, which account for about one-quarter of the arteriovenous CO_2 difference, than do the proteins of the plasma. This is done according to this reaction:

$$Hb - N\overset{\displaystyle H}{\underset{\displaystyle H}{\Big\langle}} + CO_2 \rightarrow Hb - N\overset{\displaystyle H}{\underset{\displaystyle COO}{\Big\langle}} + H^+$$

In the lungs, the reverse of the above processes takes place. Because it is highly soluble in an aqueous media, carbon dioxide diffuses rapidly into the alveoli and the partial pressures of carbon dioxide in the pulmonary capillary blood and the alveolar air equilibrate promptly. In contrast to what happens at the tissues, some Cl^- leaves the red blood cell and HCO_3^- enters it. This reverse chloride shift in the pulmonary capillaries is important, for otherwise it would be impossible for the bicarbonate to enter the red blood cells from the plasma. On entering the red blood cells, the HCO_3^- combines with H^+ to form H_2CO_3, and this in turn is **dehydrated** to carbon dioxide and water. It is this carbon dioxide that passes through the plasma into the alveoli. At the same time, the osmotic equilibrium between the red blood cells and the plasma is once again maintained by the movement of water, this time out of the red blood cells into the plasma.

The capacity of the blood to carry carbon dioxide is expressed in the CO_2 **dissociation curve,** which is illustrated in Figure 46. Unlike the oxyhemoglobin dissociation curve, the CO_2 dissociation curve is almost linear in the

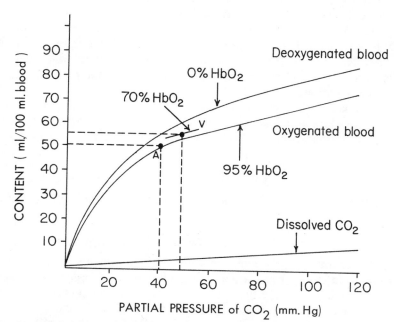

Figure 46. The *in vitro* CO_2 dissociation curve. The upper two curves show total CO_2 content in deoxygenated and oxygenated blood. The arterial point (A) and the venous point (V) indicate typical values obtained in normal resting man.

physiologic range of P_{CO_2}, especially when the effect of oxygenation of hemoglobin is taken into account.

ACID-BASE BALANCE

In addition to carbon dioxide, which is a volatile acid, nonvolatile acids, such as H_2SO_4 and H_3PO_4 are generated by tissue metabolism. The hydrogen ions that dissociate from the nonvolatile acids are buffered and then slowly excreted by the kidney. However, only about 60 to 80 mEq of nonvolatile (often called fixed) acids are excreted each day, under normal circumstances. On the other hand, as we have seen, carbon dioxide is rapidly eliminated by the lungs, and the CO_2 equivalent of about 15,000 mEq of carbonic acid is normally eliminated by the lungs in a day. Clearly then, through the control of carbon dioxide elimination the respiratory system plays an important role in the regulation of acid-base balance of the body.

Before describing the role of the respiratory system in acid-base balance, it is important to explain the terms used in discussing acid-base relationships. The terms *acid* and *base* are usually applied to proton (or hydrogen ion) donors or acceptors. It is customary to express the acidity or alkalinity of a solution by its pH, which is the negative logarithm, to the base 10, of the hydrogen ion concentration. (This means that a decrease or increase of a pH unit represents a tenfold change in the opposite direction of the hydrogen ion concentration.) Pure water, which is neutral, has a hydrogen ion concentration of about 10^{-7} moles/l., so that its pH is 7.0. By convention, a solution that has a hydrogen ion concentration greater than 10^{-7} moles/l. (i.e., pH less than 7.0) is called an acid solution, and one that has a concentration lower than 10^{-7} moles/l. (i.e., pH greater than 7.0) is called an alkaline solution.

The capacity of an acid-salt mixture to resist changes in pH is called its buffer action, and a mixture that can do this is called a *buffer*. The reaction of a solution that contains both acid and salt can be expressed by the equation

$$pH = pK + \log \text{(buffer anion/undissociated buffer)}$$

where pK is a constant that varies depending on the types of acid and salt involved.

HENDERSON-HASSELBACH EQUATION

The relationship between carbon dioxide (carbonic acid) and the anion bicarbonate in the plasma, which is reflected in the *Henderson-Hasselbach equation,* is quantitatively the most important buffering system of extracellular fluid. This equation is used clinically to establish the existence and the severity of an acid-base disturbance:

$$pH = pK + \log (HCO_3^-/H_2CO_3)$$

The pK for blood at body temperature is 6.10, and since the concentration of H_2CO_3 is a thousand times less than that of dissolved carbon dioxide and this, in turn, is proportional to the partial pressure of CO_2, the equation may be rewritten

$$pH = 6.10 + \log (HCO_3^-/0.0301 \times P_{CO_2})$$

The balance between the bicarbonate and the dissolved carbon dioxide (i.e., carbon dioxide tension) in arterial blood is normally maintained at about 20 to 1 (Fig. 47). In healthy individuals, the bicarbonate level is about 24 mM./l., the dissolved carbon dioxide about 1.2 mM./l., the pH about 7.40 (range 7.35–7.45) and the hydrogen ion concentration about 40 nM./l.

ABNORMALITIES OF ACID-BASE BALANCE

Before discussing abnormalities of acid-base balance, it is important to distinguish between the acid-base state of the blood and the abnormal process that led to the primary disturbance. The abnormal acid-base states of the blood are *acidemia,* in which the hydrogen ion concentration (cH^+) is high and the pH low, and *alkalemia,* in which the cH^+ is low and the pH high. The abnormal processes that lead to acid-base disturbances are *acidosis,* in which either a strong acid is gained or HCO_3^- is lost in excessive amounts, and *alkalosis,* in which either a strong base is gained or a strong acid is lost.

The terms *acidosis* and *alkalosis* are further qualified according to the nature of the process that led to the primary disturbance. In a *respiratory acidosis,* the alveolar ventilation is not sufficient to cope with the rate of metabolic CO_2 production, so that *hypercapnia* is present. This is equivalent to the retention of the strong acid H_2CO_3. In a *respiratory alkalosis,* the alveolar ventilation is excessive in relation to the metabolic CO_2 production, so that *hypocapnia* is present. This is equivalent to the loss of a strong acid. A *metabolic acidosis* is characterized by a primary gain of strong acid by the extracellular fluid (e.g., organic acids from metabolism, or exogenous

NORMAL ACID-BASE BALANCE

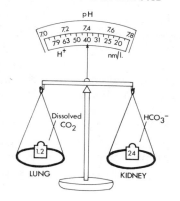

Figure 47. The balance between bicarbonate (24) and dissolved CO_2 (1.2 or P_aCO_2 = 40) is normally 20:1, and this is usually associated with a pH of about 7.40 and a H^+ concentration of about 40 mM./l.

acids such as NH_4Cl) or a primary loss of HCO_3^- from the extracellular fluid via the kidney or the gastrointestinal tract. A *metabolic alkalosis* is characterized by a primary gain of strong base by the extracellular fluid (e.g., due to administration of exogenous bicarbonate) or a primary loss of strong acid from extracellular fluid, such as loss of HCl from the stomach.

An acidosis will at first lead to *acidemia,* and an alkalosis to *alkalemia.* This calls secondary processes into play to compensate for the primary disturbance. The degree of compensation may be complete or incomplete, and this is judged on the basis of whether the H^+ ion concentration (or the pH) has returned to normal value.

In simplified terms, the H^+ ion concentration or the pH can be looked upon as the balance between metabolic (i.e., HCO_3^-) and respiratory (i.e., Pco_2) functions. Thus, the acid-base balance is altered by nonrespiratory disturbances, more traditionally called metabolic disturbances, in which the rate formation of hydrogen ions or their excretion by the kidney changes, or by respiratory disturbances that lead to changes in the carbon dioxide tension (i.e., the alveolar ventilation is unable or more than able to cope with the rate of carbon dioxide production). Whenever the balance of HCO_3^- to Pco_2 is disturbed, the other system (either metabolic or respiratory) is called into play in an attempt to restore the balance and return the ratio of bicarbonate to dissolved carbon dioxide to normal. In the completely compensated state, the primary disturbance, i.e., the acidosis or alkalosis, will still be present, but the acidemia or alkalemia will have been ameliorated.

Respiratory Acid-Base Disturbances

A respiratory acid-base disturbance is present whenever the P_aco_2 deviates from the normal level of 40 ± 5 mm. Hg at sea level. As we have seen, the alveolar (and the arterial) Pco_2 at any given point in time is related to the ratio of the alveolar ventilation to the carbon dioxide production.

$$Pco_2 = (\dot{V}co_2/\dot{V}_A) \times 0.863$$

The situations in which respiratory disorders of acid-base balance occur are summarized in Table 4. When the respiratory acid-base disturbance is the primary event, compensation is brought about by a physiologically induced metabolic disturbance (usually renal), an alkalosis to correct a respiratory acidosis, and an acidosis to correct a respiratory alkalosis.

Respiratory Acidosis. When the alveolar ventilation is inadequate relative to the carbon dioxide production, the P_aco_2 rises above the normal range *(respiratory acidosis)* and the bicarbonate/dissolved carbon dioxide ratio falls below 20:1. As a result, the hydrogen ion concentration rises (pH falls); i.e., there is a *respiratory acidemia* present (Fig. 48A). An acute reduction in minute ventilation, or an increase in physiologic dead space without a compensatory rise in minute ventilation, in the absence of a proportionate reduction in carbon dioxide production will lead to acute respiratory acidosis and acidemia. A respiratory acidosis will also develop if

TABLE 4. Respiratory Disorders of Acid-Base Balance

DISORDER	GENERAL MECHANISM	SPECIFIC MECHANISM	EXAMPLES	BLOOD PICTURE
Respiratory acidosis	Inadequate alveolar ventilation relative to carbon dioxide production	Airway obstruction	Upper airway, large airways, COPD, asthma	$P_{a_{CO_2}}$ high
		Respiratory center depression	Brain disease, primary?; administration of anesthetics, narcotics, sedatives; chronic CO_2 retention; compensation for metabolic alkalosis	pH low
				HCO_3^- normal (acute) high (compensated)
		Neuromuscular impairment	Myopathies, neuropathies, administration of muscle relaxants	Cl low if compensated
		Chest wall disease	Kyphoscoliosis, obesity, tight binders, etc.	K normal or high
Respiratory alkalosis	Increased alveolar ventilation relative to carbon dioxide production	Exogenous administration of respiratory stimulants	Salicylates, progesterone	$P_{a_{CO_2}}$ low
		Iatrogenic	Excessive mechanical ventilation	pH high
		Increased respiratory center activity	Psychogenic (emotion), brain disease, fever, arterial hypoxemia, reflex from lung receptors?; compensation for metabolic acidosis	HCO_3^- normal (acute) low if compensated
				Cl high
				K low

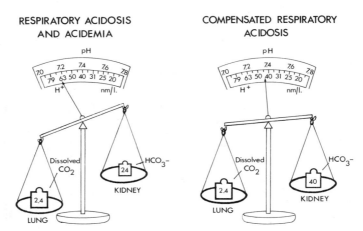

Figure 48. An elevated P_aCO_2 means respiratory acidosis. In the acute situation the balance between HCO_3^- and dissolved CO_2 is less than 20:1, so that the pH is low (acidemia) and the H^+ concentration is elevated. With compensation by the kidney, bicarbonate is retained, so that the HCO_3^-/dissolved CO_2 ratio is closer to 20:1 and the pH and H^+ ion concentration are almost normal (but on the acidemic side).

the metabolic production of carbon dioxide rises without a proportionate increase in alveolar ventilation. This is particularly true when the work of breathing is excessive, because, under such circumstances, any increase in ventilation may be associated with the production of more carbon dioxide than can be eliminated by the lungs.

When respiratory acidosis and acidemia develop, the kidney increases its excretion of hydrogen ions and the renal tubular cells reabsorb and release HCO_3^- back into the blood. There is also an increased elimination of chloride in the form of HCl or NH_4Cl, and the plasma Cl^- decreases by the same number of mEq./l. that the plasma HCO_3^- increases. This compensatory process begins immediately, but it may take days or weeks before the bicarbonate/dissolved carbon dioxide ratio, and hence the pH, are restored to within the normal range (Fig. 48*B*).

Respiratory Alkalosis. When the alveolar ventilation is increased relative to the CO_2 production, there is excessive elimination of carbon dioxide, so that the P_aCO_2 is low *(respiratory alkalosis)*. Although the pH is protected to some extent by a reduction in the amount of renal reabsorption and generation of bicarbonate, the bicarbonate/dissolved carbon dioxide ratio rises above 20:1. As a result, the H^+ ion concentration falls (pH rises); i.e., *respiratory alkalemia* is present (Fig. 49*A*). Respiratory alkalosis may develop because of direct or reflex stimulation of the central chemosensitive centers, following the ingestion of a drug that stimulates respiration (such as salicylate), a cerebrovascular accident or stimulation of the peripheral chemoreceptors by hypoxemia. It may also be seen occasionally in highly emotional or apprehensive individuals without any organic cause.

When a respiratory alkalosis develops, the kidney begins to excrete

RESPIRATORY ALKALOSIS
AND ALKALEMIA

COMPENSATED RESPIRATORY
ALKALOSIS

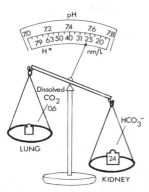

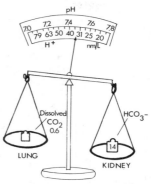

Figure 49. A reduced P_aCO_2 means respiratory alkalosis. In the acute situation the balance between HCO_3^- and dissolved CO_2 is greater than 20:1, so that the pH is high (alkalemia) and the H^+ concentration is low. With compensation by the kidney, bicarbonate is excreted, so that the HCO_3^-/dissolved CO_2 ratio is closer to 20:1 and the pH and H^+ concentration are closer to normal (but on the alkalemic side).

more HCO_3^- and excess cations while chloride ions are conserved, so that plasma Cl^- is elevated and HCO_3^- is lowered. As a result, the bicarbonate/dissolved carbon dioxide ratio is lowered, and the pH tends to return toward the normal range (Fig. 49*B*). Whether the kidneys are capable of compensating completely for a chronic respiratory alkalosis is still controversial, but it is generally considered that the compensation that takes place is incomplete, so that the pH remains slightly elevated.

Metabolic Acid-Base Disturbances

At a given level of alveolar ventilation (or PCO_2), the total number of positively charged cations (sodium, potassium, calcium and magnesium) must equal the total number of negatively charged anions (chloride, bicarbonate, phosphate, sulfate, lactate, pyruvate, proteinate and organic acids). The H^+ ion concentration rises (i.e., pH falls) if their rate of formation increases, their excretion via the kidney diminishes, or loss of bicarbonate from the gastrointestinal tract increases because of diarrhea. The hydrogen ion concentration falls (i.e. pH rises) whenever there is an excessive loss of hydrogen ions from the stomach because of vomiting or there is accumulation of bicarbonate because of excessive ingestion.

The situations in which a metabolic disorder of acid-base balance occurs are summarized in Table 5. When a metabolic disturbance is the primary event, compensation is brought about by a physiologically induced respiratory disturbance, an alkalosis to correct a metabolic acidosis, and an acidosis to correct a metabolic alkalosis.

Metabolic Acidosis. When there is an excess of hydrogen ions, as in diabetic ketosis, they react with bicarbonate to form carbonic acid. As Figure

TABLE 5. Metabolic Disorders of Acid-Base Balance

DISORDER	GENERAL MECHANISM	SPECIFIC MECHANISM	EXAMPLES	BLOOD PICTURE
Metabolic acidosis	Gain of strong acid by extracellular fluid	Exogenous agents that induce hyperchloremic acidosis	NH_4Cl, argenine chloride, lysine, HCl, acetazolamide	
		Exogenous agents that lead to production of endogenous acids	Salicylates, ethylene glycol, methyl alcohol	HCO_3^- low pH low
		Increased production of non-volatile acids due to incomplete oxidation of fat	Diabetic ketoacidosis, starvation, alcoholism (acute and chronic)	
		Increased production of non-volatile acids due to incomplete oxidation of carbohydrate (anaerobic metabolism) – lactate acidosis	Primary lactate acidosis (idiopathic, or in association with leukemia, diabetes, and liver disease; circulatory insufficiency (drug induced – phenformin)	$P_{a_{CO_2}}$ normal (acute); low as compensation
	Loss of HCO_3^- from the extracellular fluid	Via kidneys	Acute and chronic renal failure, renal tubular acidosis, compensation for respiratory alkalosis	Cl normal or high K high, unless associated with K depletion
		Via intestines	Diarrhea or loss of small intestinal alkaline content	

Metabolic alkalosis			
Gain of HCO_3^- from the extracellular fluid	Excess alkali intake	Ingestion of absorbable antacids ($NaHCO_3$), infusion of alkali; milk-alkali syndrome	HCO_3^- high
	Oxidation of salts of weak organic acids Via kidneys	Ingestion or infusion of lactate, citrate, or acetate Compensation for respiratory acidosis	pH high
Loss of acid from the extracellular fluid	Loss of HCl	Vomiting, gastric suction, diarrhea, gastrocolic fistula	$P_{a_{CO_2}}$ normal (acute) slightly elevated as compensation
	Potassium depletion	Diuretics, vomiting, diarrhea, fistulas, low intake, steroid therapy, Cushing's syndrome, primary aldosteronism, potassium-losing enteropathy, potassium-losing nephropathy	Cl low K usually low

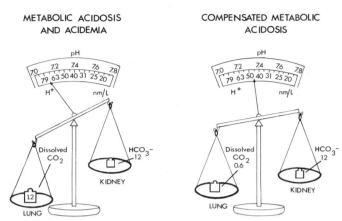

Figure 50. A reduced HCO_3^- means metabolic acidosis. In the acute situation the balance between HCO_3^- and dissolved CO_2 is less than 20:1, so that the pH is low (acidemia) and the H^+ concentration is high. With compensation by the respiratory system, CO_2 is eliminated, so that the HCO_3^-/dissolved CO_2 ratio is closer to 20:1 and the pH and H^+ concentration are closer to normal (but on the acidemic side).

50A demonstrates, when the bicarbonate level falls acutely (i.e., a ***metabolic acidosis*** is present), the bicarbonate/dissolved carbon dioxide ratio is less than 20:1 and there is an elevated H^+ ion concentration and a low pH (***metabolic acidemia***). The increased H^+ ion concentration stimulates ventilation, so that more carbon dioxide is eliminated from the lungs, and the P_aCO_2 is secondarily lowered. In this way, the bicarbonate/dissolved carbon dioxide ratio tends to be returned toward normal, although it appears that the respiratory response is never sufficient to completely restore the pH to normal (Fig. 50B).

Metabolic Alkalosis. When excess OH^- is present in the blood, it reacts with carbonic acid so that the bicarbonate level rises (i.e., a ***metabolic alkalemia*** is present) and the bicarbonate/dissolved carbon dioxide ratio is increased. As is illustrated in Figure 51A, there is a resultant reduction in hydrogen ions and rise in pH (***metabolic alkalemia***). The concentration of chloride usually falls in association with the increase in bicarbonate.

As might be expected, compensation for a metabolic alkalosis is brought about by a depression of ventilation due to the reduced H^+ ion concentration, so that the P_aCO_2 rises (Fig. 51B). Under normal circumstances, however, the P_aCO_2 does not rise above 50 mm. Hg no matter how severe the metabolic alkalosis, so that compensation is usually not complete.

Mixed Acid-Base Disturbances

Pure acid-base disturbances such as we have described occur only briefly. Compensatory measures are introduced rapidly, and each of the four primary disturbances is usually encountered with varying degrees of compensation. In addition, more than one disturbance of acid-base balance, and combina-

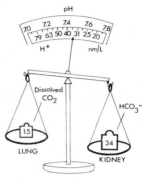

METABOLIC ALKALOSIS
AND ALKALEMIA

COMPENSATED METABOLIC
ALKALOSIS

Figure 51. A raised HCO_3^- means metabolic alkalosis. In the acute situation the balance between HCO_3^- and dissolved CO_2 is greater than 20:1, so that the pH is high (alkalemia) and the H^+ concentration low. With compensation by the respiratory system, CO_2 is retained, so that the HCO_3^-/dissolved CO_2 ratio is closer to 20:1 and the pH and H^+ concentrations are closer to normal (but on the alkalemic side).

tions of acute and chronic disorders, may occur, particularly in very ill people. For instance, it is not uncommon to find that the pH is disproportionately low in patients with respiratory failure, particularly when shock or severe anemia is also present. Under these circumstances, it may not be possible, on the basis of the blood data alone, to determine whether the hypercapnia is relatively acute and there has been little compensation, or whether the hypercapnia has been present for some time and there has been compensation, but an acute metabolic acidosis, such as a lactic acidosis, is superimposed on the underlying defect. Conversely, the pH may be found to be abnormally high in a patient with an elevated PCO_2; i.e., a metabolic alkalosis exists along with the respiratory acidosis. This may be because the metabolic alkalosis is the primary event, with respiratory compensation, or because the respiratory acidosis is the primary event, and the concomitant metabolic alkalosis has been induced by the administration of diuretic agents or corticosteroids. The dominant disorder in mixed disturbances is often reflected by the status of the pH, but it is usually the clinical evaluation that serves as the guide to the major disturbance.

4

CONTROL OF BREATHING

Most cardiopulmonary diseases, and some medications, affect the way we breathe, and hence gas exchange, through their effects on the nerves and the respiratory muscles. In addition, ventilation is frequently altered to compensate for metabolic acid-base disturbances. Thus, an understanding of the control of breathing is important.

In this chapter, we will present a review of current thinking about the regulation of respiration. Much of our knowledge of the chemical influences on respiration has been derived from study of humans. However, it is not possible to give a complete description of the neural mechanisms involved in human respiration, as the experiments that would provide the pertinent information cannot be carried out. Instead, we will use the information that has been derived from animal experiments and then emphasize its relevance to human respiration.

RESPIRATORY CENTERS

Although it is useful to refer to the central connections of respiratory nerves as the respiratory centers, this is actually a term of convenience, for there are no clearly defined "nuclei" concerned with respiration. The nerve cells that participate in the central regulation of respiration are widely dispersed and may be found in the cerebral cortex, hypothalamus, pons and medulla. They can be stimulated or inhibited voluntarily, by reflex action, or by chemical stimuli.

The cells in the cerebral cortex are concerned with the voluntary changes of respiration and with those involuntary acts that require high levels of integration, such as talking, laughing and crying. Clearly, one can alter one's breathing voluntarily, as is exemplified during voluntary hyperventilation or breath-holding. There are many other situations in which ventilation is affected presumably by involvement of the higher centers, such as when we experience pain, apprehension or excitement, all of which may be associated with augmented respiration. The higher centers also appear to play a role in the hyperpnea of exercise.

The cerebral cortex is not essential for the maintenance of rhythmic respiration; this function appears to be carried out by nerve cells located in the medulla. There are inspiratory neurones, which are mostly located in the posterolateral parts of the medulla, and expiratory neurons, which are apparently in the internal and rostral parts. Functionally, it has been suggested that the inspiratory neurones of the *tractus solitarius* generate the central inspiratory drive and are responsible for initiating inspiratory flow. There are other pools of inspiratory neurones, which are located in the *nucleus ambiguus* and *nucleus retroambiguus,* and these are thought to receive volume-related information via the vagal afferents and *pneumotaxic center.* They apparently act by inhibiting the tractus solitarius through a complex network. These pools of cells are influenced by impulses coming to them from the pons, the glossopharyngeal and vagus nerves, and other locations in the brain stem, such as the reticular activating system. The pons is thought to influence the medullary cells to facilitate inspiration, which, if uncontrolled, results in prolonged inspiratory spasms, which is called *apneustic breathing.* The *pneumotaxic centers,* which are located in the upper third of the pons, may also play a role in the rhythmicity of respiration in that they periodically inhibit inspiratory activity and therefore govern the timing mechanism. Apneusis is thought by some to represent the effect of activity of the reticular system and by others to be the result of the activity of a discrete *"apneustic center."*

RESPIRATORY REFLEXES

The respiratory reflexes involved in the regulation of breathing that have received the most attention are those in which the afferents arise in the lungs, the central chemosensitive areas and the peripheral chemosensitive areas.

REFLEXES ARISING IN THE LUNG

The Inflation or Stretch Reflex

In 1868 Hering and Breuer showed that maintained distension of the lungs of anesthetized animals will cause a decrease in the frequency of respiratory effort. This *"Hering-Breuer reflex"* was shown to be mediated by afferent vagal fibers. The receptors for this reflex are probably located in the bronchi or bronchioles, and the afferent impulses travel in a particular type of vagal fiber that is temperature-sensitive. The impulses traveling in these fibers are thought to be inhibitory, because inflation of the lungs results in an increased frequency of impulses in the afferent fibers and a simultaneous decrease of electrical activity in inspiratory muscles.

Earlier physiologists felt that this reflex played a major role in the regulation of respiration and that it was responsible for terminating inspiration, by exciting tonic inhibition of the respiratory center. The reflex is well developed in animals, and it also appears to be active in newborn babies. By contrast, it appears to be relatively inactive in adults, since blocking the vagi has little effect on the normal pattern of breathing, although there is some effect if the tidal volume is greater than one liter.

Head's Paradoxical Reflex

In 1889, Head demonstrated that inflation of the lungs of rabbits causes an additional reflex inspiratory effort if the Hering-Breuer reflex inhibition of respiration is prevented by a partial vagal block. The phenomenon has been termed *Head's paradoxical reflex* or, more simply, the *gasp reflex*. The receptors for this reflex lie in the lungs, and their activity appears to be augmented by progressive collapse of alveoli so that a tidal inspiration becomes sufficient to produce a "positive feedback" and a self-augmented gasp or "complementary" cycle. Newborn animals, including human neonates, also exhibit a "gasp reflex," but it appears to disappear in the human after the first week of life. This vagally mediated reflex may underlie the sighs or self-augmenting cycles seen in adults in situations associated with a tendency for lung collapse.

Other Reflexes Arising in the Lung

Bilateral vagotomy prevents the hyperpnea and hyperventilation that are associated with marked deflation of the lung such as may occur with an atelectasis, a pneumothorax or vascular congestion. This suggests that the hyperventilation occurring under these conditions may be reflex in nature. There is some evidence that the response is mediated by receptors in the lung that respond to deflation and to changes resulting from pulmonary embolism or congestion. Lung receptors are also thought to contribute to the unpleasant sensation of breathing CO_2, or breath-holding, since the breath-holding time is prolonged by vagal block.

REFLEXES ARISING IN THE TRACHEOBRONCHIAL TREE

In response to irritants, mechanoreceptors in the subepithelial regions of the airways give rise to hyperpnea and cough and, in addition, may produce bronchoconstriction and systemic hypertension. Similar effects may be produced by the injection of histamine or serotonin. The relative contribution of mechanoreceptors in the airways to the tachypnea seen in pulmonary conditions is difficult to judge at present. However, there is substantial evidence to suggest that these receptors may become hypersensitive and that they play a major role in the pathogenesis of airways hyperreactivity.

REFLEXES ARISING IN CENTRAL CHEMORECEPTORS

An elevation of the arterial CO_2 tension is thought to stimulate the chemosensitive areas located near the ventrolateral surface of the medulla close to the roots of the ninth and tenth cranial nerves. The central chemosensitive areas are thought to be activated by an increase in the H^+ ion concentration of the extracellular fluid, which is presumed to be in direct contact with these areas. Since the precise location of the central chemosensitive areas as well as their relative contribution to overall central chemosensitivity is not known, it is probably best to refer to them as the "central component of chemosensitivity" rather than as "central chemoreceptors."

REFLEXES ARISING IN PERIPHERAL CHEMORECEPTORS

Two main collections of receptor cells, which lie outside the central nervous system, are stimulated by chemical stimuli. One collection of chemoreceptors is in the carotid body, which lies in the bifurcation of the common carotid artery; the other chemoreceptors lie above the aortic arch between the subclavian and common carotid arteries bilaterally, below the arch between the aorta and pulmonary artery. Impulses arising in the carotid body reach the central nervous system via the glossopharyngeal nerve, and those arising in the aortic chemoreceptors are carried in the vagus. Stimulation of these chemoreceptors causes an increase in the rate and depth of breathing. They are stimulated particularly by a low arterial oxygen tension, but an increased arterial CO_2 tension or an elevated H^+ ion concentration is also stimulatory. Similarly, a decrease in blood supply relative to their metabolic needs and an increase in blood temperature cause an increase in respiratory rate and depth. There may be interaction of several of these stimuli, and it is likely that the response of the peripheral chemoreceptors to a given stimulus depends on the coincident levels of the other stimuli.

The cardiovascular effects of the carotid and aortic chemoreceptor reflexes differ in that stimulation of the aortic receptors produces tachycardia and systemic vasoconstriction, whereas stimulation of the carotid receptors produces bradycardia, a rise in pulmonary vascular resistance, increased bronchiolar tone and increased secretion from the adrenal cortex and medulla.

Peripheral and Central Chemosensitivity

Under ordinary circumstances, the peripheral chemoreceptors do not play a major role in the control of respiration. Hypoxic stimulation of the peripheral chemoreceptors results in an increase in minute ventilation and in alveolar ventilation, although acute hypoxia depresses ventilation if the peripheral chemoreceptors are denervated. If hypoxemia is sustained, however, there is a delayed increase in respiratory rate and fall in tidal volume, and this persists for some time after the hypoxemia is eliminated. The net effect of this delayed respiratory stimulation under these circumstances is an increase in total ventilation but not in alveolar ventilation. The effects of an increase in H^+ ion concentration on the aortic and carotid bodies are similar to those seen in response to a low Po_2. Metabolic acidemia and alkalemia act directly on the peripheral chemoreceptors and stimulate or depress ventilation over a range of arterial pH between 7.3 and 7.5. Below 7.3, and possibly above 7.5, it is thought that changes in H^+ ion concentration likely affect the intracranial chemoreceptors directly.

In contrast to the peripheral chemoreceptors, impulses arising from the central chemoreceptors are sometimes essential for breathing. A significant reduction of the arterial Pco_2 in anesthetized humans and in animals leads to apnea. In conscious humans the results are variable, but apnea may follow voluntary hyperventilation, particularly if the peripheral chemoreceptor drive is eliminated by high levels of Po_2. The stimulus for continued breathing in subjects who fail to manifest apnea presumably arises from other inputs to the respiratory center, such as those arising in the reticular activating system.

REFLEXES ARISING IN OTHER RECEPTORS

Baroreceptors

Receptors in the adventitial coat of the aortic arch and the carotid sinus that are sensitive to alterations in the blood pressure chiefly influence the cardiovascular system, although they also affect respiration to a lesser extent. The impulses arising from these receptors are inhibitory; a rise in the systemic blood pressure inhibits ventilation, and a fall in blood pressure increases ventilation, presumably by reducing a pre-existing inhibitory influence. These responses are only moderate in degree, and their role in the control of respiration in humans is not clear.

Receptors in Muscles and Joints

Afferent activity from any receptor, particularly those involved in muscle activity, will influence the tone or level of excitability of many, if not all, of the anterior horn cells. It would not be surprising, therefore, to find that the respiratory movements are influenced by tension and stretch receptors in the muscles and joints of the extremities, or, for that matter, anywhere in the body. The change in ventilation that is associated with passive movements of the limbs has been attributed to some such mechanism. In addition, it is believed that receptors in the muscles, tendons and joints of the extremities reflexly contribute to the hyperpnea of exercise.

It has also been suggested that "act of breathing" involves the participation of motor control mechanisms that adjust the tension developed by the inspiratory muscles so that they change in length by the amount appropriate to the tidal volume demanded, despite changes in mechanical conditions. It has been postulated that the tension development in the inspiratory muscles is adjusted by an interplay between the "alpha" motor neurones, which innervate them, and the "γ" motor system, which controls the intrafusal fibers of the muscle spindles. If the shortening of the inspiratory muscle is impeded while the intrafusal muscle continues to contract, then the tension in the annulospiral receptor of the muscle spindle will rise and result in an increase in afferent discharge. This is relayed to the alpha motor neurones and results in an increase in the force of contraction of the inspiratory muscles, thereby compensating for the effect of any increase in load.

Thermoreceptors

There are receptors that are sensitive to variations in blood temperature in the anterior hypothalamaus and others that respond to alterations in surface temperature in the skin. Thermoregulatory centers in the hypothalamus receive impulses from these thermoreceptors and discharge the appropriate impulses over the somatic and visceral motor nerves to control the production and elimination of heat. In animals, at least, it is assumed that there are connections between the thermoregulatory centers and the respiratory centers. For instance, the respiratory passages constitute a very important means of heat elimination in dogs. This mechanism of temperature regulation is relatively unimportant in humans, but sustained fever or an artificial elevation of the body temperature does lead to hyperventilation. However, since both the H^+ ion concentration and the solubility of carbon dioxide in the body fluids are directly affected by changes in temperature, the hyperventilation that occurs under these circumstances may be influenced by these factors.

RESPIRATORY CHEMOSENSITIVITY IN MAN

Under normal circumstances, breathing is primarily regulated by chemical stimuli, and ventilation is affected particularly by changes in the blood carbon dioxide level but also by the hydrogen ion concentration and occasionally by blood oxygen levels.

CARBON DIOXIDE STIMULATION

A rise in the arterial carbon dioxide tension is the most potent of all of the known chemical influences on ventilation. If increasing percentages of carbon dioxide are inhaled, the ventilation increases in a relatively linear fashion, reaching a maximum of approximately 70 to 90 l./min. at a concentration of about 15 per cent carbon dioxide. This is primarily because of stimulation of the chemosensitive areas in the medulla by the increase of hydrogen ions in the extracellular fluid. This happens because carbon dioxide can diffuse easily from the blood into these areas, but the blood-brain barrier does not allow hydrogen ions or bicarbonate to enter. Thus, when the carbon dioxide tension of the blood is raised, carbon dioxide diffuses readily into the chemosensitive areas, whereas bicarbonate cannot; so the hydrogen ion concentration rises in the extracellular fluid. However, an elevated blood P_{CO_2} resulting from either alveolar hypoventilation or the inhalation of carbon dioxide also causes the cerebral blood vessels to dilate, and this in turn leads to an increased removal of carbon dioxide. The resultant lowering of the P_{CO_2} in the cerebral tissues tends to counteract the effect of hypoventilation on the composition of the extracellular fluid in the brain. Thus, the ventilatory response to a change in arterial P_{CO_2} represents the integrated effect of several influences.

When the arterial P_{CO_2} is lowered acutely below the normal range, ventilation is depressed, and if the hypocapnia is marked, apnea may ensue. On the other hand, persistence of a low carbon dioxide tension for a lengthy period, as in a patient who is being ventilated, will lead to adaptation, and spontaneous ventilation may be stimulated at lower-than-normal levels of P_aCO_2. This adaptation to a chronically low P_{CO_2} involves a gradual reduction of the HCO_3^- concentration in the central chemosensitive areas so that the hydrogen ion concentration becomes almost normal. Under these circumstances, any rise in P_{CO_2} results in an exaggerated increase in H^+ ion concentration. Thus, if CO_2 is inhaled under these circumstances, there is usually a greater ventilatory response than might normally be seen at the same P_{CO_2}. For the same reason (i.e., the low HCO_3^-), a patient who has been made chronically hypocapnic will suffer from severe acidemia because of the rise in P_aCO_2 that follows cessation of ventilation.

When the arterial P_{CO_2} is chronically elevated, as may be the case in some patients with chronic respiratory disease, the HCO_3^- concentration of the extracellular fluid in the central chemosensitive areas is also increased, so that the local H^+ ion concentration may be virtually normal. Under these circumstances, rapid lowering of the P_aCO_2 by mechanical ventilation may induce deleterious effects. Since carbon dioxide is freely diffusible across the blood-brain barrier, the P_{CO_2} in the central chemosensitive areas will also fall rapidly when the arterial P_{CO_2} is lowered. However, because the blood-brain barrier is impermeable to HCO_3^-, its concentration in the chemosensitive areas will remain high. Consequently, the hydrogen ion concentration in the chemosensitive areas will fall markedly, and this will depress ventilation. The respiratory alkalosis will also cause cerebral vasoconstriction, and, as a result, cerebral blood flow may be seriously impaired and coma may ensue. Clearly then, the reduction of P_aCO_2 in patients with chronic hypercapnia should proceed slowly to allow sufficient time for the active processes, which are involved in lowering the HCO_3^- concentration in the chemosensitive areas, to become operative.

The ventilatory response to inhaled carbon dioxide is frequently used to assess the status of the respiratory center. Because the ventilatory response is frequently reduced in patients suffering from chronic carbon dioxide retention, it is thought that the sensitivity of the respiratory center is diminished in these patients. Indeed, a reduced ventilatory response can also be demonstrated in normal subjects who have been exposed to an environment of carbon dioxide for some time. In both instances, the diminished ventilatory response is likely related to the increased buffering capacity of the blood and extracellular fluid, so that a given increase in P_{CO_2} does not produce the expected rise in hydrogen ion concentration. On the other hand, it has been shown that the introduction of an artificial resistance (i.e., an increase in work of breathing) limits the ventilatory response to carbon dioxide in healthy subjects and that the response is increased in patients with chronic obstructive lung disease following the inhalation of inhaled bronchodilator (i.e., a reduction in work). Clearly then, the ventilatory response to CO_2 reflects the response of the total respiratory system, and a lower-than-expected response does not necessarily mean that the respiratory center has lost its sensitivity.

Ideally, to assess the sensitivity of the respiratory center, it would be desirable to measure the number of impulses coming from the centers in response to a given stimulus, but this is clearly difficult to accomplish. Nevertheless, investigators have used changes in the diaphragmatic electromyogram and, more recently, the airway pressure developed by the inspiratory muscles against an occluded airway during the first 100 sec. of inspiration ($P_{0.1}$) as indices of the respiratory center output. In the airway occlusion technique, the pressure developed in the airway is independent of the compliance and resistance of the respiratory system, because there is no airflow and essentially no volume change (except for some decompression of alveolar gas) during this short period of occlusion. Thus, the $P_{0.1}$ is considered to be representative of the respiratory drive.

One usually determines the response to CO_2 by having the subject rebreathe from a small bag or a spirometer that initially contains a volume of gas (6–7% CO_2 in O_2) that is about one liter greater than the subject's vital capacity. Breathing takes place through a mouthpiece-valve arrangement that allows inspiration through one tube and expiration through another. During the procedure, the end-tidal carbon dioxide tension ($P_{A CO_2}$) and ventilation, which increase at a relatively constant rate while CO_2 is rebreathed, are measured continuously, whereas the inspiratory $P_{0.1}$ is determined randomly at 15-to-30 second intervals. When average values for $P_{A CO_2}$ and minute ventilation ($\dot{V}_E$) or $P_{0.1}$ are plotted against one another, a linear relationship is usually obtained. A reduced relationship between $P_{A CO_2}$ and $P_{0.1}$ is considered to reflect an impaired respiratory drive. However, a change in the shape of the chest wall during occlusion will affect the pressure developed, so that the $P_{0.1}$ may not reflect central inspiratory drive when compared with that of a healthy subject if the interruptions occurred at different lung volumes, e.g., hyperinflation.

It has also been suggested that respiratory flow per se can be used as an index of inspiratory drive. This is based on the following considerations.

Ventilation ($\dot{V}_E$) is the product of tidal volume (V_T) and respiratory frequency (f):

$$\dot{V}_E = V_T \times f$$

In addition, the duration of a breath (t_{TOT}) is the total time taken for both inspiration (t_i) and expiration (t_e):

$$t_{TOT} = t_i + t_e$$

and

$$1/t_{TOT} = f$$

Therefore,

$$\dot{V}_E = V_T(1/t_{TOT})$$

or

$$\dot{V}_E = V_T/t_i \times (t_i/t_{TOT})$$

In such an analysis, V_T/t_i is considered to represent inspiratory flow and thus the central inspiratory drive; t_i/t_{TOT} is thought to represent the timing mechanism that starts and stops inspiration. However, even with this technique, it must be recognized that the inspiratory flow that results from the pressure developed by the respiratory muscles will be affected by changes in resistance or compliance of the respiratory system.

HYDROGEN ION STIMULATION

As we have seen earlier, the respiratory system brings about compensation for metabolic disturbances of acid-base balance by altering the level of ventilation. It is thought that ventilation is stimulated through a direct effect on the peripheral chemoreceptors when the pH falls to 7.3 and that it is depressed if the pH rises to 7.5. The central chemoreceptors are stimulated when the pH is below 7.3 and are depressed if it is above 7.5. The hyperpnea that is induced by an acute metabolic acidemia leads to a fall in P_{CO_2} in the brain extracellular fluid and the arterial blood. The resultant low hydrogen ion concentration in the brain reduces the central drive to ventilation and thereby offsets the full action of the peripheral chemoreceptors. After about 24 hours, the hydrogen ion concentration in the brain is almost normal because of a proportionate reduction in HCO_3^-. When this occurs, slight increases in P_{CO_2} will increase ventilation, because they will be associated with greater changes in hydrogen ion concentration. The converse of this sequence of events is seen in a metabolic alkalosis, which occurs clinically with excessive vomiting.

HYPOXEMIC STIMULATION

Hypoxemia increases ventilation through stimulation of the carotid body and aortic chemoreceptors. If an exceedingly brief period of hypoxemia is induced by the inhalation of a few breaths of a hypoxic gas mixture, the ventilation increases as soon as the oxygen tension falls below 90 mm. Hg. If the same hypoxic gas mixture is breathed for a more prolonged period of time, ventilation barely increases until the concentration of oxygen falls to about 14 per cent, i.e., until the P_aO_2 falls to approximately 60 mm. Hg., which is the equivalent of an altitude of 10,000 feet. On the other hand, if a hypoxic gas mixture is breathed for a still longer period of time, the ventilation is often increased even more. The difference in response between the exceedingly brief and the prolonged periods of exposure to hypoxic gas mixtures is probably explained by the compensatory mechanisms that take place when the gas mixtures are breathed for a prolonged period, and it is likely similar to what happens when one is exposed to altitude. Initially, the fall in arterial oxygen tension stimulates the carotid and aortic chemorecep-tors, so that hyperventilation ensues. As a result, the arterial and brain PCO_2 as well as hydrogen ion concentration fall. This results in inhibition of the central chemosensitive areas, partially offsetting the effect of impulses originating from the peripheral chemoreceptors. After a few days at altitude, the central H^+ ion concentration is restored to a virtually normal level, because the HCO_3^- falls. The level of ventilation is elevated as a consequence of an increased peripheral chemoreceptor activity, even though the central chemoreceptor activity is normal. When fully adapted to altitude, both the blood and the central H^+ ion concentration are normal, so that the hyper-ventilation induced by the low PO_2 is unopposed by alkalosis of either the blood or the brain. This explains why prolonged hypoxemia may be a more potent stimulus to breathing than acute hypoxemia.

Moving from altitude to sea level fails to restore breathing to normal immediately. Alleviation of the hypoxia does lead to a drop in ventilation, but this causes the PCO_2 to rise, so that the central hydrogen ion concentration increases and ventilation is stimulated. To compensate for the elevated PCO_2, the central HCO_3^- rises over a period of days (presumably by active transport mechanisms), so that the hydrogen ion concentratioin, and hence ventilation, are restored to normal.

In persons born at high altitude the ventilatory response to acute hypoxia has been shown to be reduced, and this is not corrected by subsequent residence at sea level. Conversely, those born at sea level who later live at an altitude for prolonged periods have an intact response to acute hypoxia. These observations suggest that the acute hypoxic response is irreversibly determined early in life, although the mechanisms by which this comes about are unknown.

THE REGULATION OF VENTILATION IN RESPIRATORY DISEASE

In most patients with respiratory disease, the minute ventilation is increased because of stimulation of either the central chemosensitive areas or the peripheral chemoreceptors. In healthy individuals, hypoxemia and the peripheral chemoreceptors seem to play a minor role in the control of breathing. In patients with chronic respiratory disease, on the other hand,

TABLE 6. The Alterations in Chemical Agents During Various Conditions

Condition	Arterial pH	Arterial P_{CO_2}	Arterial P_{O_2}
Inhalation of 5 per cent CO_2 in oxygen	↓	↑	↑
Inhalation of 10 per cent O_2 in nitrogen	↑	↓	↓
Voluntary hyperventilation	↑	↓	↑
Acute alveolar hypoventilation	↓	↑	↓

hypoxemia may become an important stimulus to respiration. As has been pointed out, chronic hypercapnia may reduce the sensitivity of the medullary respiratory centers to carbon dioxide in some patients suffering from chronic obstructive lung disease; hypoxemia then becomes the primary stimulus to ventilation, and the peripheral chemoreceptors the principal regulators of the respiratory drive.

Aside from laboratory experimentation, it is unusual to find that only a single chemical stimulus is altered in patients with respiratory disease. Table 6 demonstrates that when ventilation is altered in response to a particular stimulus, other respiratory stimuli are also affected, and each contributes to the total ventilatory response. For instance, in many patients with respiratory disease, where hypoxemia is present because of mismatching of ventilation and perfusion, the ventilatory stimulation induced by the hypoxemia may be counteracted to some extent by the presence of hypocapnia as well as alkalemia. In addition, as we have seen earlier, the activity of the respiratory centers appears to be modified when the work of breathing is high. In respiratory disturbances, the body apparently tolerates hypercapnia rather than expending the amount of effort necessary to keep the arterial P_{CO_2} at a normal level. Indeed, it has been suggested that the work required to lower the P_aCO_2 might require so much oxygen that little would be available for nonventilatory muscular work. In any case, these findings suggest that an elevated P_{CO_2} is not as potent a stimulus to respiration when the work of breathing is increased.

The work of breathing also influences the respiratory rate and depth at which a patient breathes. As indicated in Chapter 1, the respiratory pattern is frequently adjusted to the level at which the least amount of work or force will bring about the body's required alveolar ventilation. Thus, the respiratory frequency is frequently increased in obese subjects and in patients with kyphoscoliosis, where the compliance of the "chest wall" is low, or in pulmonary fibrosis, where the compliance of the lungs is reduced. Although these considerations would cause one to predict that the respiratory frequency would be decreased when the flow resistance is high, the respiratory pattern is often also frequently rapid and shallow in patients suffering from obstruction to airflow. This paradox has been attributed to the increased FRC in these conditions, which may also be an important determinant of the respiratory pattern. Clearly, alterations in chemical stimuli play a role in the respiratory pattern as well, so that the rate and depth of breathing seen in pulmonary disorders are the net result of all stimuli.

PERIODIC BREATHING

In view of the many interrelated factors that affect respiration, and their variability, one wonders how regular breathing ever occurs. Nevertheless, periodic breathing, in which the respiratory pattern is markedly irregular, occurs in only a small number of clinical conditions. Healthy infants born at less than 37 weeks of gestation frequently exhibit periodic respirations, and irregular respirations occur occasionally in healthy persons residing at a high altitude, or even at sea level, during light sleep. Breathing also becomes irregular under conditions in which there are rapid changes in the neural drive to respiration or interference with the feedback of information from the respiratory apparatus to the "respiratory centers."

One can induce variations in the pattern of breathing experimentally. For instance, when a subject begins to breathe through a long dead space, the carbon dioxide concentration waxes and wanes. Initially, rebreathing of the carbon dioxide, which accumulates in the dead space, stimulates ventilation; as a result, carbon dioxide is washed out of the dead space and the inspired gas contains less CO_2, so that the ventilation decreases. This then results in reaccumulation of CO_2 in the dead space, which once again increases ventilation. This "hunting" process continues until the subject comes into equilibrium with the expired carbon dioxide in the dead space and reaches a "steady state." This irregular pattern of breathing is particularly evident when room air is breathed through the dead space. If oxygen is inhaled through the dead space, the oscillations in breathing pattern are reduced.

Alternate waxing and waning of ventilation is also seen when the circulation time to the brain is increased, because the distance through which blood travels on its way to the brain from the heart is lengthened. Under these conditions, the sensing of changes in blood gas tensions by the central chemoreceptors is delayed, so that the ventilatory response lags behind the changes in arterial blood gas tensions. Thus, a rise in P_{CO_2} will not be sensed immediately, and it may rise to high levels. This increases ventilation and thus lowers the P_{CO_2}. Because the circulation is delayed, the low P_{CO_2} is not detected immediately, so the ventilation continues to be elevated and the P_{CO_2} continues to fall. When the hypocapnic blood finally reaches the chemoreceptors, ventilation may cease. This raises the P_{CO_2}, but again this will not be sensed immediately, and ventilation will remain depressed, allowing the P_{CO_2} to rise to high levels. This cyclic change in gas tensions and ventilation therefore continues to be perpetuated.

The commonest form of periodic breathing encountered clinically is known as ***Cheyne-Stokes respiration,*** in which the respirations wax and wane, each sequence of breaths being interrupted by a period of apnea. As indicated earlier, Cheyne-Stokes respirations are seen often in patients suffering from sleep disorders, particularly obese individuals and newborn infants. This form of periodic breathing is also encountered clinically in patients with congestive heart failure, presumably because of the increased circulation time to the brain, as well as in patients who have cerebral damage due to trauma or those suffering from an increased cerebrospinal fluid pressure. Although the presence of Cheyne-Stokes respirations is considered to be an ominous sign, it need not be, for it can be reversed, particularly if it is caused by congestive heart failure. As in healthy individuals breathing through a dead space, administration of oxygen frequently abolishes the periodic breathing in such patients.

5

RESPIRATION UNDER STRESS

This chapter will deal with the response to exercise and exposure to artificial atmospheres. They are discussed together because both exercise and altitude constitute challenges to the oxygen transport system. Both can be associated with a fall in tissue oxygenation in the absence of homeostatic responses. A second reason for linking exercise and altitude in a book on respiratory disorders is that the limitations to human existence at an altitude or in coping with respiratory impairment include both the ability to withstand hypoxia as well as the ability to work and move about. In addition, many patients with respiratory disease who are hypoxemic often complain of limited exercise tolerance and some only experience symptoms on effort. Indeed, in some patients, abnormalities in cardiorespiratory function may be undetected at rest and only manifest themselves during exercise.

EXERCISE

Exercise may be classified in various ways, but the two most important factors that determine an individual's response to work are the type of exercise being performed (i.e., large muscle groups vs. small muscle groups or weight bearing vs. movement) and the duration of the exercise. The type of exercise that will be discussed in this chapter is that which employs large muscle groups and movement, such as those involved in running, cycling and swimming. The extent of the exercise load that is being undertaken can be expressed as the *power,* which is the amount of work performed per unit time. Many physiologists use the unit of *kilopond meters,* which is equivalent to a mass of 1 kg moved through a vertical distance of 1 meter; about 600 kpm./min. is equivalent to 100 watts.

The ability to carry out an exercise depends on the capacity of the respiratory and circulatory systems to increase the transport of oxygen to the exercising muscles and the amount of extraction by the exercising muscles. For most of the activities that one undertakes in ordinary daily life, the exercise period usually lasts for only a few seconds or a few minutes. During these short periods, the respiratory, circulatory and metabolic changes occur very rapidly, and a steady state is not achieved. The capacity to perform short bursts of exercise does not depend on the immediate ability of the circulatory and respiratory system to meet the oxygen requirements of the tissues, but rather on being able to meet the energy costs during the recovery phase. For these brief periods of exercise, the oxygen requirments of the tissue are usually not met immediately, and we "exercise now and pay later." The amount of oxygen that is repaid after an exercise is measured by determining the amount of oxygen consumed in excess of the resting oxygen consumption following the cessation of exercise. This *oxygen debt* is used to replenish the high energy stores within the muscles and to remove substances (chiefly lactic acid) that were formed in the anaerobic pathways of energy metabolism.

At the start of any given exercise, the ventilation increases abruptly and then levels off at a steady state value. At low levels of work, the increased ventilation is due mainly to an increase in tidal volume, but the respiratory frequency rises as well. The cardiorespiratory response to exercise in a normal subject while pedaling on a cycle ergometer for 10 minutes at each of several intensities of exercise is shown in Figure 52. Ventilation (primarily tidal volume) and cardiac output (primarily heart rate) increase linearly with the oxygen consumption and carbon dioxide production during increasing exercise loads up to power outputs of about 60 per cent of the maximal. In other words, ventilation and cardiac output appear to respond proportionately to the intensity of the work or the metabolic requirements.

The increase in oxygen utilization during exercise is achieved through an increase in ventilation, greater diffusion of gases across the alveolocapillary membrane, greater blood flow (cardiac output) and increased extraction of oxygen by the tissues. The amount of increase in blood flow is related to the size of the individual and the level of physical fitness.

The ratio of ventilation to O_2 consumption (ventilatory equivalent for O_2, ventilation coefficient) rises during particularly heavy work. Increases in work intensity above about 60 per cent of the maximal are associated with a lesser increases in O_2 consumption, and the ventilation now becomes more closely related to carbon dioxide production. Above the level of work at which this happens, which has been called the *anaerobic threshold,* lactic acid accumulates in the blood, and further increases in ventilation are associated with a rise in the respiratory quotient.

MAXIMAL OXYGEN CONSUMPTION

The increase in oxygen consumption that occurs during exercise is a reflection of the muscular effort expended. Maximal exercise is usually described in terms of the maximal oxygen consumption, i.e., the state

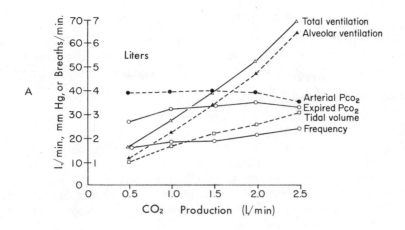

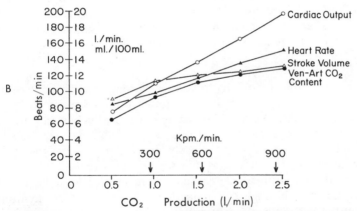

Figure 52. Changes in cardiorespiratory variables during exercise at three intensities on a cycle ergometer. Average values for respiratory parameters **(A)** and cardiovascular parameters **(B)** are shown. (From Campbell, E. J. M.: Exercise Tolerance. The Scientific Basis of Medicine Annual Reviews. University of London, The Athlone Press, 1967. By permission.)

beyond which further increments in work load fail to elicit a further rise in oxygen uptake.

One can predict the maximal oxygen uptake ($\dot{V}O_{2\,max}$) for an individual using the following equations:

For males: $\dot{V}O_{2\,max}$ (l./min.) = 4.2 − 0.032 age

or $\dot{V}O_{2\,max}$ (ml./kg. min.) = 60 − 0.55 age

For females: $\dot{V}O_{2\,max}$ (l./min.) = 2.6 − 0.014 age

or $\dot{V}O_{2\,max}$(ml./kg. min.) = 48 − 0.37 age

THE HYPERPNEA OF EXERCISE

The hyperpnea of muscular exercise is associated with changes in many variables that may stimulate breathing, and it is the interaction of these influences that is believed by many to account for the ventilatory response.

Neurogenic Factors

The neurogenic factors that may be involved in the hyperpnea of exercise include reflexes, which originate in proprioceptors or muscle spindles in the exercising muscles, as well as impulses from higher brain centers. Examination of the change in ventilation that occurs immediately on starting or stopping exercise, before there are any changes in chemical stimuli, indicates that as much as 40 per cent of the ventilatory drive during exercise can be related to movement-related factors. However, the interpretation of the ventilatory transients at the beginning or end of exercise is complicated by "learned" responses. Anxiety or conditioned reflexes from higher levels of the brain could account for the rest of the rapid increase in ventilation at the onset of exercise. Such transients may thus be influenced by cortical factors as well as by reflexes arising in the periphery.

Chemical Factors

The main chemical stimulus to ventilation during exercise is thought to be the hydrogen ion concentration. Although the changes in hydrogen ion concentration during moderate exercise may be relatively small, they correlate positively with changes in ventilation. The hydrogen ion concentration and ventilation are even more closely correlated during the anaerobic metabolic acidosis that develops during heavy exercise. These findings suggest that the hyperpnea of muscular exercise is at least in part due to acid-base changes, although the major locus of action of the hydrogen ion during exercise has yet to be determined.

The role of hypoxia in the hyperpnea of exercise is difficult to establish. In healthy persons, the arterial P_{O_2} does not change during exercise. Nevertheless, a single breath of oxygen during exercise is sufficient to produce, within a few seconds, a 10 to 15 per cent drop in ventilation, and this has been attributed to a lessening in peripheral chemoreceptor drive. It has been postulated that the sensitivity of the peripheral chemoreceptors is increased by the change in hydrogen ion concentration during exercise so that even normal levels of P_{O_2} are associated with an increased impulse traffic. In individuals whose response to a hypoxic stimulus has been removed or at least markedly reduced as a result of carotid body resection, ventilation fails to increase with exercise.

The influence of P_{CO_2} on ventilation during exercise is also difficult to assess, because it is often normal or low rather than increased. It has been proposed that the arterial P_{CO_2} may act as a fine controller of the ventilatory drive during exercise and that, when other ventilatory drives are excessive with respect to metabolic CO_2 production, the low P_{CO_2} acts centrally to check the excessive ventilation.

The role of body temperature in stimulating ventilation is also contro-versial. The temperature rises, sometimes by more than 2°F during exercise, and a change of this magnitude is known to stimulate ventilation at rest. However, if one assumed the same degree of response to temperature during exercise, it would still only account for 10 to 15 per cent of the total ventilation response.

If one can extrapolate from the resting response to these stimuli to the condition of exercise, then it would appear that the level of ventilation achieved during steady state exercise can be almost entirely accounted for by an increase in blood hydrogen ion concentration, by muscle movement and by the change in body temperature. The residual portion still unac-counted for may be due to the inappropriateness of such an extrapolation or to other factors that are as yet not perfectly understood.

THE CIRCULATORY RESPONSE TO EXERCISE

The circulatory response to exercise serves to provide an increased supply of oxygen to the working muscles, to remove carbon dioxide and acid metabolites from the tissues and to dissipate heat. The response involves an increase in cardiac output, vascular dilatation in the working muscles and diversion of blood flow away from the nonworking organs, so that there is an increase in the fraction of the cardiac output that goes to the working skeletal muscles.

Cardiac Output

The increase in cardiac output that occurs during exercise is linearly related to the oxygen uptake. At the onset of the exercise, the stroke volume increases because of a shift of blood from the periphery into the thorax. There is an increased filling of the heart during diastole and greater systolic emptying because of an increased force of contraction that is adrenergically mediated. In the average male, the stroke volume increases from about 80 ml./beat in the resting state to 120 to 150 ml. during exercise. Once the stroke volume has reached its exercise level, further increases in cardiac output are the result of an increase in heart rate.

Heart Rate

The heart rate increases almost linearly with work intensity (oxygen consumption) and reaches a maximum of about 200 beats/min. in youth. This maximum heart rate declines with advancing age according to the following formula:

$$\text{Max. H.R.} = 210 - 0.65 \times \text{age (years)}$$

Peripheral Blood Flow

Blood flow is diverted from nonworking areas because there is vasocon-striction in the splanchnic vascular beds and a fall in the vascular resistance of the working muscles. The fall in resistance is due to both arteriolar dilation and a hundredfold increase in the number of open capillaries. The arteriolar dilatation occurs almost immediately when exercise begins, suggesting that a reflex inhibition of vasomotor tone may be involved. As work continues, the accumulation of vasodilator metabolites and the increased temperature also contribute to the decrease in vasomotor tone. This promotes diversion of a greater proportion of the cardiac output away from the nonworking areas to the exercising muscles. In addition, as the core temperature increases during exercise, cutaneous vasodilation occurs because of hypothalamically mediated decreases in vasomotor tone. In hot environments, cutaneous blood flow increases at the expense of flow to the working muscles, so that the amount of work one can perform is reduced.

THE METABOLIC RESPONSE TO EXERCISE

The metabolic response to an exercise lasting more than a few minutes is characterized by an increased utilization of both fat and carbohydrate. With prolonged exercise in a fasting person, the ventilatory exchange, i.e., the respiratory quotient (R), declines toward 0.7 and plasma free fatty acid and glycerol concentrations increase, suggesting that fat mobilization and utilization are the main mechanisms for providing energy. With heavy work loads and in the presence of anaerobic metabolism, the R value rises, often to values greater than 1.0. This high ventilatory exchange ratio does not reflect the tissue respiratory quotient but rather the accumulation of lactic acid in the blood. The amount of carbon dioxide that is eliminated from the lungs increases, because the carbon dioxide that is released from the bicarbonate stores is eliminated along with the carbon dioxide that is produced by tissue metabolism. When the respiratory quotient rises to high levels during exercise, it reflects the degree of metabolic acidosis that is present and, by extension, indicates the presence of anaerobic metabolism.

EXERCISE TOLERANCE AND PHYSICAL FITNESS

The ability to perform exercise depends on factors that are related to motivation as well as the functional capacity of the oxygen transport system. *Physical fitness* implies optimal usage of the oxygen transport mechanisms and energy by the exercising muscles, so that one can perform work without discomfort. In general, it has been found that the aerobic working capacity (i.e., the work intensity at which the oxygen consumption reaches its maximum) correlates well with the sense of well being. In addition, regular exercise improves the oxygen transport system. The oxygen utilization of the exercising muscles and the work output and maximum oxygen consumption increase when one becomes fit, while the heart rate at submaximal work loads decreases. The level of anaerobic metabolism, i.e., the blood lactate level, is lower in fit subjects than in untrained individuals. Continuous work for an hour in an untrained subject cannot be carried out at more than 50 per cent of that subject's maximal oxygen uptake, whereas highly trained subjects are able to maintain a work intensity of 80 to 90 per cent of their maximal oxygen consumption.

The factors that lead normal subjects to stop exercising during maximum effort are extremely difficult to evaluate. For the same exercise and for different types of exercise, subjective "reasons" for stopping vary from one person to another. The physiologic event that leads to the breaking point when maximal work is carried out for a few minutes is an inadequate supply of oxygen to the working muscles. This does not occur because the level of ventilation or the oxygen diffusing capacity is inadequate, since the arterial blood gases and the $P_{(A-a)}O_2$ are normal. Instead, it appears that it is a circulatory factor, such as the amount of blood flow to the working muscles and their ability to transfer the necessary oxygen, that limits exercise tolerance under normal circumstances.

EXERCISE TOLERANCE IN PATIENTS WITH RESPIRATORY DISEASE

Clearly, exercise tolerance may be impaired in respiratory disease by a variety of mechanisms. In patients with severe disturbances in gas exchange, exercise impairment may result from an inadequate oxygen supply to the exercising muscles because of hypoxemia or because an excessive proportion of the oxygen consumption is expended by the respiratory muscles in overcoming the resistances to ventilation. In patients with cardiac insufficiency, oxygen transport during exercise may be impaired by a restricted cardiac output. When exercise is limited by ventilatory impairment, the alveolar and arterial PCO_2 rise, and the alveolar and arterial PO_2 fall. The application of exercise tests to the assessment of patients with respiratory disease will be considered further in Chapter 7.

Limitation of exercise tolerance because of ventilatory impairment is relatively uncommon, and limitation due to invalidism or physical unfitness is more frequently encountered. Despite marked disturbances in respiratory function, considerable improvement in exercise tolerance can usually be achieved through a program of exercise training. The training effect is most often not due to improved ventilatory function but rather to improved circulatory function, particularly improved distribution of blood flow to the working muscles.

ALTITUDE

The response to altitude is, in essence, the response to hypoxia, and this has already been considered, in part, in Chapter 4. The respiratory adaptation to altitude includes stimulation of ventilation by the hypoxemia, with an initial decrease in blood and central hydrogen ion concentration due to the low arterial P_{CO_2}; this is gradually offset by active processes that lowers the bicarbonate concentration. Hyperventilation is not as common in natives of high altitude, who are chronically hypoxemic, and this is thought to be due to a blunted ventilatory response to hypoxia. Apparently this blunting of the response to hypoxia requires a period of time, because the ventilatory response is greater in children at altitude than it is in adults.

Just as at sea level, the ventilation and oxygen consumption during exercise at altitude are linearly related to work intensity. On Mt. Everest, which is 29,000 ft. high, the inspired oxygen tension is only 73 torr, or about half that at sea level; the maximum oxygen consumption of climbers is about half of that present at sea level.

Although the ventilatory response to altitude hypoxia is the major adaptation of the respiratory system, there are also changes in lung volume. The residual volume, functional residual capacity and vital capacity are apparently increased in natives at high altitudes. The increase in gas reservoir of the lungs is advantageous, in that short periods of breath-holding or hypoventilation do not result in as great a drop in alveolar P_{O_2} or rise in P_{CO_2} as would occur if the lung volume were small. The diffusing capacity for oxygen is also said to be increased in individuals who have become acclimatized to altitude, perhaps because of polycythemia, and this may be an important factor affecting their exercise performance.

In contrast to the respiratory responses that persist, the circulatory adaptations to altitude, such as tachycardia and increased cardiac output, are transient. However, there are changes in the oxygen transport system. In acutely acclimatized persons, the oxyhemoglobin dissociation curve remains normal when the acid-base changes are taken into account, whereas in natives at altitude, the dissociation curve is shifted to the right, indicating a diminished affinity for oxygen. The amount of circulating hemoglobin increases as a result of the hypoxic stimulation of erythropoiesis, so that the arterial oxygen content is increased to values near to those found at sea level, even though the arterial P_{O_2} is reduced. In addition, the transfer of oxygen to the tissues occurs along the steep portion of the hemoglobin dissociation curves. These two facts mean that the required amount of oxygen can be unloaded to the tissues at altitude without the development of a capillary P_{O_2} that is so low that the oxidative potential of the tissue is impaired.

ARTIFICIAL ATMOSPHERES

The effects of exposure to excessive concentrations of carbon dioxide and carbon monoxide have been considered previously. These gases may accumulate in closed system environments, and the nature of their toxicity is well established. As the range of human activities has broadened to encompass aerospace and undersea environments, knowledge of the effects of excessive pressures of oxygen and inert gases have permitted people to create suitable artificial atmospheres to meet the demands of these environments.

HYPEROXIA

Excessive pressures of oxygen may result in deranged function in two general ways: by replacement of the inert gas, nitrogen, in the lung; and by direct chemical toxicity. Because of nitrogen, the gas volume reservoir in the lungs and other gas-containing spaces in the body is normally maintained. When the communication between the airways and alveoli and the external environment is blocked, oxygen and carbon dioxide are rapidly absorbed from the alveoli, but nitrogen is absorbed slowly, because it is poorly soluble in body fluids. However, if the oxygen concentration of the inspired gas is increased (i.e., the nitrogen concentration is reduced), the development of airway obstruction can lead to rapid collapse of the lung (i.e., atelectasis).

The direct chemical toxicity of oxygen is manifested mainly in the lungs and the central nervous system. The pulmonary effects include bronchial irritation, cough and a fall in vital capacity after 24 hours of exposure to 80 per cent oxygen. Higher concentrations and longer exposures may lead to bronchopneumonia, pleural effusion, impairment of the mechanical properties of the lung and altered gas exchange. In particular, hyperoxia in the acutely ill individual may result in alveolar epithelial and capillary endothelial injury in the lung (ARDS), and this, in turn, may progress to interstitial fibrosis and collagen deposition.

Pressures of oxygen in excess of 2 atmospheres produce central nervous system toxicity. This means that a depth of 30 feet is the practical limit for diving when pure oxygen is being breathed. If a gas mixture containing oxygen in helium is inhaled rather than pure oxygen, the equivalent depth limit is considerably increased. The manifestations of central nervous system toxicity are neuromuscular irritability progressing to generalized convulsion. The appearance and severity of central nervous system effects depend on the oxygen pressure, the duration of exposure and the activity of the subject. They are aggravated by increased CO_2 concentrations.

Hyperoxia also leads to contraction of the visual fields in adults, but the most serious ophthalmic effects are seen in premature infants, who can develop severe vascular changes (*retrolental fibroplasia*) leading to blindness when they are given high concentrations of oxygen to breathe. The use and abuse of increased pressures of oxygen in the treatment of hypoxemic states will be considered in more detail later.

INERT GASES

The effects of the inhalation of inert gases under excessive pressure are both direct and indirect. The direct effects are the result of involvement of the excitable tissues, narcosis being the most dramatic manifestation in humans. The threshold for narcosis with inert gases falls with increasing molecular weight, being lowest for radon, highest for helium, and intermediate for nitrogen. The indirect effects of inert gases result from rapid decompression of the body, which may occur following compression of divers, caisson workers and subjects in pressure chambers. Compression in a person breathing a gas mixture containing an inert gas such as nitrogen increases the partial pressure of nitrogen in the lungs, so that additional nitrogen is dissolved in the body fluids. If decompression occurs rapidly, the nitrogen may come out of solution and form bubbles of gas in the tissues and small vessels, where they may obstruct blood flow. The symptoms produced are called *decompression sickness,* or *bends,* and include joint pains, paralysis, sensory loss, paraplegia and dyspnea. The symptom pattern depends on the sites at which the bubbles are formed or trapped.

6

SPECIAL ASPECTS RELATED TO THE NEWBORN INFANT

The dramatic events at the time of birth continue to intrigue the physician as well as the layman. Within a few moments following birth, the lung must replace the placenta as the organ of gas exchange, and thereafter it must continue to function efficiently for many decades. This sudden adaptation to extrauterine life also requires rapid circulatory adjustments to provide the necessary nutrients to the tissues. To understand the vital events associated with adjustment to the external environment, one must have a knowledge of some aspects of lung development.

DEVELOPMENT OF THE FETAL LUNG

By the sixteenth week of gestation, there are already about 20 generations of branches in the bronchial tree. Thereafter, the respiratory bronchioles and the alveolar ducts continue to increase in number until adulthood, when there are about 23 generations of airway branches. In contrast to the early development of airways, the gas-exchanging, or respiratory, portions of the lung (i.e., the alveolar sacs and alveoli) do not begin to form until the fetus is about 24 weeks of age. In fact some morphologists feel that truly recognizable alveoli do not develop until about two months after birth. Initially, the terminal air spaces are lined by cuboidal epithelium, but as term approaches (40 weeks), the epithelium becomes flattened. At term, the terminal air spaces consist of large saccules and primitive "alveoli" that are shallow out-pouchings from the saccules. Even at term the total number of saccules and primitive alveoli is only about 10 per cent of the total number of alveoli in the adult lung.

The pulmonary capillary network develops from the pulmonary mesenchyme at 20 weeks, and by 28 weeks it has proliferated in close proximity to the developing airway. The fetus is not viable before the twenty-eighth week of gestation for several reasons. First, the pulmonary capillary bed is not sufficiently developed to accommodate the entire cardiac output; second, the pulmonary capillaries are separated from the alveolar sacs by mesenchymal tissue until the twenty-eight week, so that adequate pulmonary gas exchange is not possible.

The internal surface of the airways is lined by cells at all phases of lung development. Ciliated cells, goblet cells and brush cells are found in the trachea and bronchi by the fifteenth week of gestation. Ciliated cells are also found in the bronchioles, but the goblet cells are replaced by columnar cells with small apical secretory droplets. The first evidence of bronchial gland formation is epithelial invaginations or buds, which are seen at about 13 weeks. They are found at term in only the central airways. The glands in the more peripheral airways appear after birth.

The lining cells of the most terminal air spaces are particularly specific to the lung and are the last to appear in lung development. Two types of alveolar cells are present: the Type I cell, which has a thin, attenuated cytoplasm, and the Type II cell, which has a bulky cytoplasm containing many mitochondria, osmophilic inclusions and other organelles. These latter cells appear in the alveolar epithelium at about the twenty-fourth week of gestation and become more numerous until about the thirty-second week. The fact that the appearance of surfactant is coincident with the proliferation of Type II cells is evidence in favor of the theory that the Type II cell is responsible for surfactant production.

The fetal lung is not in a collapsed state in utero, but rather it is distended with a volume of liquid that is almost equal to the functional residual capacity of the lung in the newborn infant. The liquid originates in the lung itself and represents an ultrafiltrate of plasma with a protein content of about 0.3 gm./100 ml. There is evidence that active sodium transport occurs, and it has been suggested that the lung liquid may be formed against a considerable osmotic gradient. At one time it was thought that intrauterine respiratory movements were necessary for normal lung development and that the liquid within the lung represented aspirated amniotic fluid. This is now known to be untrue, since it has been demonstrated that the fetal lung will develop normally and become distended with liquid even if the trachea is ligated in utero. Nevertheless, the fetus does gasp occasionally, and bursts of regular respiratory activity interspersed with apneic periods may occur, particularly during REM sleep. However, a regular rhythmic respiratory pattern is apparently not established before birth.

PERINATAL CIRCULATION

Before birth the placenta acts as the nutritive, respiratory, digestive and renal organ of the fetus. The fetal circulation is adapted to serve these functions of the placenta, and when the fetus and placenta are separated at birth, rapid and dramatic circulatory changes must occur before adequate gas exchange can proceed in the lungs.

The blood flow to the lungs during fetal development is only a small proportion of the total cardiac output. Oxygenated blood from the placenta comes to the fetus via the umbilical vein. Figure 53 illustrates that there are two important extracardiac channels through which blood is shunted in the fetus. The first is the ***ductus venosus,*** through which oxygenated blood from the placenta bypasses the portal system and enters the inferior vena cava on its way to the right atrium. About 50 per cent of the inferior vena caval flow is diverted through the ***foramen ovale*** to the left atrium and left ventricle. There it mixes with the small proportion of the cardiac output that passes through the lungs. It is this blood, which has a relatively high oxygen content, that perfuses the fetal brain. The second extracardiac shunt is the ***ductus arteriosus.*** Venous blood coming from the inferior and superior vena cava to the right atrium passes into the right ventricle and then the pulmonary artery. This poorly oxygenated blood bypasses the lungs, because it is shunted through the ductus arteriosus and enters the descending aorta. Thus, the umbilical arteries deliver poorly oxygenated, hypercapnic blood from the fetus to the placenta.

Because both the right and left sides of the heart contribute blood to the systemic circulation, measurement of separate ventricular output has little meaning in the fetus. Cardiac output is therefore expressed as the combined right and left ventricular outputs and is approximately 300 ml./kg.

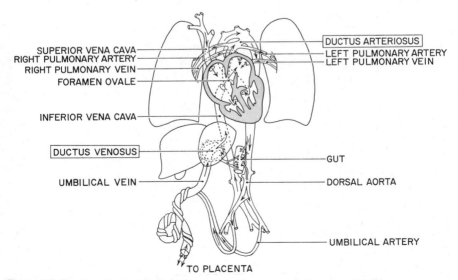

Figure 53. The fetal circulation. Note the extracardiac channels through which blood is shunted. (From Avery, M. E.: The Lung and Its Disorders in the Newborn Infant, 2nd ed. W. B. Saunders Co., Philadelphia, 1964, p. 32. By permission.)

The distribution of this combined ventricular output depends upon the relative distribution of vascular resistance in the various beds of the fetal circulation.

PULMONARY VASCULAR RESISTANCE

The mean pressure in the pulmonary artery of the fetus is a few mm. Hg above the aortic pressure (about 60 mm. Hg), and that is why the blood flows from the right to the left through the ductus arteriosus. The pulmonary vascular resistance is high because of the marked tortuosity and kinking of the vessels, the proportionately large smooth muscle mass in the arterioles and the vasoconstriction in response to the low PO_2 (30 mm. Hg) of the intrauterine environment.

RESPONSE OF FETAL AND NEONATAL PULMONARY CIRCULATION TO GASES AND DRUGS

The fetal and neonatal pulmonary circulation appears to be exquisitely sensitive to vasoconstrictor agents such as hypoxemia, acidosis, epinephrine, norepinephrine and serotonin. These agents produce a prompt and marked increase in pulmonary vascular resistance. The response to vasodilator agents depends on the level of the pulmonary vascular resistance, but acetylcholine, histamine, isoproterenol and bradykinin all produce a marked fall in pulmonary vascular resistance. The qualitative responses are similar in the fetal, neonatal and adult pulmonary circulations, but the quantitative effects of vasoactive stimuli differ in the three groups.

THE INITIATION OF RESPIRATION AT BIRTH

In utero, the fetus exists in an environment that isolates it from tactile, thermal, visual and other stimuli. At birth the newborn infant is suddenly bombarded by the sensory stimuli of a new environment. In addition, the process of birth markedly interferes with placental gas exchange, and as a result, the fetus becomes hypoxemic and hypercapnic. Consequently, both central and peripheral chemoreceptors are stimulated. The initial inflation of the lung may be aided by Head's paradoxical reflex, or the *"gasp reflex,"* which is mediated by the vagus nerves (see Chapter 4). This reflex is apparently present in the human neonate, but then disappears a few weeks after birth. It is believed that the large airways become distended by the first inspiration and that this stretch triggers a reflex augmentation of the first inspiration. It is the combination of these chemical and nonchemical stimuli that results in the initiation of respiration within moments of birth.

Clearly, the lung liquid must be cleared rapidly if the lung is to function efficiently as an organ of gas exchange within a few moments after birth. About one third of the liquid is squeezed from the thorax and out of the oropharynx as the infant passes through the birth canal. About one-half of the remaining two-thirds of the lung liquid is absorbed into the capillaries, and the remainder is removed by the pulmonary lymphatics. Thus, within a few moments after the onset of respiration, the liquid is replaced by air and the volume of gas in the lungs (FRC) is almost at a normal level, so that the internal surface area of the lungs is sufficient for adequate gas exchange.

To initiate the first inflation of the lungs after birth, the fetus must develop a very high transpulmonary pressure. This is necessary to move air and a column of liquid in the lungs and to overcome the viscosity of the liquid in the tracheobronchial tree. This liquid is about 100 times more viscous than air, and, as pointed out earlier, may amount to the size of the FRC, or about 40 per cent of the TLC. The forces of surface tension at the interface of the air and liquid in the small airways must also be overcome. Although the liquid within the lung clearly increases the viscous forces that must be overcome during inspiration, it also acts to distend the small airways and to keep the radius of curvature of the air-liquid interface relatively large. As we have seen, according to the LaPlace formula (see Chapter 1), this helps to reduce both the surface forces that resist inflation and the tendency toward atelectasis. Figure 54 illustrates transpulmonary pressures that were recorded from a human infant during the first three breaths after

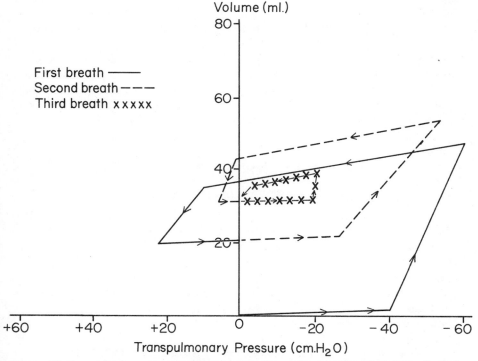

Figure 54. Transpulmonary pressures developed in the newborn human infant during the first three breaths after birth. (Modified from Avery, M. E.: The Lung and Its Disorders in the Newborn Infant, 2nd ed. W. B. Saunders Co., Philadelphia, 1964, p. 29. By permission.)

birth. Note that virtually no air began to enter the lung until a transpulmonary pressure of -40 cm. H_2O was present transiently. Transpulmonary pressures of -80 cm. H_2O may be produced during the first few breaths, and occasionally peak transpulmonary pressures of as much as -100 cm. H_2O are achieved. Note that not all of the air inspired is completely exhaled, and some of the air is retained with each of the first few breaths.

The inspiration of air into the airless lung does not produce uniform expansion of the alveoli, because some of the alveoli remain full of liquid and the airway resistance varies throughout the lung. Further expansion of the lung with breathing is also asynchronous; groups of alveoli become fully distended, and other areas of the lung remain atelectatic. After a short period of time, however, practically all of the air spaces are inflated to some extent. At the end of the first expiration, then, the lungs contain a small volume of air; subsequent inspirations encounter less impedance, and the fetus must develop transpulmonary pressures of decreasing magnitude. During the first few expirations the pleural pressure may be positive, because expiration is made against a partially closed glottis. Expansion of alveoli and retention of air in the lungs after expiration depends on the presence of pulmonary surfactant, which lowers the surface tension in the terminal lung units, thereby allowing alveoli to remain open at a low transpulmonary pressure.

The aspiration of meconium, blood or mucus during the first few breaths may result in airway obstruction and lead to complications. When this happens the newborn must develop a high and prolonged transpulmonary pressure in order to overcome the bronchial obstruction, and this may result in overdistention and rupture of some patent alveoli. Indeed, the highest incidence of spontaneous pneumothorax in the neonatal period occurs in those infants who demonstrate evidence of aspiration of foreign material.

ADJUSTMENT OF CIRCULATION AT BIRTH

PULMONARY VASCULAR RESISTANCE

Expansion of the lung with air at birth results in a local increase in Po_2 and a decrease in Pco_2 and hydrogen ion concentration. Concomitantly there is an immediate and dramatic fall of the pulmonary vascular resistance. However, the pulmonary vascular resistance remains higher in the neonate than it is in the adult, and the pulmonary arterial pressure may be about 40 mm. Hg after birth. With time, the pulmonary vascular resistance gradually decreases, the pulmonary artery pressure falling to normal adult levels at about 1 to 2 weeks after birth.

CLOSURE OF THE FORAMEN OVALE AND DUCTUS ARTERIOSUS

At birth, *functional closure of the foramen ovale* occurs, because cessation of the umbilical circulation leads to a fall of inferior vena caval blood flow and a concomitant fall in the right atrial pressure. The left atrial pressure rises because of the increased pulmonary blood flow. *Anatomical closure of the foramen ovale* may not occur for some time, and indeed in 25 per cent of adults the foramen ovale remains "probe patent."

Closure of the ductus arteriosus at birth is thought to be due to vasoconstriction, which is brought about by an increase in arterial PO_2. However, a number of other agents probably play a role in the closure. It has been demonstrated that bradykinin (a vasoactive polypeptide) is released from the lung during its initial inflation. This substance is capable of producing profound vasoconstriction of the ductus arteriosus and the umbilical artery when the arterial PO_2 is above 40 mm Hg. Other substances, such as serotonin and prostaglandin, have also been implicated in the constriction of the ductus at birth. In full-term human infants a small bi-directional ductal shunt may be present until about 6 hours of age, and then a small left-to-right shunt may be present until about 16 hours of age. The ability of the ductus to close at birth apparently depends on the degree of maturation, because the lower the gestational age at birth, the higher the incidence of persistent patency of the ductus.

POSTNATAL GROWTH AND FUNCTION OF THE LUNG

A comparison of the infant and adult measurements of pulmonary anatomy and the function of the lung is shown in Table 7. The number of airways down to the level of the terminal bronchioles does not increase after birth, but the length and diameter of the airways do increase proportionately

TABLE 7. Comparison of Infant and Adult Measurements of Pulmonary Anatomy and Function

	Infant	Adult
Body weight (kg.)	3	70
Lung weight (gm.)	50	800
Lung surface area (m.^{2})	2.8	75
Alveolar diameter	150	300
Number of alveoli	24×10^6	296×10^6
Number of airways	155×10^6	14×10^6
Calories/kg./hr.	2	1
$\dot{V}O_2$ (ml./kg./min., STPD)	7	3
$\dot{V}CO_2$ (ml./kg./min., STPD)	6	3
$\dot{V}_E$ (ml./min.)	525	6000
f	35	12
$\dot{V}_T$ (ml.)	15	500
$\dot{V}_A$ (ml./kg.)	120	60
V_D (ml.)	5	150
$\dot{V}O_2/\dot{V}_A$	0.06	0.06
FRC (ml.)	70	3000

over the years. The bronchioles beyond the eighteenth generation of airways are disproportionately narrow in children younger than 5 years of age. This is exemplified by the relatively small change in conductance of the central airways with increasing age, whereas conductance of the peripheral airways increases markedly at about 5 years of age. Thus, disease of the small airways in young infants (e.g., bronchiolitis) may be severe and life threatening.

The number of alveoli increases some tenfold, but adult values are reached only by about 8 years of age. Although the surface area of the infant lung is approximately equal to that of the adult, the oxygen requirements of the infant are nearly twice that of the adult when compared on the basis of body surface area or body weight. Thus, the pulmonary reserve of the infant is considerably less than that of the adult.

Because of the asphyxial insult that occurs at the time of birth, most newborn infants have a combined metabolic and respiratory acidosis. However, by 12 hours of age, the arterial pH returns to normal values as the arterial P_{CO_2} falls. It is of interest that in children up to 2 years of age, the serum bicarbonate is slightly lower and the arterial P_{CO_2} is about 5 mm. Hg less than that of normal adults, whereas the arterial pH is in the normal adult range of 7.35 to 7.45. The arterial P_{O_2} averages only· 70 mm. Hg at sea level in healthy newborn infants when they are 24 hours of age, but it increases to adult values within the next 48 hours. These low values in the first 24 hours represent the persistence of fetal circulatory pathways and the considerable right-to-left shunting that occurs through the foramen ovale and the ductus arteriosus.

Studies of the chemical control of respiration in newborn infants have indicated that there is a very active ventilatory response to hypoxia and carbon dioxide. There do not appear to be any major differences in ventilatory control mechanisms between term infants and adults.

7

APPLICATION OF PULMONARY PHYSIOLOGY TO PULMONARY FUNCTION TESTING

There are a variety of tests that may be used to detect disturbed respiratory function, and used judiciously, they are an essential component of the clinical assessment of a patient with respiratory complaints, particularly in evaluating the severity of impairment and the extent of disability present. With repeated assessments, the physician is able to prescribe proper therapy and assess its effects objectively, as well as follow the progress of the disease. When surgery, particularly removal of lung tissue, is planned for someone with pulmonary disability, such tests help to assess the patient's ability to tolerate anesthetics, narcotics or the removal of lung tissue; they also serve as a guide to the preparation and the postoperative care of the patient. Since only one aspect of pulmonary function may be altered by some diseases, assessment of function may occasionally assist in establishing the correct diagnosis of the respiratory condition.

The degree of sophistication and complexity of the pulmonary function tests that are used varies widely, depending on local circumstances. In the majority of patients, simple spirometry will provide an adequate assessment of function. In a number of patients, definitive interpretation of an abnormality of even the forced vital capacity and evaluation of the benefits of therapeutic intervention require knowledge of the absolute lung volume at which these parameters were determined, so that these patients may have to be referred to a laboratory for further assessment.

In this chapter, we will confine the discussion to those tests of function that are simplest, most widely used and most helpful. These tests fall into two general groups: those that relate to the ventilatory function of the lungs and chest wall and those that relate to gas exchange. However, before discussing these tests, it is important to stress that *no* measurement or

125

calculation of function is meaningful, and consequently no interpretation justified, unless one is satisfied that the performance of the technician is optimal, the equipment used has been carefully calibrated (particularly when electronic circuitry is involved), and the variability and reproducibility of each test have been validated in each particular laboratory. This is true of even the simplest of tests. One must ensure that a recording spirometer measures volume and time accurately; a flow meter, the flow rates; and a gas analyzer, gas concentrations. A calibration curve must be derived for each piece of equipment, and this should be checked at regular intervals. When several sensing devices are used simultaneously in order to derive a particular parameter (such as thoracic gas volume or the mechanical properties of the lungs), one must ensure that the frequency response of the various instruments is adequate and that there is no phase lag between the electronic responses. When the measurements are related to prediction equations, it is important that the predicted values be derived in the same unit or at least with the same equipment, if they were derived elsewhere.

VENTILATORY FUNCTION

In clinical practice, simple spirometry provides an adequate assessment of the status of function in a patient with respiratory complaints and reflects the status of the mechanical properties of the lung and chest wall. Ventilatory function tests are affected primarily by the elastic resistance of the lungs and chest wall and the factors that limit airflow.

ELASTIC RESISTANCE

In practice, the status of the elastic properties (compliance) of the lungs and chest wall is estimated by quantitation of the total lung capacity (TLC) and its subdivisions. Indeed, valid interpretation of measurements of the elastic or flow-resistive properties of the lungs or, as we shall see, of even simple spirometric tests requires knowledge of the absolute lung volume at which these parameters were determined. The absolute volume of the TLC and its subdivisions depends on the balance between the elastic forces of the thorax and the respiratory muscles. Thus, a change in lung volume compartments is indicative of either an alteration in the compliance of the lungs or the chest wall or of respiratory muscle weakness.

Examples of the alterations in lung volume that are encountered in respiratory disease are shown in Figure 55. When the distensibility of the respiratory apparatus is reduced (i.e., a **restrictive pattern** is present), the TLC and its subdivisions are lower than expected for a given age, sex and size. This may be due to a reduced compliance of the lungs (as in pulmonary fibrosis or congestion) or of the chest wall (as in obesity or kyphoscoliosis). However, it must be pointed out that whereas measurement of the functional residual capacity (FRC) by gas dilution or in a body plethysmograph requires

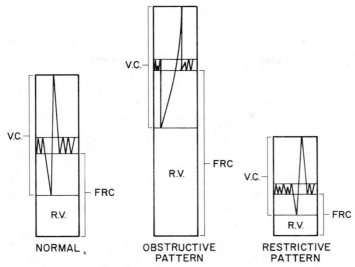

Figure 55. Lung volume and its subdivisions in normal subjects, patients with airway obstruction and patients with restricted movement of the lung or thorax.

only a minimum of cooperation from the patient, calculation of the TLC (and RV) requires maximum cooperation; one must take in as big a breath as possible (i.e., an inspiratory capacity) to calculate TLC, and blow out as far as possible to determine RV. Thus, if respiratory muscle strength is reduced or if the patient has not cooperated fully, the TLC will be lower than expected (and RV will be higher than expected). Since several of the components of the TLC are derived separately, it is important that the alterations of the different subdivisions be consistent with one another before one assumes that an abnormality is present.

A greater-than-expected TLC and its subdivisons indicate overdistension of the lungs (*an obstructive pattern*). The overdistension may be due to an increased resistance to airflow (as in asthma or chronic bronchitis), a loss of lung elastic recoil (as in emphysema), or both.

The size of the vital capacity (VC), which varies normally with age, body size and sex, may also provide a useful index of the distensibility of the respiratory apparatus. However, as can be seen in Figure 55, the VC can be lower than expected in patients suffering from an obstructive disorder, as well as in restrictive disorders. In a restrictive disorder, the low VC is associated with a reduced RV and TLC, whereas in an obstructive disorder, it is associated with an increased RV and RLC.

To determine the mechanisms underlying a change in lung volume, it is often necessary to evaluate the status of the elastic properties of the lung. As was described in Chapter 1, the elastic resistance (compliance) of the lungs and the chest wall, either together or separately, can be determined by assessing the relationship between the distending pressure and the resultant change in lung volume at times when there is no airflow. If these are determined during breathing, one can calculate the *dynamic compliance* of the lungs. However, since the pressure-volume relationship over the entire range of the lung volume is not linear, the calculated lung compliance will depend on the lung volume at which it was determined, so that the calculated compliance is corrected for the lung volume at which it is determined, i.e., the *specific compliance*.

As pointed out earlier, to properly evaluate the elastic properties of the lung, one must assess the shape of the curve relating the static transpulmonary pressure to lung volume over the range of the expiratory vital capacity (i.e., the pressure-volume relationship of the lung). From such curves, it is possible to determine whether overdistension of the lungs and an obstructive disorder are associated with a loss of lung elastic recoil (as in emphysema), or chronic airway disease (as in asthma or bronchitis). As we have seen in Figure 15, the curve is shifted upward (lung volume is greater), and to the left (pressure is lower at any lung volume) in both patients with emphysema and those with asthma. However, in the patient with emphysema the slope of the pressure-volume curve is increased, indicating that the lung is easier to distend (i.e., its elastic resistance is low or compliance is high), whereas in the patient with asthma, the shape of the curve is essentially the same as that in a healthy individual. Similarly, it is possible to determine whether a restrictive disorder is due to a reduced compliance of the lungs (as in fibrosis) or of the chest wall (as in obesity). In both the patient with pulmonary fibrosis and the obese individual, the pressure-volume curve is shifted downward (lung volume is less) and to the right (pressure is greater at any lung volume). In the patient with fibrosis, the slope of the curve is decreased, indicating that the lung is difficult to distend (i.e., the elastic resistance is high, or compliance is low), whereas in the obese individual, the slope of the curve is essentially the same as that in the healthy individual.

FLOW RESISTANCE

The flow resistance of the lungs during breathing is assessed from simultaneous measurements of the pressure within the lung and the rate of airflow at the mouth. As was discussed in Chapter 1, one may derive airflow resistance in a body plethysmograph or from simultaneous measurements of airflow, volume and transpulmonary pressure. As we saw in Figure 21, flow resistance varies with lung volume, so that it must be corrected for the lung volume at which it was determined. The reciprocal of the resistance to airflow, *conductance* is linearly related to the lung volume (i.e., it is greatest at high lung volume, where the bronchi are widest), so that it is also expressed with reference to the lung volume at which it is measured, this is called the *specific conductance*.

The Forced Vital Capacity

Considerable information about the flow-resistive properties of the respiratory system may be obtained from determination of the rate at which air flows out of the lungs during a forced expiration, i.e., a *forced expiratory vital capacity* maneuver (FVC). Thus, this simple test is part of the physical examination and a part of the assessment of all patients.

Analysis of the FVC can be carried out in several ways (Fig. 56). The commonest way is to calculate the volume of air expelled during a certain period of time, in particular the amount expired in the first second, i.e., the *forced expiratory volume in one second* (FEV$_1$). Other commonly used calculations are the *peak expiratory flow rate* (PEFR); the *forced expiratory flow between 25 and 75 per cent of the FVC* (FEF$_{25-75}$), which is the mean rate of airflow during the middle half of the forced expired vital capacity (what used to be called the MMFR); and the *maximal expiratory flow rate* (MEFR), which is the length of time taken to expire 1.0 liter after the first 200 ml. have been expired. Not all of these analyses are equally informative, and most investigators prefer to use the FEV$_1$ or the FEF$_{25-75}$ as indices of expiratory resistance to airflow. This choice is determined by the fact that at high lung volumes maximal flow is subject to wide variability and is very dependent on patient effort, whereas over the lower two-thirds of the lung volume, maximum flow is not as dependent on maximal effort (see Fig. 22). Clearly then, any assessment of flow resistance that is based predominantly on analysis of the expiratory flow rate at high lung volumes, such as FEV$_{0.5}$, or PEFR, may be unreliable, because the value obtained may be related more to patient cooperation and effort than to alterations in pulmonary mechanics. Even the FEF$_{25-75}$ is fraught with problems, because it is clearly dependent on the size of the FVC and will be affected by early cessation of the FVC maneuver.

The FEV$_1$/FVC ratio can provide a useful index of expiratory airflow limitation. In patients suffering solely from a restrictive disorder, this ratio is

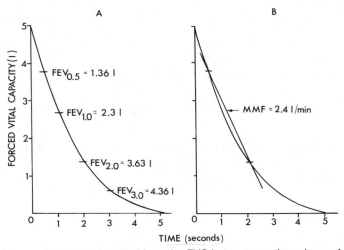

Figure 56. Flow resistance is assessed from the FVC in two ways: the volume of air expired in a particular period of time (**A**), such as ½, 1, 2, or 3 seconds; or the mean rate of air flow during the middle half of the FVC (**B**).

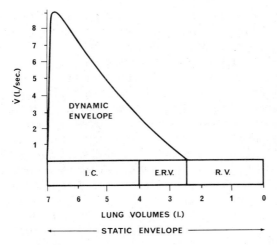

Figure 57. The lung volume ("static envelope") and the flow volume relationship during a forced expiratory vital capacity ("dynamic envelope") in a healthy subject.

usually within the upper range of normal linits, whereas it is markedly reduced in patients suffering from an obstructive disorder. However, once again, anything that will affect the patient's ability to inspire or expire fully, such as dyspnea, pain, or poor effort, may lead to a less-than-maximum FVC in a patient with an obsturctive disorder, and consequently the ratio may appear to be higher than it actually is.

THE INTERPRETATION OF VENTILATORY FUNCTION TESTS

The approach to the interpretation of the FVC or its parameters can be best understood if considered in light of the relationship between lung volume and the instantaneous flow rates during the forced expiration, i.e., the maximum expiratory flow-volume relationship. This is illustrated in Figure 57, where the flow-volume relationship (the "dynamic envelope") in a healthy subject is pictured on the absolute lung volume (the "static envelope") at which the FVC was carried out.

Table 8 compares the patterns of abnormality of ventilatory function in patients suffering from a restrictive pulmonary disorder and those with an

TABLE 8. Patterns of Ventilatory Function Abnormality in Restrictive and Obstructive Pulmonary Disorders

Test	Obstructive	Restrictive
VC	↓ ⟷	↓
FEV_1	↓	↓
FEV_1/FVC	↓	⟷
FEF_{25-75}	↓	↓ ⟷
FRC	↑	↓
TLC	↑	↓

obstructive pulmonary disorder. The finding of a low FEV_i or FEF_{25-75} in patients with a restrictive disorder may suggest concomitant airflow limitation. However, visualization of these measurements in the light of the two envelopes allows differentiation of a restrictive ventilatory pattern from an obstructive ventilatory pattern (Fig. 58).

RESTRICTIVE VENTILATORY PATTERN

In the patient suffering from a restrictive pulmonary disease, such as pulmonary fibrosis, the total lung capacity and its compartments are reduced. The FEV_1, FEF_{25-75} and $\dot{V}_{max}$ at a particular lung volume may be lower than predicted, but, as indicated in Figure 58, this can be explained by the low lung volume. In fact, the expiratory flow rates, though low in absolute terms, are usually higher than expected at this lung volume, because the driving pressure (lung elastic retractive force) is increased. As a corollary, however, if the $\dot{V}_{max}$ is not greater than expected at a particular lung volume in a patient suffering from a restrictive disorder, then it is likely that flow resistance is also increased.

OBSTRUCTIVE VENTILATORY PATTERN

In obstructive pulmonary disease, such as emphysema or asthma, the TLC and its components are increased, and the FEV_1, FEF_{25-75} and $\dot{V}_{max}$ at a particular lung volume are lower than expected, indicating overdistension and flow limitation.

Postbronchodilator Studies

When an obstructive pattern of abnormality is seen, the potential reversibility of the flow limitation should be determined by repeating the FVC maneuver after the inhalation of an adequate dose of nebulized

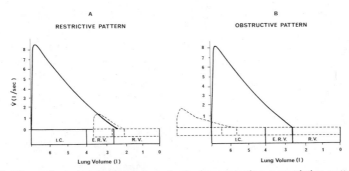

Figure 58. Flow-volume relationships in patients demonstrating a restrictive pattern (**A**) and an obstructive pattern (**B**) are graphed. The observed values are indicated by the interrupted lines. In the restrictive pattern, the static and dynamic envelopes are reduced but the flow rates are consistent with the fact that the lung volume is reduced. In the obstructive pattern, the dynamic envelope is again reduced but the static envelope is increased. Here the flow rates are considerably less than expected at the increased lung volume.

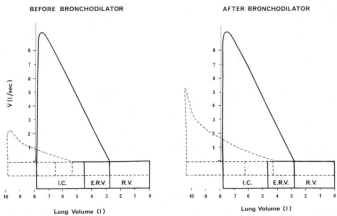

Figure 59. The effect of a nebulized bronchodilator on the flow-volume relationships in a patient with obstruction to air flow. Note that following the bronchodilator, the VC has increased (and RV decreased), the dynamic envelope has increased, and flow rates are higher at equivalent lung volumes.

bronchodilating agent. Improvement of the FVC and $\dot{V}_{max}$ at any lung volume after use of an inhaled bronchodilator is illustrated in Figure 59.

It is important to point out that lack of improvement in flow parameters following use of an inhaled bronchodilator may not indicate lack of reversibility, for any change in lung volume must be taken into account. Figure 60 presents two examples of how measurements of expiratory airflow alone may

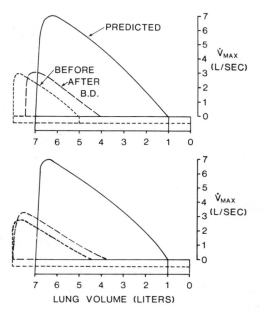

Figure 60. The effect of an inhaled bronchodilator agent (B.D.) on the lung volume and flow-volume relationship in two patients with chronic airflow limitation. In one patient, there is no change in the size of the forced vital capacity but the TLC and RV fall so that airflow is increased at any particular volume. In the other patient, TLC is unchanged following B.D. but the FVC increases so that RV is reduced. Flow at 50 per cent of the FVC is unchanged, but it is determined at a different lung volume than before B.D. (because FVC is larger), and in reality $\dot{V}_{max}$ is higher at all lung volumes after B.D.

provide misleading information. In both cases, the maximum expiratory flow rates were unchanged following the use of an inhaled bronchodilator. However, it can be seen that when the flow-volume relationship is considered relative to the absolute lung volume, there is evidence of improvement in both patients. In one patient, the FVC was unchanged following bronchodilator use, but the TLC and RV both fell. In the other patient, the TLC was unchanged, but RV fell (i.e., VC increased). In both cases, the calculated FEF_{25-75} or $\dot{V}_{max}$ at 50 per cent of the FVC was unchanged following bronchodilator inhalation, and yet the flow rates at equivalent lung volume (isovolume) were significantly increased. Clearly then, interpretation of the benefit, or lack of it, of a nebulized bronchodilator is valid only if the flow rates in a particular individual are compared at equivalent lung volumes. Equally important, one should not withhold bronchodilators on the basis of lack of improvement of $\dot{V}_{max}$, FEF_{25-75} or FEV_1 after bronchodilator inhalation, unless these values have been assessed at isovolume.

UPPER AIRWAY OBSTRUCTION

Although the maximal inspiratory flow rates may yield important information about the flow resistance during inspiration, they are much more effort dependent. Thus, the finding of low inspiratory flow rates is not necessarily due to alteration of the mechanical properties of the respiratory system, and such rates may merely be a reflection of inadequate effort. Nevertheless, provided that maximal effort is ensured, measurements of inspiratory flow are particularly useful in assessing upper airway obstruction and may be diagnostic of this condition. In upper airway obstruction, expiratory flow limitation is accompanied by a marked reduction in inspiratory flow rates as well, so that the ratio of inspiratory to expiratory flow at 50 per cent of the VC is markedly reduced (Fig. 61).

BRONCHOPROVOCATION

Ventilatory function tests are also used to determine whether the patient has an increased propensity to bronchial constriction. In this case, ventilatory

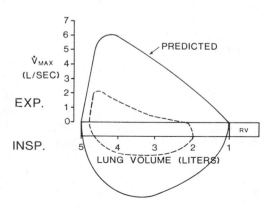

Figure 61. The inspiratory and expiratory flow-volume relationships in a patient with upper airway obstruction. Note that the flow rates at any lung volume are reduced during both inspiration and expiration.

function is assessed before and after exercise or the inhalation of a specific allergen or occupational dust, nonspecific bronchoconstricting mediators such as histamine, or neurotransmitters such as acetylcholine and its analogue, methacholine.

Inhalation challenge with an antigen is especially useful when the history is suggestive, particularly when occupational exposure is implicated. To date, a large number of chemical agents, such as toluene diisocyanate and phthalic anhydride; wood dusts, such as western red cedar; and flour, such as wheat and soybean, have been implicated in occupational asthma. Extracts of these and other agents are commercially available, but they may also be specially prepared in phosphate-buffered saline with a pH of 7.0 and containing 0.4% phenol and then used for antigenic challenge.

Bronchoprovocation should be carried out while the subject is asymptomatic and has relatively good lung function (e.g., the FEV_1 is more than 80% of the best value previously recorded). Since bronchodilators, antihistamines, anticholinergics and disodium cromoglycate may affect the bronchial response to provocation, these drugs are withheld before the procedure. A drop in FEV_1 of 20 per cent or in R_{aw} of 40 per cent following the inhalation of the specific agent or the performance of a given exercise load can be considered a positive response to bronchoprovocation. However, it is important to point out that bronchoconstriction may develop 4 to 8 hours after antigenic bronchoprovocation, whether or not there was an immediate reaction. An example of such a *late reaction* is seen in patients with **allergic bronchopulmonary aspergillosis** following inhalation of aspergillus extract. Thus, the subject should be observed closely and lung function assessed at frequent intervals over the first hour, at hourly intervals for 8 to 10 hours, and again after 24 hours in order to detect a late asthmatic response.

RESISTANCE TO AIRFLOW IN PERIPHERAL AIRWAYS

As we have seen in Chapter 1, the commonly employed indices of flow resistance, such as FEV_1, FEF_{25-75}, and even the airway resistance measurement itself, may be within normal limits, even though the resistance to airflow in the peripheral portions of the airways (i.e., those less than 2 mm. in diameter) may be markedly increased. It is possible to determine the resistance to airflow in the peripheral airways, but it is the maldistribution of mechanical time constants in the lung that is the basis of a number of tests that are thought to reflect disorders of the peripheral airways.

Upstream Resistance

Measurements of maximum expiratory airflow ($\dot{V}_{max}$) at the lower lung volumes yield valuable information about the elastic and flow resistances of the peripheral lung units. Although it is not possible to pinpoint the anatomic location of any increase in resistance in the small airways, it is possible to derive an estimate of the resistance of the airways upstream from the **equal pressure point** (EPP) during a forced expiration (see Fig. 23). A lower-than-expected $\dot{V}_{max}$ at any particular lung volume may be due to a increased upstream resistance (i.e., in airways between the EPP and the alveoli) or a lower-than-normal driving pressure (i.e., a reduced lung elastic recoil). By examining the relationship between the static lung elastic recoil pressure (P_{EL}) and $\dot{V}_{max}$ at equivalent lung volumes, it is possible to determine the underlying cause(s) of low maximal expiratory flow rates (Fig. 24). The static pressure–flow curve is shifted to the right (i.e., the pressure required to produce a given flow is greater) when the upstream resistance is increased. On the other hand, a normal slope of the static pressure–flow relationship, but a lower maximal pressure than would be expected in the healthy individual, indicates that the low $\dot{V}_{max}$ is due to a loss of lung elastic recoil. Clearly, there are also situations in which a low $\dot{V}_{max}$ is due to both an increase in upstream resistance and a loss of lung elastic recoil, which would be the interpretation if the curve were shifted to the right and the maximum lung elastic recoil pressure were also lower than expected.

Air-Helium Flow-Volume Curves

Performance of a forced vital capacity while the subject breathes first air and then a helium-oxygen mixture has also been used to assess the status of the peripheral airway resistance. Failure of the $\dot{V}_{max}$ to increase to the same extent as that of healthy individuals at almost all lung volumes when the FVC is performed after inhaling the helium-oxygen gas mixture suggests that the length of the airway segment in which laminar flow is increased (i.e., the small airways) is narrowed. Thus, when the difference in $\dot{V}_{max}$ at 50 per cent of VC ($\Delta\dot{V}_{max\ 50}$) is less than expected, or when the volume at which the airflow is equivalent with both gases ($V_{iso\ \dot{V}}$) is greater than expected, "small airways" obstruction is thought to be present.

Frequency Dependency of Compliance

This test is generally considered to be the "gold standard" for evaluating small airway disturbances. A drop in dynamic lung compliance below 80 per cent of the static compliance at an equivalent lung volume with increasing respiratory frequency is indicative of a maldistribution of the time constants within the lung (i.e., the product of the compliance and flow resistance of each unit). Unlike an abnormality of the two tests described above, which is indicative of an increase in small airway resistance, the dynamic compliance will be frequency dependent if the alveolar compliances or the small airway resistances are dissimilar in the lung. When *frequency dependence of compliance* is present and the static compliance, airway resistance and spirometric measurements (such as the FEV_1) are normal, "small airway" disease is thought to be present. On the other hand, it clearly could also be due to a variation of alveolar compliance throughout the lung.

Single-Breath Nitrogen Curves

Abnormalities of tests of gas distribution such as the single-breath nitrogen test, the index of intrapulmonary mixing, or the mixing efficiency

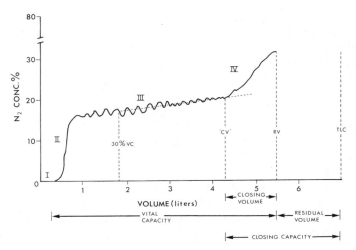

Figure 62. The single-breath N_2 curve. From this curve the anatomic dead space residual volume, total lung capacity, closing volume, closing capacity, and the slope of the alveolar plateau (Phase III) are frequently calculated.

are also indicative of regional variations of mechanical time constants. A typical example of the single-breath nitrogen curve in a healthy individual is shown in Figure 62. It can be seen that the expired N_2 can be separated with several components, representing gas coming from the dead space (Phase II), from emptying alveoli (Phase III) and from alveoli and airways remaining open while other airways have closed (Phase IV).

SLOPE OF PHASE III. Although it has been suggested that the slope of the alveolar plateau (Phase III) of the single-breath nitrogen curve is primarily influenced by the elastic properties of the peripheral air spaces, the fact that it improves following smoking cessation suggests that it primarily reflects the uniformity of time constants in the lung. Whatever the mechanism, the *slope of Phase III* appears to be a sensitive indicator of abnormalities in the lung, and it has recently been suggested that an abnormal slope may be predictive of those individuals whose FEV_1/FVC ratio will deteriorate at an increased rate.

CLOSING VOLUME AND CLOSING CAPACITY. The *closing volume* (CV) and *closing capacity* (CC) are nonspecific tests that are affected by both airway and parenchymal changes. An increase in closing volume/vital capacity (CV/VC) or closing capacity/total lung capacity (CC/TLC) ratios indicates premature airway closure, presumably at the base of the lung, and this in turn may be due to increased narrowing of the lumen of small bronchioles, as in bronchitis or asthma, or to a loss of radial traction on the airways, as in emphysema.

CHEMICAL REGULATION OF VENTILATION

In those patients suffering from alterations of gas exchange, it may be very important to assess the chemical regulation of ventilation. Assessment of the response to both inhaled carbon dioxide and a hypoxic gas mixture may be particularly important when one is attempting to determine the mechanism underlying sleep disorders or alveolar hypoventilation.

Response to Carbon Dioxide

The finding of a lower-than-normal ventilatory response to inhaled carbon dioxide has been thought to be indicative of a diminished sensitivity of the central chemosensitive areas. However, the ventilatory response of even healthy individuals falls when breathing through an artificial airway obstruction, and the inhalation of a bronchodilator often increases the response in a patient with chronic airflow limitation, so that a reduced ventilatory response to carbon dioxide may be another reflection of ventilatory impairment. In recent years, the mouth occlusion pressure developed in the first 100 milliseconds after inspiration is initiated from FRC (i.e., $P_{0.1}$) in response to a rising P_{CO_2} has been used to assess the respiratory drive. In this case, a lower-than-expected $P_{0.1}$ for a given P_aCO_2 is thought to reflect a diminished responsiveness of the respiratory center.

Response to Hypoxemia

Like the response to carbon dioxide, the ventilatory response to hypoxemia can be affected by ventilatory impairment as well as an alteration of chemoreceptor sensitivity. Again, using the $P_{0.1}$, it may be possible to distinguish the status of the respiratory drive in response to a given P_aO_2. A lower-than-expected $P_{0.1}$ response to hypoxemia suggests that the chemical responsiveness is diminished, this time in the peripheral chemoreceptors.

GAS EXCHANGE

Assessment of the status of gas exchange in the lungs requires sampling of the arterial blood gas tensions and calculation of the alveolo-arterial oxygen tension gradient ($P_{(A-a)}O_2$). The gas exchange function of the lung is said to be normal when the blood leaving the lungs has approximately the same gas concentrations as the alveolar gas and the values for arterial P_{O_2} and P_{CO_2} are within the normal range. Gas exchange is abnormal when the arterial P_{O_2} is less than expected, with or without an abnormal P_{CO_2}, or there is an increased $P_{(A-a)}O_2$.

It is now generally accepted that assessment of arterial blood gases and pH is necessary in individuals suffering from acute respiratory insufficiency. However, since many patients only experience symptoms during exertion, assessment of gas exchange and acid-base balance at rest and during exercise is equally necessary in any patient suffering from chronic respiratory insufficiency. In addition, an exercise load can be used as a bronchoprovocation test when hyperreactive airways are suspected.

THE ALVEOLO-ARTERIAL OXYGEN TENSION GRADIENT

The alveolar to arterial O_2 tension gradient $(P_{(A-a)}O_2)$ can be derived by calculation of the effective alveolar oxygen tension, using a simplified alveolar air equation:

$$P_AO_2 = P_IO_2 - P_ACO_2/R$$

In practice, one substitutes the arterial PCO_2 for P_ACO_2 and assumes an R of 0.8 if the patient was breathing room air or 1.0 if an oxygen mixture was being breathed.

Thus, when the patient is breathing air the $P_{(A-a)}O_2$ becomes

$$P_{(A-a)}O_2 = P_IO_2 - (P_aCO_2 \times 1.25) - P_aO_2$$

and if breathing oxygen,

$$P_{(A-a)}O_2 = P_IO_2 - P_aCO_2 - P_aO_2$$

As we have seen earlier, the $P_{(A-a)}O_2$ is normally 5 to 10 mm. Hg, even in healthy individuals, because there is always some mismatching of ventilation and perfusion in the lung, and because there is some admixture of venous blood with arterialized blood via the thebesian and bronchial veins, which empty into the left side of the heart and the pulmonary veins, respectively.

Hypoxemia (a low P_aO_2) may be due to a number of disturbances: increased mismatching of ventilation and perfusion in the lung, true venous admixture, a diffusion defect, alveolar hypoventilation or a combination of these disturbances. The salient features of the different mechanisms underlying abnormal gas exchange are presented in Table 9. It can be seen that the $P_{(A-a)}O_2$ is elevated only in the first three of these disturbances.

TABLE 9. Disturbances of Gas Exchange

Parameter	V/Q Mismatch		Venous Admixture	Diffusion Defect	Alveolar Hypoventilation	
	(a)	(b)	(c)	(d)	(e)	(f)
$\dot{V}_E$	↑	↑	↑ ←→	↑	←→ ↑	↓
V_D	↑	←→	←→	←→	↑	←→
$V_D/V_T (\%)$	↑	←→	←→	←→	↑	↑
$P_{(A-a)}O_2$	↑	↑	↑	↑	←→	←→
P_aO_2 (room air)	←→	↓	↓	↓	↓	↓
$P_aO_2 (O_2)$	> 500	> 500	< 500	> 500	> 500	> 500
P_aCO_2	↓ ←→	↓ ←→	↓ ←→	↓ ←→	↑	↑

VENTILATION/PERFUSION MISMATCHING

Increased mismatching of ventilation and the perfusion in the lungs is the most common cause of an elevated $P_{(A-a)}O_2$. This may be due to well-ventilated alveoli that are poorly perfused (i.e., the ventilation/perfusion ratio is high) or poorly ventilated alveoli that continue to be well perfused (i.e., the ventilation/perfusion ratio is low).

Dead Space–Like Ventilation

The physiologic dead space/tidal volume (V_D/V_T) ratio is normally less than 30 per cent in young individuals and rises to about 40 per cent in older subjects. An elevated V_D/V_T ratio indicates ventilation of alveoli that are poorly perfused or, in the extreme case, not perfused at all. The gas entering these alveoli takes little part, if any, in gas exchange, so that the gas concentrations are virtually the same as those in the inspired air; this is called *dead space–like ventilation.* If this is the only condition present, the blood leaving these alveoli is fully oxygenated and often excessively depleted of carbon dioxide. Under these circumstances, then, the P_aO_2 is usually normal, the P_aCO_2 normal or low, and the $P_{(A-a)}O_2$ elevated (Table 9,*a*).

Venous Admixture–Like Perfusion

Blood leaving inadequately ventilated alveoli, or in the extreme case, nonventilated alveoli, is only slightly aerated, if at all, and this poorly aerated blood mixes with "arterialized blood" that is coming from well-ventilated, well-perfused alveoli. Under these circumstances, the $P_{(A-a)}O_2$ is elevated and the P_aO_2 is low (Table 9,*b*). In most cases, there is sufficient hyperventilation of other well-perfused alveoli, so that the P_aCO_2 is usually normal or even low. However, because of the shape of the oxyhemoglobin dissociation curve, the hyperventilation does not significantly correct the hypoxemia.

TRUE VENOUS ADMIXTURE

As we have seen earlier, a small part of the $P_{(A-a)}O_2$ is normally due to the admixture of venous blood into the systemic arterial blood via the thebesian and the bronchial veins. The amount of admixture or shunt increases in certain congenital heart diseases and when there are abnormal pulmonary arteriovenous communications. Under such circumstances, the $P_{(A-a)}O_2$ is elevated and the P_aO_2 reduced, whereas the P_aCO_2 is usually lower than normal, because the hypoxemia induces hyperventilation.

It is possible to obtain a qualitative assessment of the amount of venous admixture or shunt present by sampling arterial blood while the patient is breathing 100 per cent oxygen. If there is excessive shunting, the P_aO_2 will fail to rise above 500 mm. Hg at sea level (Table 9,*c*). The P_aO_2 may also fail to rise above 500 mm. Hg if there is significant polycythemia, even without increased shunting. In addition, continued perfusion of lung regions that are not ventilated at all, as in atelectasis, pulmonary edema or consolidation, will simulate an increase in true venous admixture. In these conditions, intravenous injection of a marker such as green dye, which is used to determine cardiac output, may help to delineate whether there is an anatomic shunt. The dye will appear in a peripheral artery earlier than expected if the shunting is due to an increase in true venous admixture, and in a normal period of time if there is perfusion of nonventilated areas.

DIFFUSION ABNORMALITY

In practice, a diffusion defect is rarely responsible for hypoxemia. The single-breath diffusing capacity of carbon monoxide ($D_L CO$) is often used to assess the status of the alveolocapillary membrane, but a low $D_L CO$ is usually the result of a mismatching of ventilation and perfusion. Nevertheless, a diffusion defect is theoretically possible during heavy exercise if there is a marked reduction in the alveolar surface available for diffusion. In this situation the $P_{(A-a)}O_2$ will be elevated and $P_a O_2$ and $P_a CO_2$ low (Table 9,*d*).

ALVEOLAR HYPOVENTILATION

When the alveolar ventilation is inadequate relative to the CO_2 production (i.e., alveolar hypoventilation), the $P_a CO_2$ is elevated (hypercapnia) and the $P_a O_2$ low (unless oxygen is being inhaled). As is seen in Table 9,*e* and *f*, when the alveolar hypoventilation is uncomplicated, the $P_{(A-a)}O_2$ remains within normal limits, because the gases in the alveoli equilibrate with those in the pulmonary capillary blood. Clearly, the finding of a low $P_a O_2$ and a high $P_a CO_2$, which is associated with an elevated $P_{(A-a)}O_2$, indicates that the hypoxemia is not solely due to alveolar hypoventilation and that one or more of the other physiologic disturbances must also be present.

Alveolar hypoventilation develops as a result of a disproportionately high work of breathing or total body metabolism for a given alveolar ventilation, as is encountered in obesity, excessive dead space–like or wasted ventilation (as in emphysema), or when the minute ventilation falls (as in barbiturate poisoning or muscular paralysis).

ACID-BASE BALANCE

Since the respiratory system, through its effect on the $P_a CO_2$ plays an important role in acid-base balance, its determination is an important component of the assessment of pulmonary function. The characteristic findings in the blood in the acid-base disorders that are encountered clinically have been illustrated and the underlying mechanisms and clinical examples described in Chapter 3.

In patients with a restrictive disorder, and in the earlier stages of chronic airflow limitation, an alkalemia (pH > 7.45) may be present, because the hyperventilation induced by hypoxemia has induced hypocapnia. If the hyperventilation has been present for some time, then compensatory elimination of bicarbonate by the kidneys in response to the low P_aCO_2 will raise the hydrogen ion concentration toward or into the upper range of normality.

When the work of breathing becomes excessive, particularly in patients suffering from airflow limitation, so that the alveolar ventilation is insufficient to cope with the CO_2 production, the P_aCO_2 rises and the P_aO_2 falls. An acutely elevated P_aCO_2 results in an acidemia, i.e., a pH < 7.35. If alveolar hypoventilation persists for some time, then compensatory retention of bicarbonate by the kidneys lowers the H^+ concentration toward or into the lower range of normality.

ASSESSMENT OF ACID-BASE STATUS

Analysis of the acid-base status from an arterial blood sample can be approached in many ways. Whichever approach is adopted, it should proceed in an orderly fashion. A relatively simple approach is to start with the pH.

If an acidemia is present (pH < 7.35), one must then determine whether the primary disturbance is respiratory or metabolic. If the P_aCO_2 is greater than 45 mm Hg, then a ***respiratory acidosis*** is present; otherwise, a ***metabolic acidosis*** is present.

If an alkalemia is present (pH > 7.45) one must again determine whether the primary disturbance is respiratory or metabolic. If the P_aCO_2 is less than 35, then a ***respiratory alkalosis*** is present; otherwise, a ***metabolic alkalosis*** is present.

In some patients, especially if the disturbances are chronic and varied medications have been administered, interpretation of the acid-base status may be difficult. If the pH is normal (between 7.35 and 7.45) but the P_aCO_2 and HCO_3^- are abnormal, then the acid-base disturbance is chronic and probably due to several disturbances. In such cases, proper clinical evaluation and elucidation of the duration of the problem, as well as the patient's therapy, may be the only guide to the major defect present. However, the level of the pH once again provides a valuable clue; if the pH is below 7.40, the major disturbance present is probably an ***acidosis***; if the pH is above 7.40, it is probably an ***alkalosis***.

Calculation of the unmeasured anions (the ***anion gap***) in the case of a metabolic acidosis may be helpful in establishing the cause. This is determined by subtracting the sum of the plasma bicarbonate and cloride levels from the plasma sodium concentration. If the anion gap is less than 12 mM./l. then a hyperchloremic acidosis is present, likely as a result of intestinal loss of bicarbonate or the administration of ammonium chloride, arginine chloride lysine or acetazolamide. An anion gap greater than 12 mM./l. is typical of an increased production of nonvolatile acids, as in renal failure and poisoning by salicylates, ethylene glycol and methyl alcohol.

EXERCISE TESTING

Since most patients develop symptoms during or after exercise, determination of the cardiorespiratory response to exercise is essential. Exercise testing provides an insight into the extent of exercise tolerance and the factors that may limit it and is also a useful method of determining whether hyperreactive airways are present.

ASSESSMENT OF EXERCISE TOLERANCE

Many cardiopulmonary parameters are altered during exercise, even in healthy individuals. As we have seen in Chapter 5, there is an increase in oxygen consumption ($\dot{V}O_2$), carbon dioxide production ($\dot{V}CO_2$), respiratory quotient (R), ventilation ($\dot{V}_E$), tidal volume (V_T), respiratory frequency (f), physiologic dead space (V_D), cardiac output and arteriovenous O_2 content difference during heavy exercise in healthy individuals. Conversely, the V_D/V_T ratio (i.e., dead space–like ventilation) and the amount of venous admixture–like perfusion decrease, whereas the $P_{(A-a)}O_2$ and arterial blood gas tensions are little altered in moderately heavy exercise. When the exercise load is so great that there is an increased oxygen debt and production of lactic acid, a metabolic acidosis develops.

MECHANISM OF EXERCISE LIMITATION

A variety of mechanisms, both respiratory and nonrespiratory, may limit exercise performance in patients. Table 10 indicates that the alterations that develop during exercise when there is cardiovascular impairment are different from those present when there is respiratory impairment.

A greater-than-expected heart rate and ventilation at a particular exercise load, as well as a rise in respiratory quotient above 1.0 or a fall in pH (without a proportionate rise in P_aCO_2), suggest that the oxygen delivery to the exercising muscles is unable to cope with their energy demands during the exercise. This will occur if the cardiovascular system is unable to cope

TABLE 10. Gas Exchange Abnormalities During Exercise

Parameter	Cardiovascular Impairment or Physical Unfitness (a)	Pulmonary Vascular Disorder (b)	Ventilatory Impairment (c)	$\dot{V}/\dot{Q}$ Mismatch (d)
$\dot{V}_E$	↑	↑	↑	↑
R	↑	↔	↔	↔
V_D/V_T (%)	↔ ↓	↑	↓ ↔	↑ ↔
$P_{(A-a)}O_2$	↑ ↔	↑	↔	↑
P_aO_2	↓ ↔	↓ ↔	↓	↓
P_aCO_2	↓ ↔	↓ ↔	↑	↓ ↔ ↑
pH	↓	↑ ↔	↓	↑ ↔ ↓

with the increased demands of the tissues during the exercise or if the individual is not physically fit (Table 10,*a*).

A marked increase in ventilation and a rise in physiologic dead space or V_D/V_T ratio with little if any other alteration (Table 10,*b*) suggests that there is a disorder of lung perfusion, i.e., pulmonary vascular disease.

A rise in P_aCO_2 accompanying a fall in P_aO_2 during the exercise indicates that the patient is unable to increase alveolar ventilation sufficiently during the exercise load to cope with the increased metabolic production of carbon dioxide (Table 10,*c*). Thus, these findings suggest that exercise performance is limited by ventilatory impairment.

A fall in P_aO_2 and rise in $P_{(A-a)}O_2$ during the exercise (Table 10,*d*) indicates a deterioration in gas exchange caused by increased mismatching of the blood and gas distribution in the lungs (predominantly perfusion of poorly ventilated alveoli) or, in rare cases, a diffusion defect. Conversely, a rise in P_aO_2 and fall in $P_{(A-a)}O_2$ during exercise indicates that the matching of ventilation and perfusion throughout the lungs has improved during exercise.

ASSESSMENT OF AIRWAY REACTIVITY

Exercise testing is also an important bronchial "challenge," and it is frequently used to assess the state of bronchial reactivity. Assessment of latent airway hyperreactivity may be particularly important in patients suffering from allergic rhinitis, frequent bronchitis or unexplained chronic cough.

Bronchoconstriction following short-term exercise (exercise-induced bronchoconstriction, or EIB) is characteristic of hyperreactive airways. Although the range of response to exercise is wide, the maximum broncho-constrictive response is typically characterized by the onset of cough, shortness of breath, chest tightness and wheezing about 7 to 15 minutes after the exercise. The degree of EIB is generally proportional to the severity and type of exercise as well as its duration. In addition, the response is affected by the temperature and humidity of the inspired air during the physical activity. In the majority of individuals, spontaneous recovery occurs in 30 to 35 minutes.

In general, a 20 per cent decrease in FEV_1 or FEF_{25-75} or a decrease in specific airway conductance of 35 per cent or more is indicative of exercise-induced bronchoconstriction. Since a forced expiration, of itself, may induce bronchoconstriction, measurements of airway resistance and thoracic gas volume should always precede spirometry. However, it is important to recognize that failure to determine whether lung volume has increased in association with the development of exercise-induced bronchospasm (the opposite of what is shown in Fig. 61) may not allow recognition of this disturbance. If the bronchi are found to be hyperreactive, one should assess the effectiveness of acute or chronic medications in preventing the development of symptoms.

SUMMARY

It is important to assess the functional disturbances present in any patient who has respiratory symptoms, and assessment of the forced vital capacity is an integral component of the clinical evaluation. The extent of further testing necessary to elucidate the disturbances present depends on the problem being evaluated. Repeated assessments allow one to determine the progress of the condition and to evaluate the effect of various therapeutic interventions.

DEFENSES OF THE RESPIRATORY SYSTEM

The respiratory apparatus, which is perfectly designed for gas exchange, is also a major source of contact between man and the environment. The inhaled air is contaminated by inert dust particles; particulate matter emanating from animals and plants; gases liberated by combustion of fossil fuels; infectious agents, such as viruses and bacteria; and droplets expelled from the respiratory tract by sneezing, coughing, talking and even laughing. Since the average adult inhales approximately seven liters of air in a minute and about 10,000 liters in a day, a section devoted to the basic mechanisms of respiratory disease would be incomplete without considering the very active and effective defense mechanisms that normally protect the tracheobronchial tree and alveoli from injury by foreign substances, that prevent the accumulation of secretions, and that bring about repair, all of which are extremely important in the pathogenesis of disease.

Pulmonary disorders often develop when these extensive defenses of the respiratory system break down. Indeed some disorders may even be the result of the activity of the defense mechanisms. In addition, the pulmonary defenses can be depressed by certain agents, and this may predispose an individual to the development of pulmonary disease. For instance, chronic alcohol intoxication predisposes one to frequent episodes of acute bacterial infections, cigarette smoke and air pollutants to chronic bronchitis and emphysema, and occupational irritants to hyperreactive airways or interstitial pulmonary fibrosis.

THE UPPER RESPIRATORY TRACT

The nasal passages are designed to protect the airways and the delicate alveolar structures from inhaled foreign materials. The external openings of the nasal passages, **the nares**, constitute the first line of defense against inhaled particles. The long hairs at the nasal openings filter out the larger particles in the air; those greater than 10 μ in diameter that pass the external nares are largely trapped in the mucus coating the nasal mucous membrane and are propelled mouthward by ciliary movement so that they can be swallowed or expectorated.

The upper respiratory tract plays another important role in the defense of the respiratory system because it warms, humidifies and filters the air as it is inspired through the nasal passages. The **nasal turbinates**, highly vascular structures, act as radiators of heat and warm the inspired air as it flows past them, and the mucous glands of the nasal mucosa supply about 650 ml. of water per day to moisten the inspired air. No matter how cold or dry the inspired air may be, under normal conditions it is almost at body temperature and practically saturated by the time it reaches the carina of the trachea. If the air entering the trachea is not properly humidified and warmed by the upper respiratory tract, as may occur in patients who are intubated or have a tracheostomy, airway secretions may become dry and crusted.

THE SNEEZE REFLEX

Irritant materials are also cleared from the upper respiratory tract by means of a sneeze. Stimulation of the sensory receptors of the trigeminal nerves in the nasal mucosa as a result of irritation results in a deep inspiration, which is then followed by a violent expiratory blast that, as long as the mouth is closed, is discharged through the nose.

THE LARYNX

The larynx acts like a vigilant watchdog, in that it usually prevents the aspiration of foreign material into the tracheobronchial tree. This is best exemplified during the act of eating, food being prevented from entering the trachea when we swallow. There are times, however, when the larynx lets us down. For instance, it has been shown that during sleep nonirritating radiopaque material is readily aspirated into the depths of the lungs, even in healthy individuals. Secretions draining from the upper respiratory tract likely follow the same course, and since the upper repiratory tract is not sterile, the lung may be continually contaminated by organisms. When one cosiders the complexity and tortuosity of the respiratory tract, which invites trapping and pocketing, it is a marvel that the lung is not a cesspool of suppuration.

THE LOWER RESPIRATORY TRACT

The filtering system of the upper respiratory tract and the larynx is not perfect, and some potentially harmful agents bypass these protectors of the lower respiratory tract. The foreign material that does manage to evade the barriers of the upper respiratory tract and larynx meets up with other defense mechanisms. Most of it is trapped in a layer of sticky mucus that lines the entire respiratory tract, propelled mouthward in the respiratory tract by mucociliary clearance, and then eliminated by the cough mechanism.

The damage that occurs following the inhalation or aspiration of foreign material depends on whether the agent is gaseous material or particulate matter and on the site of deposition. In the case of gases, this depends on the extent of absorption in the tracheobronchial tree, which, in turn, is related to the chemical composition and solubility of the gas in question. The lungs are protected from soluble gases, such as sulfur dioxide, by the extensive absorptive capacity of the mucous blanket of the upper airways and the tracheobronchial tree. However, insoluble gases, such as nitrogen dioxide and ozone, or oxygen in high concentrations are not absorbed by the mucous blanket and can penetrate to the alveoli, where they may produce an inflammatory response. The response is not as great as it could be, however, because there is a concomitant outpouring of plasma from the alveolar capillaries into the alveolar spaces and this tends to dilute the gas and neutralize its acidity.

The site of deposition of particulate matter that has penetrated into the tracheobronchial tree depends on the matter's size, shape and concentration. The size is particularly important, as about 90 per cent of the particles between 2 and 10 μ in diameter settle out on the mucociliary blanket of the tracheobronchial epithelium. The majority of the particles that are less than 2 μ in diameter penetrate to the alveolar ducts and alveoli, where they are deposited by gravitational forces and, to a lesser extent, by Brownian movement. The effectiveness of the respiratory tract as a whole in defending against injury from foreign material is related to the uniqueness of its epithelium and its mucociliary activity, as well as the cough reflex.

MUCOCILIARY CLEARANCE

Foreign agents are eliminated from both the upper and lower respiratory tract by a thin film of mucus with elastic and adhesive properties, which is normally propelled mouthward by ciliary action. In the upper respiratory tract, mucus is propelled from the nose and sinuses to the pharynx; in the tracheobronchial tree, mucus is propelled upward toward the glottis.

Respiratory Epithelium

The nonrigid areas of the upper and lower respiratory tracts, such as the oropharynx and the terminal and respiratory bronchioles, are lined by *cuboidal epithelium*. The rigid, noncollapsible areas of the respiratory tract, such as the nose, the paranasal sinuses, the trachea and the larger bronchi are lined by *ciliated columnar epithelium*. Plump elongated cells, the *goblet cells*, are situated either singly or in groups between the ciliated epithelial cells. The goblet cells are abundant in the proximal part of the tracheobronchial tree, particularly at the bifurcations of the larger bronchi, and are more sparse peripherally. They are innervated by the autonomic nervous system, and acetylcholine serves as the chemical mediator in their control. In addition, there are *mucous glands* in the submucosa just below the epithelial layer in the nasal passages, paranasal sinuses and the large airways that contain cartilage. The mucous glands, which are innervated by the cholinergic nervous system, are approximately 40 times as numerous as goblet cells.

Respiratory Mucus

The epithelial lining of the upper and lower respiratory tract is covered by a thin, transparent film of mucus. It has been estimated that 100 ml. of mucus is produced in the tracheobronchial tree of a healthy person every day. The mucus contains about 95 per cent water, the remainder being a mixture of mucoproteins, mucopolysaccharides and some lipid. It is derived partly from the capillaries, seeping out between the epithelial cells in the bronchi; the remainder is secreted by the mucous glands and the goblet cells. The mucus layer is made up of an internal and an external component. The internal thin water layer is approximately 3 to 4 μ thick and completely covers the surface of the ciliated columnar epithelium. Since the cilia beat in this internal layer, its high aqueous content helps to conserve energy. The external layer is approximately 1 to 2 μ thick and lies on top of the internal layer. It is very viscous, elastic and sticky, so it serves as a trap for foreign matter, and it probably also protects the respiratory epithelial cells against loss or gain of water.

The rate of movement of mucus in the tracheobronchial tree is affected by its viscosity: if this is reduced, it will move faster; if it is increased, it will move slower. In addition, the movement of mucus is slowed if the mucus layer becomes greater than 5 μ thick, and it may stop moving entirely if it becomes 25 μ thick.

Cilia

The movement of the respiratory mucus blanket in the respiratory tract is carried out by the whiplike action of the cilia on the surface of the epithelial cells. The cilia in the large airways beat in a constant, rhythmic manner at approximately 1000 times a minute, but the ciliary beat becomes slower the further one goes down in the tracheobronchial tree.

Normally, the ciliary beat resembles that of the oars of a boat: there is a rapid forward motion, the cilium becoming almost upright, and a slow return to a curved and backward leaning position. The rapid forward motion is about three times as fast as the backward recoil, so that the mucus flows toward the glottis, at a rate of approximately 20 mm./min., or approximately a mile per week. However, clearance is slower in the peripheral portions of the tracheobronchial tree. Ciliary activity is influenced by numerous agents. It is stimulated by acetylcholine, inorganic ions, weak acids, beta agonists, and low concentrations of local anesthetics. It is inhibited by low humidity, alcohol, cigarette smoke or other noxious gases.

Examination of the ultrastructure of a cilium indicates that it consists of an outer fibrous sheath, which surrounds dynein arms of nine outer microtubular doublets, and radial spokes, which join the microtubules. Recently a syndrome has been described in which there are variable defects of the axonemal components (i.e., the dynein arms, the microtubular structure or the radial spokes) that are associated with an altered function of the cilia. In this condition, the cilia may be totally immotile for periods of time; they may only beat about 200 times a minute; the pattern of the beat may be abnormal; and they may vibrate or rotate in a circular fashion, bend at or near their base or move like a windshield wiper. The altered ciliary function markedly impedes the movement of mucus, and this may be associated with a variety of respiratory tract infections and bronchiectasis (Kartegener's syndrome). In addition, infertility is commonly associated in the male; this is apparently because of immotile sperm that have the same structural defects.

THE COUGH REFLEX

A cough helps to protect the tracheobronchial tree from the entry of foreign substances or the accumulation of bronchopulmonary secretions. It can be induced by irritation of either the sensory endings of the vagus nerve in the larynx, trachea and larger bronchi or the afferent fibers of the pharyngeal distribution of the glossopharyngeal nerve. Cough may also be stimulated by impulses arising from nerve endings in the mucous membrane of the pharynx and esophagus, the pleural surfaces and the external auditory canal. The impulses are transmitted to the "cough center" in the medulla, which in turn sends impulses to the muscles of the chest and the larynx, and a cough results. The stimuli may be inflammatory, such as an infection; mechanical, such as smoke, dust or foreign bodies; chemical, such as irritating gases; or thermal, such as cold air. Thermal stimulation, however, probably occurs only if the tracheobronchial tree has already been irritated by other agents.

The act of coughing differs from a sneeze, in that it is less explosive and easier to control voluntarily. As is illustrated in Figure 63, it is comprised

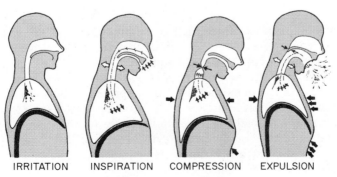

IRRITATION   INSPIRATION   COMPRESSION   EXPULSION

Figure 63. The cough reflex.

of four separate and distinct phases. Irritation (the first phase) induces a deep inspiration (the second phase). During the short third phase, the glottis closes and the intercostal and abdominal muscles contact forcibly, so that the intrathoracic and intra-abdominal pressure rise (the "compressive phase"). When the intrathoracic pressure reaches a very high level, the glottis suddenly opens slightly, so that the intrapulmonary pressure falls. Because of the very high intra-abdominal pressure that is produced by the contraction of abdominal muslces, the diaphragm then ascends sharply, likely in a passive fashion, although it may actively help to regulate the expulsive force of the cough by controlling the upward push of the abdominal viscera. The forceful ascent of the diaphragm results in a violent, explosive movement of air from the lungs (the "expulsive phase"). Because the nasopharynx is closed off by the soft palate when the glottis opens, the foreign material that is expelled from the respiratory tract enters the mouth and can be expectorated.

Using radiopaque materials, it has been demonstrated that the intrathoracic airways are compressed concurrently with the onset of the expiratory blast of air, so that the airflow velocity becomes jetlike, and any foreign material is expelled much like a bullet from the barrel of a pistol. The cough has little effect on foreign material that is in the smaller bronchioles, because the air blast of the expulsive phase is very feeble at this level. Particles deposited distal to the ciliated columnar epithelium (i.e., in the terminal and respiratory bronchioles) are phagocytosed by alveolar or interstitial macrophages and then are transported to the mucociliary blanket in the airways, though some may be cleared from the alveoli by the lymphatics.

THE ALVEOLAR SURFACE

Those particles that succeed in penetrating as far as the alveolar level are subject to the phagocytic activity of alveolar macrophages and other cells. In addition, the immune system plays a major role by recognizing foreign material and then neutralizing or destroying it.

THE ALVEOLAR EPITHELIUM

The alveolar surface is designed along the same lines as other exposed surfaces: its connective tissue resembles that of other surfaces, its blood supply is rich and its epithelium is unique.

The surface epithelial cells (*type I pneumonocytes*) form the major portion of the alveolar membrane, but they appear to play only a minor role in the defense of the alveolus. Granular alveolar cells (*type II pneumonocytes*), which are characterized morphologically by the presence of membrane-bound lamellar bodies in the cytoplasm, are distributed fairly uniformly over the alveolar surface and play an important role in several aspects of lung function. The lamellar bodies are believed to be the intracellular site of storage of *pulmonary surfactant*, which is rich in phospholipid and contains some protein as well. Surfactant is crucial to the function of the lungs, because it stabilizes the alveolar surface against collapse (see Chapter 1). Derangements in its production or degradation play a role in such pulmonary conditions as the *newborn respiratory distress syndrome*, the *adult respiratory distress syndrome, oxygen toxicity* and *radiation pneumonitis*. In addition, the type II cell appears to be the progenitor of the type I cell, so that it appears to play a major role in the repair of alveolar injury.

Alveolar Macrophage

The alveolar macrophages are large mononuclear ameboid phagocytes that rest on the alveolar lining and regularly scavenge the surface of the epithelium. The role of the alveolar macrophages, like that of other phagocytes, is principally to digest any harmful foreign agents. Like the other phagocytes, the alveolar macrophages are rich in lyososmes, which attach to the phagocyte membrane surrounding ingested material and kill and digest bacteria, certain virus-infected cells, or other agents. In the case of bacteria, the net rate of clearance from the lung depends on their rate of multiplication as well as the rate of phagocytosis, bacterial killing, and physical removal by mucociliary clearance. The alveolar macrophages also participate in clearing insoluble dust and debris from the nonciliated portions of the lung, and they play an important role in inflammatory and immunologic reactions.

Clearance of Alveolar Particles

Particles that settle on the alveolar surface are handled differently from those that deposit on the airway mucosa. Most of the particles are phagocytosed by alveolar macrophages. Particles on the alveolar surface, either within alveolar macrophages or lying free on the surface, are transported to the ciliated part of the lung. The rate of removal is determined by macrophage migration and the mouthward flow of alveolar capillary transudate mixed with alveolar cell secretions. The biologic half-time for removal of insoluble particles from the alveolar surface to the ciliated surface is thought to be about 24 hours.

Some foreign particles may not be phagocytosed, and these may become sequestered in the interstitial tissue or be removed via the lymphatics. Removal of these agents is less predictable, and the biologic half-life of these particles can be weeks to years. The release into the alveolar space of particles that are within cells in the alveolar wall depends on the turnover time of the cells and their rate of desquamation into the alveolar spaces.

THE INFLAMMATORY RESPONSE

The vast majority of respiratory disorders develop as a result of an uncontrolled inflammatory response, which may be acute, subacute or chronic. The neutrophil is a major contributor to the inflammatory response in both the airways and in the alveoli, whereas the alveolar macrophage is important in an alveolar inflammatory process, particularly as it either resolves or becomes chronic.

Initially in the inflammatory response, the capillaries dilate at the site of the injury, and there is an outpouring of fluid. Shortly thereafter, neutrophils begin to cluster along the capillary endothelial cells at the site of injury, a process referred to as *margination*. It appears that cleavage of *C5* to form *C5a* and ultimately *C5a des arg* plays a role in bringing about neutrophil migration. As a result of the chemotactic effect of factors derived from these complement fragments and perhaps others released by lymphocytes and macrophages, the polymorphonuclear leukocytes migrate from the blood stream through the tight junctions of the endothelial cells. Their function is to ingest (phagocytose) and destroy any potentially injurious agents, and they are more effective at killing than are the resident macrophages.

The resident alveolar macrophages act as a surveillance system, and they can presumably discriminate between foreign agents they can ingest and those they cannot. In addition, as indicated, they secrete chemotactic factors that attract more neutrophils to the scene. Several hours later, increasing numbers of lymphocytes, along with monocytes that have been transformed into macrophages, begin to migrate. The lymphocytes also respond with specific humoral and cell-mediated reactions. Subsequently, more and more phagocytes appear on the scene, and any bacteria or other unwanted digestible material are removed. The activated (i.e., inflammatory) macrophages ingest dead neutrophils and debris along with enzymes released by the neutrophils.

The inflammatory process is perpetuated until the responsible agent has been eliminated; the phagocytic cells are continually replaced and, after accomplishing their task, either die or leave by means of the draining lymphatics. The neutrophils release proteases and oxygen radicals that in themselves may cause injury, and granulation tissue is formed. The inflammatory macrophages readily ingest neutrophils that are old and release a molecule that stimulates fibroblasts to proliferate and deposit collagen and connective tissue. In addition, when there is alveolar injury, the type II alveolar epithelial cells proliferate and then replace the injured type I cells. It has been suggested that the inhibition of type II cells or their failure to proliferate will further the development of fibrosis.

In chronic inflammation, lymphocytes, monocytes and plasma cells are present, and there is very slow turnover of phagocytes. A lesion develops in which few cells enter, few divide and few die; the process is associated with the unremitting deposition of collagen by the fibroblasts, and as a result a fibrous scar develops.

GRANULOMATOUS INFLAMMATORY REACTION

This type of reaction develops when a foreign agent is not eradicated and is retained at the site of injury; i.e., it is a chronic inflammation. The foreign material is kept more or less isolated and sequestered from the neighboring nonaffected tissues, through a process that is related to cell-mediated immunity. Classically, this type of reaction occurs with infection by the tubercle bacillus, certain bacteria, fungi and parasites or after the inhalation of certain inorganic metallic dusts, such as beryllium.

The basic granulomatous lesion consists of large epithelioid or histiocytic cells that have very poor phagocytic abilities but can secrete high concentrations of enzymes. Giant cells are prominent and are surrounded by a peripheral zone of lymphocytes, sometimes with plasma cells, and fibrous tissue. Although proliferation of fibroblasts and secretion of collagen take place early in granuloma formation, these elements are continually hydrolyzed by collagenase and lysosomal proteases that are derived from dead macrophages, so that formation of fibrous tissue is prevented. If the cause of the granuloma formation is eradicated, such as when the tubercle bacilli are destroyed, the epithelioid cells leave, and because the proteases and collagenase are absent, fibrous tissue may develop unhindered.

FIBROSIS

Fibroblastic activity, which is brought about by damage and death of macrophages, results in the deposition of fibrous tissue in the lung. The repair of the mesenchyme is directed by the alveolar macrophages, which release fibronectin, a substance that is chemotactic for fibroblasts, as well as a growth factor for fibroblasts that causes them to proliferate and increase the production and deposition of collagen. It appears that the collagen matrix that replaces the parenchyma of the lung during the repair process is markedly disordered. This may be part of a persistent inflammatory exudate, a chronic granulomatous process, as in tuberculosis, or a reaction to fibrogenic inorganic dusts such as silica and asbestos. In the latter situation, the irritant particles, after being taken up by the macrophages, destroy the membranes of the vacuoles enclosing them and are then released into the cytoplasm. This results in death of the cell, and the release of the offending crystals into the extracellular environment, where they induce increased synthesis of collagen by the fibroblasts.

PROTEASES AND ANTIPROTEASES

As indicated, polymorphonuclear leukocytes and alveolar macrophages release proteolytic enzymes (proteases) during the phagocytic process, and these have the ability to digest protein material. Many proteases, such as collagenase and elastase, are potentially harmful, because they attack elastin and all other macromolecular constituents of lung tissue and can damage basement membranes, fibronectin, collagen and proteoglycans in connective tissue.

In a healthy individual, lung tissue damage by the elastic proteases is prevented by the action of antiproteases, which inhibit protease activity. These antiproteases are formed by approximately 90 per cent of the alpha fraction of the serum proteins, the principal one known currently being alpha-1-antitrypsin, as well as bronchial mucus inhibitor, which is apparently secreted locally by the respiratory epithelium in the central airways.

Certain individuals have an inherited deficiency of alpha-1-antitrypsin in the serum. Those with a severe deficiency (homozygotes) inherit an abnormal gene from both the father and mother, and may develop a very severe and characteristic form of emphysema that is associated with an extensive destruction of the alveolar walls. The parents themselves may be "heterozygotes," each carrying an abnormal and normal gene. They and other offspring, who have inherited one abnormal gene, have intermediate levels of antitrypsin deficiency and are generally well, although a certain number develop early evidence of chronic obstructive airway disease, particularly if they are smokers and have had recurrent pulmonary infections.

It is currently considered that chronic pulmonary diseases such as emphysema, on the one hand, and interstitial lung disease, on the other, may be the consequence of an inbalance between proteases and antiproteases in the lung. The high prevalence of emphysema in cigarette smokers is related to the fact that oxidants generated from phagocytes can inactivate alpha-1-antiprotease *in vitro*. Indeed, it has been suggested that cigarette smoke contains free oxygen radicals, about one-half in the gas phase and the other half in the particulate phase, with unusually long half-lives and potentially very injurious to the lung tissue. These oxidants may inactivate alpha-1-antiproteases so that smokers may acquire a deficiency of functional alpha-1-antiproteases in the lungs, thus allowing the proteases to act uninhibited. When elastin tissue is broken down, it is excreted in the urine as desmosine, and although not yet confirmed, it is possible that lung elastic tissue breakdown may be recognized at an early stage by analysis of the desmosine levels in the urine.

THE IMMUNE RESPONSE

The skin and mucous membranes of the body generally provide an effective barrier against potentially injurious agents or infections in the environment. The immune system, which entails the action of a wide variety of cells and cell products interacting with one another, also helps to protect from the harmful effects of foreign pathogens.

Inhaled foreign agents may or may not induce an immune response. A foreign substance that is capable of provoking a specific immune response is known as an *antigen*. When a foreign substance induces an immune response, it may lead to elaboration of antibody *(humoral immune response)*, the development of *cell-mediated immunity*, or both. Both of these processes are generated by lymphocytes, which are the cornerstones of the immune process.

LYMPHOCYTES

There are two broad categories of lymphocytes, each with a distinctly different function.

The *B-lymphocytes*, so named because they differentiate in the bursa of Fabricius in birds and in bursal equivalent tissue in mammals, require a stimulus in order to replicate. Under an appropriate stimulus, such as a specific *antigen*, B-cells can differentiate into plasma cells and elaborate a specific *antibody*, which is capable of neutralizing the antigen.

The *T-lymphocytes*, so named because they are derived from the thymus gland, can interact directly with the antigen and also have the capacity of helping or suppressing the production of antibody by B-lymphocytes. In addition, by secreting a variety of biologic substances, they can recruit other T-lymphocytes, act as effector agents in such cell-mediated immune responses as graft versus host, delayed hypersensitivity, or tumor rejection, and transform resting macrophages into highly active cells.

IMMUNOGLOBULINS

Immunoglobulins, or *antibodies*, are a series of serum proteins that are produced by B-lymphocytes and plasma cells in response to a material that the body recognizes as foreign, i.e., an *antigen*. The various immunoglobulins are classified according to their specific antigenic properties. There are five major classes of immunoglobulin (IgA, IgD, IgE, IgG and IgM) and respiratory secretions contain four of them (IgA, IgG, IgM and IgE). The first three classes are involved in the first line of defense against invading microorganisms in the lungs, and they may also help regulate the microorganisms that normally reside on the mucous membranes.

Most of the immunoglobulins in the lung are synthesized locally by the plasma cells in the submucosa of the respiratory tract; only a small portion is normally derived from serum by transudation. Protection of the host against reinfection and mucosal colonization of noninvasive viruses appears to be better correlated with the level of secretory immunoglobulins than with serum antibodies. On the other hand, the contribution from serum immunoglobulins increases markedly during an inflammatory process, when there is a profuse outpouring of vascular fluid. Conversely, as might be expected, the secretory antibody response to the application of a viral vaccine such as influenza vaccine to the respiratory mucosa is considerably greater than if it were administered parenterally.

Secretory IgA is the predominant immunoglobulin in respiratory secretions. It has been shown to possess virus-neutralizing activity, but, because it is unable to fix complement, its role in protecting against bacterial infections is unclear at present. It is made up of two molecules of serum IgA and a small glycoprotein component, the *secretory piece*, which is linked to the serum IgA molecules by covalent disulfide bonds. There is some evidence to suggest that the secretory piece facilitates the capability of the secretory IgA molecule to function as an antibody in secretions because its resistance to degradation by proteolytic enzymes is high. When individuals suffer from a deficiency of secretory IgA, such as occurs in ataxia telangiectasia, they are prone to develop recurrent sinopulmonary infections.

IgG is the most abundant of the immunoglobulins in the blood and is thought to contribute to immunity against many infectious agents. *IgM* is the largest of the immunoglobulin molecules and is capable of agglutinating particulate antigens such as red cells and bacteria. It appears to be of greatest importance in the first few days of the primary immune response. This immunoglobulin is present only in trace amounts in the respiratory mucus of the healthy lung, but it increases substantially when inflammation occurs. Both possess antiviral and antibacterial properties, and because they can fix complement, they facilitate the opsonization and phagocytosis of particles by macrophages.

IgE, which is present in only trace amounts in both the serum and the respiratory mucus in healthy individuals, has a characteristic property of binding to mediator cells such as mast cells or basophils. The IgE level is considerably increased in the allergic individual, where it plays a most important role in the development of immediate hypersensitivity reactions.

IMMUNE REACTIONS

Although generally protective, the immune response may overreact, particularly when re-exposure to a foreign substance occurs. This sensitized reaction, which may have a genetic basis, is termed "atopy," which actually means a strange disease but is frequently used synonomously with the terms "allergy" and "hypersensitivity." Atopic individuals may be particularly sensitive to a variety of organic and inorganic materials, such as household mites, pollen, molds, and animal danders.

The *humoral,* or *immediate hypersensitivity, reaction* is antibody mediated and depends on the production of pharmacologically active mediators that are released as a result of *antigen-antibody* interaction. The *cell-mediated,* or *delayed, reaction* depends on immunologically activated lymphoid cells that release substances known as *lymphokines.*

The immune response has been further classified by Coombs and Gell into four broad groups: an immediate or anaphylactic type of hypersensitivity, which is dependent on IgE (*Type I*); a type related to the tissue-damaging effects resulting from the reaction between specific tissue cytotoxic antibodies and cells, which is dependent on IgG and IgM *(Type II)*; a hypersensitivity resulting from the toxic effects of antigen-antibody immune complexes, which is dependent on IgG *(Type III)*; and one that is a cellular response to specific antigens and is mediated by cells *(Type IV)*. However, most pathologic processes are not that simple and clear-cut and are a response to mechanisms belonging to several or all of these categories.

Immediate (Type I) Hypersensitivity

The *immediate hypersensitivity* reaction is characterized by a rapid onset (a few minutes or even seconds) after exposure to an antigen. The development of asthma and hay fever in atopic individuals are classic examples of immediate hypersensitivity, and the most rapid reaction is known as *anaphylaxis*. The mast cells, which are chiefly concentrated in the connective tissue surrounding the bronchi and bronchioles and the pulmonary capillaries, are the cornerstone of the immediate hypersensitivity reaction. It involves a reaction between allergens and specific *immunoglobulin E (IgE) antibodies* on the surface of the tissue *mast cells* or circulating *basophils* and the subsequent release of chemical mediators.

Since contact between allergens and the respiratory system must occur by inhalation, allergens are thought to come in contact with the *IgE antibodies* on the surface of *mast cells* on the very superficial layers of the respiratory mucosa. Indeed, cells containing basophilic granules with ultra-structural characteristics identical to mast cells have been described on the surface of the bronchial mucosa. It is thought that release of chemical mediators from the superficial mast cells alters tissue permeability, thereby allowing the inhaled allergens to diffuse into the deeper layers of the respiratory mucosa and react with more mast cells there.

The chemical mediators that are released as a direct result of the IgE-mediated immunologic reaction are called *primary mediators*; these include *histamine, slow-reacting substance of anaphylaxis* (SRS-A), *platelet activating factor* (PAF) and the *eosinophil* and *neutrophil chemotactic factors of anaphylaxis* (ECF-A and NCF-A). *Secondary mediators*, such as *kinins* and *prostaglandins*, are also generated as a result of tissue inflammation induced by the primary mediators.

The morphologic changes in the airways in *asthma*, which include mucosal edema, accumulation of inflammatory cells (with a predominance of eosinophils), smooth muscle contraction and hypersecretion of mucous glands are thought to be due to the action of the mediators that are released. Histamine is known to induce vasodilation, increase vascular permeability, contract smooth muscles and increase the amount of secretion of the mucous glands. Both histamine and prostaglandin $F_{2\alpha}$ ($PGF_{2\alpha}$), whose plasma levels are increased during the acute stages of antigen-induced asthma in both the human and the experimental animal, induce bronchoconstriction when inhaled. SRS-A, which is currently thought to be a *leukotriene*, induces smooth muscle contraction *in vitro* that is slower in onset and longer in duration than that induced by histamine.

Type II Hypersensitivity

This type of immunologic injury develops as a result of antibodies directed at tissue antigens, the so-called *auto-immune diseases*, and is usually mediated through the complement-fixing properties of antibody. The antibody is thought to react with the individual's own tissue and result in tissue damage. This tissue-specific antibody is usually a member of the IgG class, and the antigen may be either a foreign substance that has become attached to the surface of certain tissue cells, or it may be a part of the surface or the basement membrane of these cells. The lung tissue damage may be brought about indirectly by lysosomal enzymes that are released from leukocytes that have been attracted to the site by chemotactic factors derived from activated complement components. The damage may also be the direct effect of the activated terminal components of the complement system, which form complexes capable of causing membrane damage. The prime example of an autoimmune disease that involves the lungs is *"Goodpasture's syndrome."* This condition is characterized by the presence of antibodies that react with glomerular and pulmonary alveolar basement membranes, and is manifested clinically by repeated pulmonary hemorrhages, hemoptysis and progressive glomerulonephritis with hematuria, proteinuria, and renal insufficiency.

Type III Hypersensitivity

In contrast to the immediate, or Type I, reaction, the Type III reaction develops slowly and usually becomes manifest at about 6 to 8 hours, finally subsiding within 24 hours. The tissue injury seen in this form of hypersensitivity is caused by immune complexes, which are large aggregations of molecules formed by the union of antigen and antibody and, at times, complement. As long as the antigen persists in the circulation, these complexes are constantly being formed until certain effector mechanisms, such as phagocytosis, result in their eventual elimination from the body.

Excessively large complexes, such as those formed when there is antibody excess (as may occur in high antibody responders), are rapidly removed from the circulation by the reticuloendothelial system, and these complexes do not appear to be particularly pathogenic. Immune complexes formed when there is slight antigen excess (in modest antibody responders) are most toxic, because they are less efficiently removed from the circulation by the reticuloendothelial system. These complexes activate the complement system, so that polymorphonuclear leukocytes are attracted to the site of the antigen-antibody reaction. This eventually leads to the release of lysosomal enzymes and the development of an acute inflammatory reaction, which is associated with slowing of blood flow in the small vessels, as well as necrosis of the walls of the vessels.

The deposition of *immune complexes* is facilitated by local changes on the vascular endothelium that are induced by mediators released from mast cells (Type I mechanism) or aggregated platelets. The vascular and glomerular basement membranes, as well as serosal and synovial membranes, are the common sites of immune complex deposition, presumably because these tissues normally serve as filtration membranes. *Serum sickness* and the *glomerulonephritis* of *systemic lupus erythematosus* are examples of hypersensitivity diseases mediated by soluble antigen-antibody complexes; in the lungs, *vasculitis* and *serositis (pleuritis)* may develop.

Immune complexes may also be actively formed in the lung parenchyma as a result of the reaction between antigens delivered to the lungs through inhalation and antibodies diffusing out of the pulmonary vasculature. Because of complement activation and the participation of neutrophils in the immune reaction, these complexes may induce an inflammatory reaction in the lung parenchyma and pleura, and thus damage blood vessel walls and lead to altered permeability and hemorrhage. In *extrinsic allergic alveolitis*, inflammation of the alveolar walls follows the inhalation of identifiable specific foreign organic material, such as the *actinomycetes* and *fungal spores* in moldy hay, which are responsible for *"farmer's lung,"* or antigens derived from droppings of parakeets, pigeons and chickens, which are responsible for *"bird-fancier's lung."*

Delayed (Type IV) Hypersensitivity

In *delayed hypersensitivity*, there is an increased reactivity to specific antigens, which is mediated by T-cells. In the skin, delayed hypersensitivity is manifested by the development of a reaction that reaches its maximum intensity 24 hours after the intradermal injection of antigen into a sensitized individual. The typical histologic findings consist of focal chronic inflammatory granulomas containing lymphocytes, monocytes and plasma cells, as well as insoluble material that has been phagocytosed by macrophages or monocytes. This delayed hypersensitivity reaction of the skin to protein antigens of fungi or bacteria, such as tuberculosis, indicates prior exposure to the organisms.

The mechanisms involved in delayed hypersensitivity or cell-mediated immune reactions in the lung have not been clearly delineated. The temporal association of granuloma formation *in vivo* with parameters of cell-mediated immunity *in vitro* suggests an immunologic basis for the granuloma. There is likely an initial interaction between antigen and specifically-sensitized lymphocytes, most likely *T-lymphocytes,* which are activated to release many different soluble factors or mediators *(lymphokines)*. Some, such as *migration inhibition factor* (MIF) and *macrophage activating factor* (MAF), proteins of similar size and physical-chemical characteristics, are capable of activating macrophages. *Leukocyte inhibitory factor* (LIF) inhibits migration of leukocytes; *chemotactic factor* (CHF) attracts mononuclear phagocytes; and *lymphotoxin* (LT) can kill susceptible target cells nonspecifically. Activated lymphocytes can also destroy target cells bearing foreign antigenic determinants, such as viral antigens or tumor-specific antigens, to which they have been specifically sensitized. They can also synthesize and release immune interferon, which makes susceptible cells resistant to penetration by viruses. It is thought that under certain circumstances, normal unsensitized lymphocytes are capable of destroying target cells coated with specific antibody in a process known as *antibody-dependent cell-mediated cytotoxicity*. This is the type of reaction that may be involved in the pathogenesis of *Wegner's granulomatosis*.

METABOLISM OF THE LUNG

In addition to an elaborate defense mechanism, the lung has other non-gas exchange functions. The lung is a site of active metabolism, and it has been estimated that it normally uses as much as 10 per cent of the total oxygen consumed, and even more in some pulmonary disorders such as cancer and tuberculosis. This high level of oxygen consumption is not surprising, because cellular elements, like the type II cell, which are responsible for surfactant biosynthesis, possess high metabolic activity. In addition, alveolar macrophages that have been estimated to number 600 million have an energy requirement that is approximately ten times that of the polymorphonuclear leukocyte and three times that of the monocyte.

Another important function of the lung is its ability to influence the circulating level of certain vasoactive substances. It is capable of inactivating circulating bradykinin, prostaglandins, serotonin and histamine, but has little effect on epinephrine. The lung also contains an enzyme that is responsible for converting the relatively inactive polypeptide angiotensin I to the potent vasoconstrictor angiotensin II. This *angiotensin-converting enzyme* (ACE) is elevated in patients suffering from *sarcoidosis*.

SUMMARY

Most of the important patterns of disease affecting the respiratory system are the result of inhaled biological agents, such as viruses, bacteria, irritants or allergens, that have bypassed the defenses of the respiratory apparatus. On the other hand, the role of the non-gas exchange functions of the lung in combatting disease has only recently been receiving attention; it may be very important in the pathophysiology of pulmonary disease and in the production of signs and symptoms.

MANIFESTATIONS OF RESPIRATORY DISEASE

- PRIMARY MANIFESTATIONS OF PULMONARY DISEASE
- SECONDARY MANIFESTATIONS OF PULMONARY DISEASE

9

PRIMARY MANIFESTATIONS OF PULMONARY DISEASE

When the defenses of the respiratory tract are strained or overcome, or when disturbances in pulmonary function occur, symptoms and signs develop. In general, *"symptoms"* of a disease process are produced by disordered physical or mental function within the body. The *"signs"* are the objective evidence of the pathologic process that are elicited during the course of the physical examination. It is not always possible to make a sharp distinction between symptoms and physical signs, for some manifestations such as dyspnea, cough and cyanosis may be both subjective and objective. In this section we shall discuss the primary manifestations of pulmonary disease, i.e., those produced by the disorder itself, and the secondary manifestations caused by inadequate gas exchange, increased pulmonary vascular resistance and other extrapulmonary manifestations.

SYMPTOMS

The primary, or cardinal, symptoms of respiratory disease are excessive nasal secretions, cough, expectoration of sputum, expectoration of blood, breathlessness, wheezing and chest pain.

EXCESSIVE NASAL SECRETIONS

As we have seen, nasal secretions are normally swept backward to the pharynx by ciliary activity, and one is usually unaware of this. Infection of the upper respiratory tract, irritants or allergens that induce an allergic response characteristically produce congestion of the nasal mucosa, obstruction of the nasal passages, increased production of mucus and frequent sneezing. In allergic states, the mucosa is pale and boggy and the discharge

163

is thin and watery. With infection, the nasal mucosa is hyperemic and the discharge is usually purulent. If the paranasal sinuses are involved, pain may be felt over the corresponding areas of the face and scalp.

Nasal secretions may become excessive premenstrually or during pregnancy and in male patients who are receiving estrogens for the treatment of carcinoma of the prostate gland. In addition, excessive nasal secretions are common in persons who are exposed to very dry air in artificially heated environments or to dusts, smoke or fumes. When there are excessive nasal secretions, they may drain into the back of the throat *(postnasal drip)*, and they may induce coughing and frequent throat clearing, or "hawking." Many patients with chronic cough and sputum have a postnasal drip, and this may aggravate their symptomatology. Excessive upper respiratory tract secretions and a postnasal drip may be responsible for other manifestations of respiratory disease, particularly if the defense mechanisms of the lower respiratory tract are relatively ineffective. Even in otherwise healthy individuals, a postnasal drip per se may induce an irritative cough.

COUGH

No one goes through life without an occasional cough, and almost everyone develops a cough at some time with colds. Many adults cough or "hawk" a few times on first arising in the morning because of the accumulation of secretions in the posterior pharynx and the trachea.

A recurrent cough may simply be habitual, or it may signify the presence of a serious pulmonary disease. It therefore always deserves a thorough investigation. In addition to the recognized association with chronic bronchitis and bronchiectasis, a chronic cough may be the major symptom in patients suffering from hyperreactive airways. It is also important to remember that, although the cough reflex is usually initiated in the tracheobronchial tree, the primary cause of the cough may be nonpulmonary. For example, left ventricular failure, which causes pulmonary congestion, is often associated with a cough.

Although the cough reflex, which has been described in Chapter 8, is a prime defender of the tracheobronchial tree, certain of its inherent features may have detrimental effects. The deep inspiration that precedes the expiratory blast may occasionally drag secretions deeper into the peripheral portions of the lungs, or purulent secretions in one portion of a lung may be splattered throughout the lungs during the expulsive phase and then inhaled into new areas during the next inspiration.

Cough Syncope. Some patients may develop lightheadedness or may even faint during a coughing spell. This is because the prolonged elevation of intrapulmonary pressure that occurs during the compressive phase of a cough interferes with the venous return to the thorax and results in a fall in the cardiac output and in cerebral ischemia. Fainting or lightheadedness during a coughing spell is known as *"cough syncope."*

EXPECTORATION OF SPUTUM

Healthy individuals do not usually expectorate sputum, except when exposed to excessive irritants. On the other hand, since sputum, which is brought into the pharynx by ciliary activity or a cough, may be swallowed, one should not assume that there are no abnormal secretions just because no sputum is expectorated.

Whenever a patient produces sputum, it is particularly important to determine its source, as the search for the source is often the search for a clinical diagnosis. If most of the sputum is cleared from the throat by "hawking" rather than by coughing, it is likely that the secretions originate in the nasal passages or the paranasal sinuses rather than in the bronchial tree. The amount of expectorated sputum may provide a clue to the underlying disorder. Very profuse, purulent sputum suggests the presence of gross pulmonary suppuration. If a large volume of sputum is suddenly expectorated after a short illness, a *lung abscess* should be suspected. If the volume of sputum has gradually increased over a period of time, *chronic bronchitis* or *bronchiectasis* is the likely diagnosis.

The color of the sputum is also important; yellow sputum indicates inflammation, green sputum, which is due to the presence of verdoperoxidase that has been liberated by polymorphonuclear leukocytes in the sputum, is indicative of stagnant pus in the bronchi or sinuses. In many patients the sputum is green early in the morning, most likely because of the accumulation of secretions and the consequent liberation of verdoperoxidase during the night, and becomes yellow later.

The character and consistency of the sputum may also yield useful information. In *chronic bronchitis* the sputum is usually mucoid, sticky, and gray or white in color. Mucoid sputum that is stained a deep, pink color, the so-called currant jelly sputum, may occur with a *pulmonary neoplasm*; profuse, frothy, pink, watery material is characteristic of *pulmonary edema.* A *pneumococcal infection* is often characterized by scanty, extremely tenacious, blood-stained sputum. A foul odor practically always indicates a putrid *lung abscess* or gross *bronchiectasis.*

EXPECTORATION OF BLOOD

Blood may be mixed with sputum in varying amounts, or it may constitute the entire expectorate. The term *hemoptysis* means the expectoration of frank blood. Streaks and specks of blood in the sputum occur commonly in acute respiratory infections, particularly during episodes of *acute bronchitis,* presumably because of rupture of vessels in the congested bronchial mucosa. Some blood is frequently expectorated during acute *pneumococcal pneumonia;* this is usually mixed with very tenacious sputum that is rusty in color.

The expectoration of pure blood is a serious symptom. It may be the first manifestation of active *tuberculosis,* and often with no other associated symptoms. Aside from tuberculosis, the commonest causes of hemoptysis are *pulmonary infarction, bronchiectasis, mitral stenosis, bronchogenic carcinoma* and *pulmonary abscess.* Frank hemorrhage only occasionally accompanies the *bacterial pneumonias* and is not a feature of *viral* or *mycoplasmal pneumonias.*

Bloody sputum loses much of its significance as far as the lungs are concerned if it is associated with bleeding from a nonpulmonary source. If there is a history of bleeding from the nose or the gums, or of vomiting of blood, then it is possible that some of the blood was aspirated into the larger bronchi and later expectorated. Abnormal bleeding in other parts of the body suggests that the hemoptysis may be part of a generalized bleeding disorder.

BREATHLESSNESS

Breathlessness *(dyspnea)* or shortness of breath is the awareness of difficulty in breathing. Ordinarily one is not aware of breathing, unless attention is directed to it. However, we frequently become aware of breathing when ventilation is increased considerably, as in exercise, or when a given level of ventilation requires an increased amount of effort. In any given person, awareness of the breathing act depends to a large extent on one's past experience. For instance, a person who exercises regularly becomes accustomed to the amount of respiratory effort required for such activity, and this is not characterized as breathlessness. On the other hand, a less active person may experience dyspnea when called upon to perform an equivalent amount of exercise. The key factor appears to be whether the level of ventilation or effort is recognized as being appropriate to the activity. The mechanism by which the inappropriateness is recognized has not been established. It has been suggested that a misalignment between the intrafusal and extrafusal fibers in the respiratory muscles is responsible for the reflex response and that breathlessness is sensed when there is an altered length-tension relationship in the respiratory muscles. When the respiratory muscles have to perform an inappropriate amount of work, these receptors are thought to send impulses to the higher centers through pathways that have not yet been defined.

When assessing the significance of breathlessness, or dyspnea, it is essential to determine its mode of onset and its severity. Shortness of breath during heavy exertion is relatively normal, particularly in elderly or obese individuals or someone accustomed to sedentary habits. A sudden change in exercise tolerance has a different significance than a change that has taken place gradually over a number of years, in that it indicates that an acute process has developed.

Since dyspnea is a subjective complaint and is extremely variable among individuals, it is very difficult to quantitate. The severity of breathlessness is assessed clinically by determining the minimum level of activity that is associated with breathlessness. A convenient classification is the following:

(1) breathlessness on mild exertion, such as running a short distance or climbing a flight of stairs; (b) breathlessness while walking short distances on the level at an ordinary pace; (c) breathlessness while talking, shaving, washing, etc.; (d) breathlessness at rest; (e) breathlessness while lying down *(orthopnea)*.

Because many factors play a role in production of dyspnea, it is clearly fallacious to attempt to correlate dyspnea with any one measurement. The factors that are conducive to the subjective sensation of breathlessness are presented in Table 11. Except in advanced cases, dyspnea should be assessed while the patient is undergoing some form of stress. The most satisfactory approach is to have the patient perform a form of exercise. Clinically, one can determine the ability to climb stairs; in the laboratory one assesses the cardiopulmonary response to walking on a treadmill or pedaling a bicycle ergometer.

Increased Awareness of Normal Breathing

Awareness of the act of breathing varies in degree from one person to another and even exists in a healthy individual if one "puts his mind to it." Some patients complain of "shortness of breath" when there is no apparent organic reason, and it is possible that their threshold of awareness of the breathing act has increased. Patients who are emotionally unstable may complain of respiratory distress or "shortness of breath," and usually this is a sense of suffocation, choking or oppression in the chest, which is often accompanied by other evidences of fear. That respiratory irregularities often arise during emotional states is not surprising, since one of the chief subsidiary functions of the respiratory system is the expression of emotion.

TABLE 11. Factors Conducive to Breathlessness

A. INCREASED AWARENESS OF NORMAL BREATHING (PSYCHOGENIC)
B. INCREASED RESPIRATORY WORK
  1. Increased ventilation
    a. Exercise
    b. Hypercapnia
    c. Hypoxic hypoxia
    d. Metabolic acidosis
  2. Altered physical properties
    a. Increased lung elastic resistance, e.g., pneumonia, congestion, atelectasis, pneumothorax, pleural effusion
    b. Increased chest wall elastic resistance, e.g., kyphoscoliosis, obesity
    c. Increased bronchial nonelastic resistance, e.g., emphysema, chronic bronchitis, bronchial asthma
C. ABNORMALITY OF RESPIRATORY MUSCLES
  1. Muscular disease
    a. Muscular weakness, e.g., myasthenia gravis, thyrotoxicosis
    b. Muscular paralysis, e.g., poliomyelitis, Guillain-Barré syndrome
    c. Muscular wasting, e.g., muscular dystrophy
  2. Reduced mechanical advantage of muscles
    a. Marked inspiratory position, e.g., emphysema
    b. Marked expiratory position, e.g., obesity

Weeping, sobbing, laughing, sighing and groaning are all produced by distortion of the respiratory rhythm. Similarly, the gasp of fear or wonder, the shout of elation, the sigh of satisfaction, and the rapid breathing of anger are examples of the effects of emotions on breathing.

A very common complaint is the inability to take a full, satisfactory, deep breath. Introspective people worry about this and try to take deep breaths; the result is that they execute a series of imperfect sighs. The complaint is rarely related to organic disease, and it can almost always be readily cured by explaining that it is a habit resulting from too close attention to a function that should be unconscious and automatic. Nevertheless, some people are so obsessed by this difficulty that dizziness or faintness, along with numbness and tingling in the extremities, may develop as a result of the repeated deep inspirations. In severe or prolonged cases, the excessive elimination of carbon dioxide and consequent alkalemia may cause tetany. This *"hyperventilation syndrome"* occurs most commonly in neurotic individuals and should be suspected if hypocapnia is associated with a normal arterial oxygen tension and there are no signs pointing to organic diseases of the heart, lungs, blood or nervous system.

Increased Respiratory Work

Breathlessness is a prevalent symptom when the work of breathing is increased in diseases that affect the tracheobronchial tree, the lung parenchyma, the pleural space or the chest wall. On the other hand, in chronic respiratory conditions in which the respiratory rate and depth may have been altered for a long period of time, the subject may become accustomed to the changed pattern of breathing so that the sensation of breathlessness is absent.

Abnormality of Respiratory Muscles

Breathlessness may be experienced if the respiratory muscles are weak, paralyzed or wasted or if their ability to perform mechanical work is diminished. This also occurs when breathing takes place in an inspiratory or an expiratory position and perhaps when the muscles must function under hypoxic or ischemic conditions. As was pointed out earlier, it has been suggested that the respiratory muscles may become fatigued when the work of breathing is markedly elevated.

CHEST PAIN

Pain in the chest is a very common complaint. It very often induces considerable apprehension, because the patient thinks it is indicative of a serious disease of either the lungs or the heart. Although it is true that both heart and lung disease can cause pain or discomfort in the chest, there are many other causes of chest pain. Consequently, it is important to determine the actual anatomic source of the chest pain. This requires an understanding of the distribution of the nerve dermatomes over the chest wall.

The Dermatomes

If nerve roots are irritated by mechanical pressure or infection, pain is frequently felt over the areas of skin of the thoracic and abdominal walls supplied by the dorsal roots of the spinal cord, which are known as *dermatomes.* There is a divergence of opinion about the exact distribution of dermatomes over the chest and abdomen. Figure 64 illustrates one mode of distribution that has been described. Clearly, there is some overlapping of the individual dermatomes, but they have been simplified in this illustration. The fourth cervical dermatome encompasses the supraclavicular and infraclavicular areas of the chest wall down to the level of the second rib. The dorsal roots of the fifth to the eighth cervical and the first thoracic nerves constitute the *brachial plexus,* and their dermatomes are located over the shoulder, the arm and the hand. The second and third thoracic dermatomes lie from the shoulder tips to just above the nipple line, and the fourth thoracic dermatome overlies the nipples. The seventh thoracic dermatome lies at the level of the xiphoid cartilage, and the tenth thoracic dermatome is at the level of the umbilicus, the eighth and ninth thoracic dermatomes lying between these two. The eleventh and twelfth thoracic dermatomes supply the lower abdominal wall, the lower level of the twelfth dermatome lying about two inches above the pubis.

The Source of Chest Pain

In determining the source of chest pain, it is best to suspect and, as far as possible, to examine each component of the chest from the skin inward. In the following discussion, trauma and other obvious surgical lesions that cause pain are not considered.

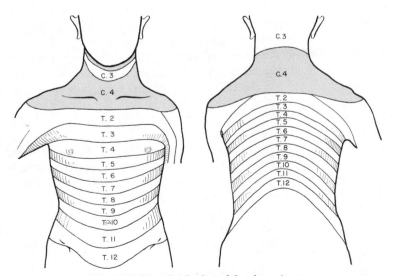

Figure 64. The distribution of the dermatomes.

The Skin. Pain is commonly localized in the skin of the chest wall. The cause may be obvious if it is due to a bruise, a boil or a carbuncle. If it is caused by inflammation of a posterior root ganglion (as in *herpes zoster*), the pain may develop long before the appearance of the characteristic vesicular skin rash which is localized to that particular dermatome. Pain due to irritation of the nerve roots is frequently accompanied by hyperalgesia over the corresponding area of the skin.

The Ribs and Cartilages. Occasionally a paroxysm of coughing may cause a *rib fracture* or a *dislocated rib cartilage.* This causes a localized pain that is accentuated by breathing and coughing, as well as tenderness over the affected area. In the *"slipping rib syndrome,"* which is thought to be caused by overriding of the tenth costal cartilage on the ninth costal cartilage and which mainly affects middle-aged individuals, the principal complaint is upper abdominal pain on one or both sides. The pain is aggravated by movement and certain postures, such as lying or turning in bed, stretching, bending forward, walking, deep breathing and coughing.

Tietze's syndrome is an uncommon cause of pain originating in a costal cartilage. This benign condition of unknown etiology may persist for years. It consists of pain over one or more costochondral or sternoclavicular junctions along with tender swelling in the affected area.

Osteomyelitis of the ribs of either tuberculous or pyogenic origin and malignant tumors involving the ribs are rare causes of chest pain. This is usually associated with tenderness, redness or swelling immediately over a rib.

The Nerves. Pain caused by disease of the intercostal nerves is hard to demonstrate, because it is difficult to know whether the pain arises in the nerves, the muscle or the connective tissue. Several diseases that involve the posterior nerve roots can lead to chest pain. *Herpes zoster,* a viral infection of the posterior root ganglions, is characterized by pain, along with exquisite hyperesthesia in the area of the distribution of the intercostal nerves, i.e., the nerve dermatomes. An eruption consisting of a cluster of small vesicles in the same area usually appears a few days after the onset of the pain. The pain, together with the hyperesthesia, may persist for a period of time after the rash has healed, but the condition may still be recognized by the brownish discoloration of the skin that is characteristic of a healed herpes infection.

Chest pain may also result from pressure on the posterior nerve root or on the nerve trunk caused by a disease of the vertebrae, such as *tuberculosis, degenerative arthritis* or a *neoplasm.* This *"root pain"* is usually referred to the peripheral distribution of its dermatome.

The Muscles. Pain originating in the thoracic muscles is often confused with pleurisy, since it is generally aggravated by deep breathing. Patients frequently become very anxious because they think that the pain originates in the heart, especially if it is over the lower left costochondral junctions, where many think the heart is located.

Provided that the ribs and costal cartilages are ruled out as the source of pain, *fibrositis* should be suspected if there is localized tenderness on deep pressure at the site of the pain or if the pain is reproduced by putting the involved muscle groups into action against resistance.

"Bornholm" disease, or *epidemic myalgia,* an acute febrile illness caused by the Coxsackie B group of viruses, is characterized by fever, profuse sweating, a frontal headache and the sudden onset of excruciating pain in the subcostal and upper abdominal regions. The pain is due to involvement of the intercostal muscles and the diaphragm, but pleural involvement has been reported in some epidemics.

The Pleura. Only the parietal layer of the pleura is a source of pain. Irritation of pain fibers in the parietal pleura is referred to the chest wall and characteristically is sharply localized, superficial, knifelike or "catching" in character. It is aggraveted by respiratory movements, particularly a deep inspiration, coughing, sneezing and yawning. A pleural origin for pain is virtually confirmed if a pleural friction rub is heard or a pleural effusion is present.

Patients suffering from a *pneumothorax* or massive *atelectasis* may occasionally have pain that is thought to be due to traction on the parietal pleura by adhesions that are attached to the moving visceral pleura. It must be emphasized that pleural pain can occur in conditions other than pleural inflammation and, conversely, that inflammation of the pleura does not always cause pain.

The Diaphragm. Pain arising from the diaphragmatic pleura is mediated through the phrenic and intercostal nerves. The central portion of the diaphragm is innervated by the third, fourth and fifth cervical nerves, so that irritation of this area results in a sharp pain that is referred to the shoulder on the same side. The pain fibers from the posterior and peripheral portions of the diaphragm travel via the fifth and sixth intercostal nerves; irritation of these areas results in pain along the costal margin; this pain projects into the epigastrium and the subchondral and lumbar regions.

The Lung Parenchyma. The lungs are usually regarded as insensitive organs. When pain is present in pulmonary disease, it is thought that the parietal pleura is likely secondarily involved. There are, however, some situations in which pain apparently originates in the lung. For instance, a pulmonary neoplasm that does not appear to be involving the pleura sometimes gives rise to a deep aching pain. Similarly, an acute atelectasis may be associated with a sudden violent pain, even though it is not associated with a pleural rub or an effusion.

The Tracheobronchial Tree. A raw burning sensation over the sternal area, which is aggravated by breathing and coughing, often occurs in persons suffering from acute tracheobronchitis.

The Aorta. A dissecting aortic aneurysm produces a severe retrosternal pain that is sudden in onset, radiates to the back, and rapidly becomes agonizing. A dissecting aneurysm may be recognized by the finding of an unequal blood pressure in the two arms.

The Heart. Pain caused by cardiac disease need rarely be confused with pleural or pulmonary pain. Ischemia or hypoxia of the myocardium leads to anaerobic tissue metabolism with the production of an excess of acid metabolites that stimulate the nerve endings in the myocardium. The resulting impulses pass through the cardiac plexus to the upper five or six thoracic sympathetic ganglia, and then through the white rami of the second to fifth thoracic nerve roots into the spinal cord, from which they reach the skeletal nerves via their respective posterior roots.

Cardiac pain is typically substernal and is brought on by exertion. *"Angina of effort"* is a central chest pain resulting from ischemia of the myocardium caused by inadequate coronary blood flow. It is often described as a heavy, viselike, squeezing or gripping sensation. It frequently radiates to the base of the neck and the jaw, over the shoulders, and the pectoral muscles, and down the arms. For some reason, the pain is referred more frequently down the left arm than the right. Anginal pain is usually relieved by rest and is also frequently relieved or prevented by nitroglycerin or beta antagonists.

The pain resulting from an occlusion of one of the coronary arteries has the same distribution as that of angina, but it is usually much more severe and "crushing." It may develop without preceding exertion and frequently occurs while the patient is resting. In contrast to angina, it does not disappear when the patient rests or takes nitroglycerin, but may continue for a long time, often requiring powerful analgesics for its relief.

The Pericardium. Inflammation of the pericardium may produce chest pain that is situated in either the substernal area or the left mammary region. The pain may vary in intensity from a dull burning discomfort to severe pressure simulating a myocardial infarction. It is frequently aggravated if the patient lies in the supine position or extends the neck. The explanation for this phenomenon is not apparent.

Neither the visceral pericardium nor the internal surface of the parietal pericardium contains any pain fibers, and only the lower part of the external surface of the parietal layer of the pericardium is sensitive. A lesion that affects the lower part of the pericardium frequently involves the adjacent diaphragmatic pleura, so that, in addition to the characteristic substernal pain of the pericarditis, pain may also be felt in the neck and shoulder.

The Pulmonary Vessels. Patients suffering from pulmonary hypertension may develop chest pain on exertion that simulates, in many respects, the pain of angina of effort. Similarly, a pulmonary embolus may cause pain that is similar to that of a myocardial infarction. It has been suggested that this pain is due to either dilatation of the pulmonary artery or ischemia of the myocardium of the right ventricle.

The Esophagus. The sensory innervation of the esophagus is derived from the vagus nerve and the visceral sympathetic nerves that arise from the inferior cervical and upper nine thoracic ganglia. Pain originating in the esophagus results from contraction of the esophageal smooth muscle, and this is often precipitated by the reflux of acid gastric contents into the esophagus. It is characteristically burning in quality and situated over the area of the sternum that overlies the affected portion of the esophagus. It can also simulate myocardial ischemic pain, and is occasionally referred to the pharynx, the lower neck, the back and the arms. It may also radiate around the chest cage along the dermatomes that correspond to the spinal segment that inervates the involved area of the esophagus.

The Abdominal Organs. A severe squeezing substernal pain may be due to distension of a hiatus hernia within the thorax. Characteristically, this pain increases in severity whenever the hernia is aggravated by an increase in the intra-abdominal pressure or by assumption of the supine position.

Psychogenic Pain. Despite the lack of obvious organic disease, a patient may complain of a nondescript chest pain or one that is much like that caused by organic disease. Such patients are frequently apprehensive about the possibility of cardiac or pulmonary disease. Anxious patients often also complain of lancinating pains in the chest which are sharp and fleeting and are often described as "stabbing." They are generally due to intercostal muscle spasm and are usually inconsequential.

CONSTITUTIONAL SYMPTOMS

Patients suffering from a pulmonary condition may complain of constitutional symptoms, such as fever, sweating, anorexia, weakness and loss of weight.

Fever

Under most circumstances, the body temperature represents a balance between the heat produced by the body and that which is lost. The body temperature is thought to be normally controlled by two thermoregulatory centers in the hypothalamus: one in the anterior hypothalamus, which prevents overheating, and one in the posterior hypothalamus, which protects the body from chilling. There are abundant neural interconnections between these two areas, and it is probable that the activity of one center tends to inhibit that of the other. The temperature rises whenever infection is present or there is degeneration of tissue or extensive trauma, probably because of both an increased heat production and a reduced heat loss. The fever may be continuous, remittent, or oscillating, or it may be intermittent with a normal temperature for varying length of time.

A protein product known as "pyrexin," which has been isolated from degenerating tissues and neutrophils, increases the body temperature when it is injected into an experimental animal. It has been suggested that the thermoregulatory centers respond to this stimulus by raising the level at which the body temperature is normally regulated. The measures that increase body temperature are similar to those that occur during exposure to cold, namely, intense vasoconstriction, the development of goose pimples or pilo-erection, the secretion of epinephrine, and shivering. This is exemplified in situations in which a patient may feel chilly even though the body temperature is normal or even above normal. "Shaking chills" may develop, along with teeth chattering and such violent shivering that the bed shakes. The skin feels cold because of peripheral vasoconstriction and a diminished peripheral blood flow. Heat loss through radiation is reduced by peripheral vasoconstriction, and heat production is increased by the increased muscle tone and activity associated with shivering.

Sweating

Under ordinary circumstances only about 600 ml. of sweat is secreted over 24 hours from special glands in the feet, hands and axillae. The heat loss caused by this insensible perspiration constitutes about one-fifth to one-fourth of the total heat loss from the body. One stimulus to increased sweating is an elevated body temperature. When the temperature of the blood rises, the thermoregulatory center in the posterior hypothalamus apparently inhibits the tonic discharge of impulses over the sympathetic vasoconstrictor fibers and results in vasodilation in the skin. At the same time, the thermoregulatory center in the anterior hypothalamus sends impulses to the sweat glands via the cholinergic, postganglionic fibers.

Profuse sweating may occur in patient suffering from a respiratory disease, and anxiety and worry about breathing difficulty may cause over-activity of the sympathetic nervous system. Occasionally there may be drenching "night or slumber sweats" in which the night clothes or pajamas become thoroughly soaked. The mechanism of this phenomenon has not been explained, but an elevated body temperature, overactivity of the sympathetic nervous system, or a resetting of the hypothalamic thermostat to a lower level all might lead to measures designed to increase heat loss during the night.

Anorexia, Weakness, Fatigue, and Weight Loss

Anorexia, weakness, easy fatiguability and weight loss are frequent complaints in patients suffering from chronic respiratory disease. These symptoms may also be encountered during acute pulmonary infections. The development of anorexia in respiratory disease is difficult to explain. In severe disease, the mere act of eating may be so tiring and energy consuming that the patient may lose all desire to eat. Consequently, a relative anorexia may exist simply because of the effort that is required for eating.

Weakness and loss of weight develop when the caloric intake does not match the expenditure of energy. In respiratory disorders, the energy expenditure is often increased because of a high oxygen cost of breathing or an increased caloric requirement resulting from fever (about 7 per cent for each degree Fahrenheit above the normal body temperature). In addition, there may be an excessive loss of protein as a result of either infection, tissue destruction, malignancy or trauma.

SIGNS

Alteration of certain properties of the lungs and chest wall by a disease process results in characteristic physical signs that can be elicited by the clinician during the physical examination. These abnormal physical signs, taken in conjunction with the patient's symptoms, help the physician to arrive at an accurate diagnosis of the underlying disease process. The most important physical signs resulting from involvement of either the lung or the chest wall by a pathologic process are due to alterations of certain properties of the thorax with respect to size, distensibility and sound transmission.

SIZE

Any alteration in the size of one lung is reflected by a shift of the mediastinum from its normal midline position within the thorax. A shift of the mediastinum may occur as a result of a disorder of the lung parenchyma, a disease affecting the pleural space, or distortion of the chest cage.

When fibrosis or atelectasis develop in one lung, the size of the affected thorax is reduced. The mediastinum is shifted toward the affected side (Fig. 65), because the end-expiratory intrapleural pressure is more negative on this side.

Conversely, if fluid or air collects in a pleural space, the size of the affected thorax is increased. The mediastinum is displaced toward the opposite side (Fig. 66), because the end-expiratory intrapleural pressure rises on the affected side. Similarly, with hyperinflation of one lung, such as occurs with a check-valve obstruction of a major bronchus, the mediastinum will be shifted to the opposite, normal side. Displacement of the mediastinum to the opposite side may also occur if abdominal contents herniate into the thoracic cavity.

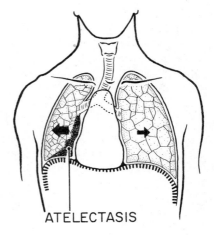

Figure 65. The mechanism of the shift of the mediastinum in atelectasis.

ATELECTASIS

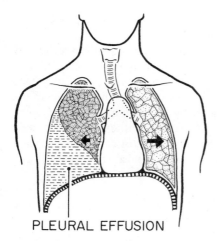

Figure 66. The mechanism of the shift of the mediastinum in a pleural effusion.

PLEURAL EFFUSION

In contrast, when a lung becomes consolidated, the alveolar air is replaced by exudate and there is little, if any, change in the size of the affected lung. As is shown in Figure 67, the mediastinum remains in its normal midline position when consolidation is present.

Distortion of the chest cage, as in severe kyphoscoliosis of the thoracic spine, generally causes displacement of the mediastinum toward the side of the lung that is compressed (Fig. 68).

If both lungs are diseased, the position of the mediastinum will depend on the lung that is most affected. Thus, if bilateral fibrosis is present, the mediastinum will be shifted toward the more-involved lung; if there is a bilateral pleural effusion or pneumothorax, it will be shifted toward the side that is least involved. Understandably, if consolidation is present in both

Figure 67. The position of the mediastinum in consolidation.

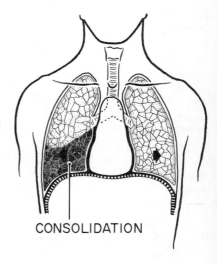

CONSOLIDATION

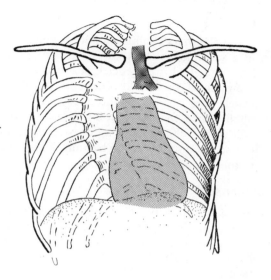

Figure 68. The position of the mediastinum in severe kyphoscoliosis.

lungs, the mediastinum will still occupy a central position. Similarly, if both lungs are equally hyperinflated as a result of emphysema, the mediastinum remains in its normal midline position.

DISTENSIBILITY

A disorder of the lung parenchyma, pleural space or chest cage alters the distensibility of the chest so that its movement is affected. Consequently, the earliest manifestation of bronchopulmonary disease is often diminished movement of that part of the chest wall which overlies the diseased area.

Chest movement is diminished when there are regional variations in the forces applied to the chest wall by the respiratory muscles, as in muscular dystrophy or poliomyelitis; when the chest cage offers an increased resistance to inflation, as in obesity or kyphoscoliosis; when there is a regional increase in the resistance to distention of the lung, as in consolidation, fibrosis and atelectasis; or when the lung is compressed by fluid or air in the pleural space. Chest movement is also reduced when the lungs are hyperinflated because of expiratory air flow limitation resulting from either an increased resistance to airflow or a loss of lung elastic recoil, as in emphysema.

SOUND TRANSMISSION

Sound consists of rapidly moving vibrations in the air. In the respiratory system, sounds are produced by phonation (vocal sounds), breathing (breath sounds), and abnormal processes (adventitious sounds); they may also be imparted to the chest by percussion. To understand how sound is transmitted, certain characteristics of sound and its production in the respiratory system must be discussed.

Pitch

The *pitch* of a musical note depends on the number of cycles of repetition in a second, which is known as the *frequency*. Low frequencies produce a low note; high frequencies produce a high note. In the respiratory system, the pitch of a sound also depends on the length and diameter of the tube in which it is produced; the shorter and narrower the tube, the higher the pitch. Since each succeeding branch of the tracheobronchial tree is shorter and narrower than its predecessor, the pitch of the sound produced within the succeeding branches become higher and higher, finally reaching a peak in the terminal bronchioles.

Intensity

The *intensity* of a sound, or its loudness, depends on both the energy with which it is transmitted and its frequency. Sound loses its intensity if it has to pass from one medium into another, such as from air into water, because the sound waves are reflected and absorbed by the fluid-air interfaces.

Timbre

The *timbre* of a sound is distinct from its pitch or intensity, because it represents its character or quality, which in turn depends on the relative proportion between the fundamental tone and the overtones. It is by means of the timbre that one is able to distinguish between sounds of the same pitch and intensity produced by different instruments.

Vocal Sounds

Voice sounds are produced by vibration of the vocal cords in the larynx, which acts like a reed instrument. The sound is carried upward into the oral cavity and the paranasal sinuses, thereby increasing its intensity and producing a particular tonal quality. The vocal sound is also carried downward through the tracheobronchial tree and lung parenchyma as far as the chest wall, causing the thorax to vibrate in unison with the laryngeal sounds. It is thought that the majority of the vibrations are conducted within the lumen of the bronchi, and the remainder are conducted down along the bronchial walls. The sound produced within the trachea has been estimated to have vibrations of approximately 400 cycles/sec., and that produced within the terminal bronchiole approximately 1700 cycles/sec.

Breath Sounds

Like the vocal sounds, most of the breath sounds that are produced within the tracheobronchial tree are conducted within the lumen of the bronchi. As is illustrated in Figure 69, eddies and turbulence are produced during inspiration when air currents strike the sharp borders of the bronchial bifurcations. During expiration, the air moving out of the small airways mixes with air currents coming from other small airways and strikes against

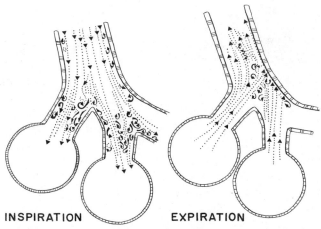

INSPIRATION   EXPIRATION

Figure 69. The production of turbulence in the airways during inspiration and expiration.

the wall of the parent bronchus, creating turbulence and small eddies, but these are presumably less than those that occur during inspiration, because fewer sharp bifurcations are encountered by the outgoing air.

It has been suggested that the lungs act as a "selective transmitter" of sound (i.e., they act like a low-pass filter, in that the high-frequency vibrations produced in the bronchial tree are dampened as they pass through the lungs), so that only sounds with a frequency of 200 cycles/sec. or less pass through to the chest wall. If the lung becomes diseased, and the number of normally functioning alveoli diminishes, its ability to act as a low-pass filter is altered and the higher frequency vibrations may be transmitted to the chest wall. In the physical examination of the chest, the transmission of sound is assessed by percussion, palpation and auscultation.

Percussion

Percussion of the chest produces vibrations of the chest wall and the underlying lung parenchyma. The heavier the percussion stroke, the deeper will be the penetration and lateral radiation of these vibrations. The pitch of the sound produced by percussion provides an indication of the ratio between air-containing tissue and solid tissue in the area underlying the percussing finger. Percussion over normal lung tissue produces slow vibrations, and the resultant sound has a low pitch that is relatively long in duration. Percussion over an area with an increased ratio of air to solid tissue, as in *emphysema* or a *pneumothorax,* produces a sound with a lower-than-normal pitch (i.e., it is hyperresonant). Conversely, percussion over an area with a reduced air-to–solid tissue ratio, as in *atelectasis* or *consolidation,* produces a high-pitched or dull sound. Clearly, percussion may not be abnormal if a lesion is deep within the lung or if the thickness of the chest wall is increased, as in the obese patient.

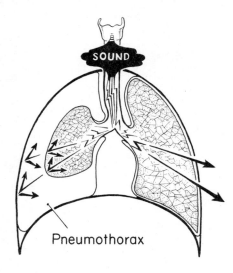

Figure 70. The reflection of sound waves at tissue-air interfaces in a pneumothorax.

Palpation

The vibrations produced over the chest wall by vocal sounds are called *vocal fremitus.* Vibrations felt by the palpating hand are known as *tactile fremitus,* and those heard with a stethoscope are known as *auditory fremitus.*

The intensity of vocal fremitus is the same over all parts of the chest wall, except over the right upper lobe, where the intensity of fremitus is increased because the large bronchi are close to the chest wall. It is normally somewhat less intense in women and children than in men, presumably because their voices are less resonant.

Vocal fremitus increases in intensity when the ability of the lungs to act as a low-pass filter is reduced, so that the higher frequency vibrations pass through the chest wall. When the alveoli are filled with inflammatory exudate, as in *consolidation,* the vibrations produced by the spoken voice are clearly felt and heard over the overlying chest wall, provided the bronchus is patent.

Vocal fremitus is decreased in intensity when there is fluid or air in the pleural space, because the vibrations passing through the underlying lung parenchyma are reflected and absorbed by the increased number of fluid-air interfaces (Fig. 70). The vocal fremitus is also diminished when the chest wall is very muscular or obese, because the sound must travel through a greater distance.

Auscultation

Breath Sounds. The breath sounds heard over the chest wall during auscultation differ considerably, both in quality and intensity, from those actually produced within the tracheobronchial tree. The breath sounds heard over the trachea are high pitched and loud, inspiration and expiration being equally affected with respect to pitch, intensity and duration. During auscultation over the chest wall, the inspiratory sound is easily heard, but the expiratory sound is fainter and approximately one-third the length of the inspiratory sound. If the breath sounds heard over the chest wall are identical to those heard over the trachea *(bronchial breath sounds),* then there must be a reduced air-to–solid tissue ratio, i.e., an area of consolidation or solid lung tissue in close approximation to a patent bronchus.

Adventitious Sounds. Adventitious sounds are produced by pathologic processes within the lungs and the tracheobronchial tree, and are never detected over healthy lung tissue.

WHEEZES. A wheeze is a prolonged musical sound that is produced within the lumen of the tracheobronchial tree as a result of turbulence and eddy formation. Since the bronchi normally shorten and narrow during expiration, wheezes are usually more pronounced during expiration. The musical character of a wheeze is related to its content of harmonic frequencies, and its pitch is determined by the lowest, or fundamental, frequency. The frequency can range from 60 to 2000 Hz. over five octaves, which corresponds to the lowest note of a bassoon and to the highest note of a flute. Experimental studies have suggested that a wheeze is produced only when an affected bronchus narrows almost to the point of closure and the bronchial wall vibrates between the closed and the barely open positions.

"Monophonic" wheezing is formed by identical notes; it is "fixed" if it is formed by a single, identical note whose pitch remains unchanged, and "random" if it consists of several identical notes, which end at different times. A fixed monophonic wheeze that is audible at the mouth as well as over the chest wall may be heard when there is stenosis and incomplete closure of a single major bronchus. If the stenosis is rigid and fixed, the wheeze is present during both inspiration and expiration; if it is flexible, the wheeze may be present during either inspiration or expiration, and its pitch may be constant or variable. Random monophonic wheezing is heard in widespread bronchial obstruction, as in *asthma*. The wheezes are numerous; occur at random during either inspiration, expiration or throughout the respiratory cycle; and are identical in pitch, but variable in duration and often overlapping one another in time.

"Polyphonic wheezing" is formed by several notes that are dissimilar with regard to pitch and harmony but that start and end simultaneously (like those forming a musical chord) and occur only during the expiration. Polyphonic wheezing indicates generalized bronchial obstruction. It is possible to determine whether the source of wheeze is in the central airways or the peripheral airways by comparing the sounds heard over the chest wall with those over the open mouth. If they originate in the large airways, then both sounds are equally loud. If they originate in the peripheral airways only, the sounds at the mouth are virtually inaudible, because they have been filtered out on their way to the mouth.

CRACKLES. A crackle is a short, explosive, nonmusical sound that is most readily heard during inspiration. Usually, crackles are best heard over the lower zones of the lungs, but if the disease is extensive, they may be heard over the middle and upper zones as well. It was originally thought that this sound was produced by the bursting of bubbles of fluid in the bronchi, and this may still explain the crackles that are heard when there are secretions in the trachea or large bronchi. Recently, however, it has been suggested that crackles originating in the peripheral airways are produced by the sudden equalization of upstream and downstream pressures or from the bursting of a film of surface material when closed bronchioles reopen. Indeed, crackles may be heard early in inspiration even in healthy individuals if they inhale from residual volume.

Crackles may not be detected during an ordinary inspiration if there is only a minimal amount of parenchymal or bronchiolar disease. However, they can often be elicited by having the patient inspire and expire deeply and then cough. Often crackles will be heard just after the cough or at the beginning of the next inspiration. These *"posttussic" crackles* are presumably produced by the sudden rush of air through bronchioles whose walls became adherent during the compressive phase of the cough.

The time at which the crackle appears during inspiration may be related to the site and type of the pathologic condition. Crackles heard only during the very early phase of inspiration suggest generalized airway disease, such as *chronic bronchitis* or *asthma.* They are typically scanty, may be loud or faint and are usually transmitted to the mouth. Late inspiratory crackles are heard in *interstitial lung disease* (often Velcro-like), *asbestosis, pneumonia,* and *pulmonary congestion.*

RUBS. A pleural rub is a coarse, creaking, leathery sound and is indicative of pleural irritation. A rub is produced when the inflamed surfaces of the pleura rub against one another during respiration, and it is therefore present predominantly during the latter part of inspiration and the early part of expiration. Since the greatest movement of the lungs, and therefore the greatest excursion of the pleural surfaces, occurs over the lower lobes, rubs are most frequently detected over the lower areas of the chest wall.

10

SECONDARY MANIFESTATIONS OF PULMONARY DISEASE

In addition to the cardinal, or primary, symptoms and signs associated with respiratory disease, there are a number of secondary phenomena that may, in turn, compromise cardiopulmonary function. The majority of the secondary manifestations of pulmonary disease are the result of alterations of gas exchange or increases in pulmonary vascular resistance. In addition, other extrapulmonary manifestations, including rare systemic derangements, may occur.

SIGNS OF INADEQUATE GAS EXCHANGE

When gas exchange becomes inadequate, hypoxemia develops, either alone or in combination with hypercapnia. Both alterations result in certain symptoms and signs and are attended by secondary effects that further compromise respiratory and cardiac function. Not infrequently, the degree of secondary manifestations present may be disproportionate to the status of the arterial blood gases while the patient is awake. In such situations, it is important to assess gas exchange during sleep.

HYPOXEMIA

Although hypoxemia does not produce a characteristic clinical picture, it occupies a central position in the pathogenesis of many of the manifestations of respiratory insufficiency. The severity of the signs and symptoms that develop depends on the degree of hypoxemia present and its duration. In some patients, mental confusion, hyperpnea, dyspnea and cyanosis may be dominant features; in others, these findings may be minimal or absent.

183

Cyanosis

Cyanosis is a diffuse, bluish discoloration of the skin and mucous membranes that develops when there is an increase in the amount of reduced or otherwise unoxygenated hemoglobin in the capillaries. It is best detected where the coverings over the capillaries of the skin or mucous membranes are thinnest and most transparent.

It has been suggested that cyanosis does not become perceptible until the mean concentration of reduced hemoglobin in the capillaries doubles. For example, in a healthy individual whose hemoglobin content is 15 gm./ 100 ml. and whose arteriovenous oxygen difference is 5 volumes per cent, the arterial and venous oxygen saturations are approximately 97 and 74 per cent, respectively. This means that the amount of reduced hemoglobin is 0.45 gm. in the arterial blood and 3.90 gm. in the venous blood. Since the average amount in the capillaries is considered to be the mean of the sum of the arterial and venous values, the amount of reduced hemoglobin is therefore $\dfrac{0.45 + 3.90}{2}$, or 2.18 gm./100 ml. of blood.

Now if, in the same individual, the arterial oxygen saturation were to fall to 80 per cent (this means an oxygen saturation of roughly 50 per cent in the venous blood), and if the arteriovenous difference remained approximately the same then there would be 3.0 gm. of reduced hemoglobin in the arterial blood and 7.5 gm. in the venous blood. The reduced hemoglobin content in the capillaries would then be $\dfrac{3.0 + 7.5}{2}$, or 5.25 gm./100 ml. of blood.

These calculations indicate that cyanosis does not develop until the oxygen saturation of the arterial blood falls to approximately 80 per cent. This means that cyanosis will not be perceived in patients suffering from respiratory disease until the arterial oxygen tension is approximately 50 mm. Hg. Clearly then, hypoxemia may be severe before cyanosis can be detected.

The severity of the cyanosis depends on the amount of hemoglobin in the blood. For a given oxygen saturation, the amount of reduced hemoglobin will be greater when the hemoglobin level is high. Thus, a polycythemic patient whose hemoglobin concentration is greater than 20 gm./100 ml. will develop cyanosis at a lesser degree of hypoxemia than does an individual with a normal hemoglobin. The converse is also important; in anemic patients, hypoxemia may be extremely severe before cyanosis develops. Clearly then, the presence of cyanosis does not necessarily indicate severe hypoxemia, particularly if polycythemia is present, and the absence of cyanosis does not rule out hypoxemia, particularly in the anemic patient.

It is important to recognize that grave tissue hypoxia may be present without the warning signs of cyanosis. For instance, it is difficult to detect cyanosis in a patient with carbon monoxide poisoning, in which a non-oxygen-carrying hemoglobin is formed. Severe tissue hypoxia may be present under these circumstances, even though the skin is pink and the blood is bright red. Similarly, in cyanide poisoning, the arterial blood may be well oxygenated, but the tissues are unable to use the oxygen that is brought to them.

Conversely, cyanosis may develop in the absence of an underlying cardiopulmonary disease or hypoxemia, particularly in the extremities. Bluish discoloration is seen when the cutaneous arterioles narrow as a result of either a cold environment or nervous influences. Vasoconstriction slows blood flow through the capillaries so that more oxygen is extracted by the tissues, and the amount of reduced hemoglobin in those capillaries is increased.

The problem is compounded by the fact that the recognition of cyanosis depends on color perception, which is subject to wide variations from one observer to another. Cyanosis is particularly difficult to detect if the skin overlying the capillaries is thickened and pigmented, or if the number and size of the capillaries are reduced. These considerations point to the many pitfalls that exist if judgment of the status of oxygenation depends entirely on the presence of cyanosis. The presence of hypoxemia can be established only by analysis of the arterial oxygen tension and oxygen saturation. As indicated earlier, this is especially true in anemic patients, who may have hypoxemia severe enough to threaten life without the clinical development of cyanosis.

Ventilatory Manifestations

Hypoxemia is a major stimulus to ventilation. Just as some clinicians use cyanosis to determine whether hypoxemia is present, others use the presence or absence of breathlessness as criteria for the diagnosis of hypoxemia. The extent to which a hypoxic ventilatory drive contributes to the breathlessness of respiratory insufficiency is difficult to ascertain. Many patients claim some relief of dyspnea and demonstrate an increased exercise tolerance when inhaling oxygen. However, the presence or absence of dyspnea or hyperpnea cannot be used as an indication of whether a patient is hypoxemic. The ventilatory response to hypoxemia varies considerably in different individuals, and in any case the P_aO_2 must fall below 60 mm. Hg (at sea level) before a noticeable increase in ventilation occurs. However, in some patients with carbon dioxide retention, hypoxemia may become the major stimulus to respiration, and the administration of oxygen may lead to hypoventilation and increasing hypercapnia.

Cardiovascular Manifestations

Hypoxemia plays an important role in the cardiovascular component of respiratory insufficiency. An increase in pulse rate is also often used clinically as an indication of the severity of hypoxemia, and this is likely a more reliable indicator than changes in respiration. An acute reduction in P_aO_2 may lead to an increase in pulse rate, even when ventilation is not stimulated. Conversely, in some cases of prolonged hypoxemia, the pulse rate may be low rather than high.

Hypoxemia causes an increase in cardiac output and dilation of peripheral blood vessels, including the cerebral vessels, but it causes constriction of the pulmonary blood vessels. Pulmonary vasoconstriction caused by hypoxemia is ordinarily readily reversible, but in some persons chronic hypoxemia may lead to considerable structural changes, with a further increase in pulmonary vascular resistance and ultimately right-sided heart failure. It is important to reiterate that the degree of hypoxemia present while awake may not be commensurate with the severity of pulmonary hypertension. In such patients, it is important to monitor the oxygen saturation during sleep.

Hematologic Manifestations

A prominent effect of hypoxemia is the development of secondary polycythemia, which is mediated by an increased erythropoietin production. Because of the increase in hemoglobin, the amount of oxygen carried to the tissues is increased. The increased oxygen-carrying capacity of the blood allows the required amount of oxygen to be given off to the tissues without producing too great a fall of the partial pressure of the oxygen in the blood. The extent of the increase in red blood cell mass is often masked by an increase in extracellular fluid and plasma volume, so the hematocrit may be normal. Unlike polycythemia vera, splenomegaly, leukocytosis and thrombocytosis are absent. The relative importance of polycythemia, either as a compensatory mechanism or as a deleterious factor that contributes to the pathogenesis of right-sided heart failure by increasing blood viscosity, is still controversial. However, just as with pulmonary hypertension, the degree of polycythemia may be excessive when related to the arterial Po_2 at rest, and the possibility of sleep hypoxemia must be considered.

Metabolic Manifestions

The metabolic changes that are operative in increasing erythropoietin production or the pulmonary vasoconstriction brought about by hypoxemia are unknown. Chronic hypoxemia apparently does not interfere with the metabolism of carbohydrate, fat or protein under resting conditions. Anaerobic metabolism, as judged by increases in blood lactate and pyruvate concentration, is increased during exercise in patients with chronic respiratory insufficiency, but whether such changes are greater than those observed in patients with similar degrees of debility caused by other chronic diseases has not been established.

Central Nervous System Manifestations

Acute hypoxemia causes visual disturbances, incoordination, dysarthria and even coma. In normal individuals, the inhalation of 10 per cent oxygen reduces the cerebral vascular resistance and increases cerebral blood flow. As a result, the oxygen tension of the cerebral tissues does not fall as much as it might otherwise. Nevertheless, symptoms related to cerebral dysfunction are the commonest manifestations of acute or chronic hypoxemia.

A patient who becomes acutely hypoxemic is usually very restless, but somnolence and lassitude or a sense of self-satisfaction and euphoria that may be associated with outbursts of hilarity or obstreperousness may also be exhibited. Neuromuscular coordination frequently suffers, as is evidenced by clumsiness and a slowed reaction time, and judgment may become impaired to such an extent that the entire clinical picture resembles one of drunkenness.

HYPERCAPNIA

In patients with respiratory insufficiency, hypercapnia is always associated with hypoxemia unless the patient is inhaling a concentration of oxygen greater than that of room air. For this reason, it is sometimes difficult to separate the effects of hypercapnia from those produced by the associated hypoxemia.

Ventilatory Manifestations

An acute rise in arterial Pco_2 is the most outstanding of all the known chemical influences on ventilation. On the other hand, acclimatization to an elevated P_aco_2 occurs in patients with chronic respiratory disease, and changes in the arterial Po_2 may become the prime stimulus to ventilation. In patients with chronic carbon dioxide retention, the ventilatory response to further increments of Pco_2 is reduced, and the sensitivity of the medullary respiratory center may be diminished. On the other hand, an increased work of breathing (and elevated CO_2 production in relation to the alveolar ventilation) may also play an important role in the apparent diminished responsiveness to inhaled carbon dioxide.

Central Nervous System Manifestations

An acute elevation of the P_aco_2 dilates cerebral vessels, increases cerebral blood flow, raises cerebrospinal fluid pressure and may result in narcosis and coma. The level of P_aco_2 at which these effects appear is highly variable. In patients with chronic respiratory insufficiency, headache on arising is a very common symptom. This is probably related to the effects of progressive hypoxemia and carbon dioxide retention during sleep. Occasionally, mental aberrations such as hallucinations, hypomania, or catatonia prompt the admission of patients with severe hypoxemia and hypercapnia to psychiatric institutions. Other unexplained neurologic manifestations include asterexis (flapping tremor), convulsions, papilledema and an apparent exophthalmos.

Cardiovascular Manifestations

As pointed out above, hypercapnia causes cerebral vasodilatation and an increase in cerebral blood flow. On the other hand, it (or more likely the acidemia associated with it) causes constriction of the pulmonary vessels, thereby aggravating and increasing any pulmonary hypertension that may be present. The response of the peripheral vasculature to carbon dioxide depends on the balance struck between its local and central effects. Although carbon dioxide normally produces peripheral vasodilatation, this is usually masked by the vasoconstriction that is produced by stimulation of the sympathetic nervous system. When carbon dioxide retention is severe, generalized vasodilatation predominates, so that hypotension is a common occurrence and the patient may be in a shocklike state.

SIGNS OF INCREASED PULMONARY VASCULAR RESISTANCE

Alterations of the pulmonary vasculature as a result of pulmonary disease increase the pulmonary vascular resistance. Although factors such as obstruction or obliteration of the pulmonary vascular bed may be prominent in pulmonary disease, pulmonary vasoconstriction plays an important role, and the level of pulmonary hypertension usually correlates well with the degree of oxygen desaturation. The main caveat to remember is that the correlation may be with the oxygen saturation during sleep rather than the awake saturation.

Examination of the lungs does not provide any indication of the presence of pulmonary hypertension; signs indicative of this abnormality are found during examination of the heart. The intensity of the second sound in the pulmonic area, which is caused by closure of the aortic and pulmonary valves, is increased when pulmonary hypertension is present. During inspiration, the second sound in the pulmonic area is often split into two parts, because closure of the pulmonary valve is delayed as a result of increased filling and prolonged systole of the right ventricle. When pulmonary hypertension is present, or when there is right ventricular failure caused by pulmonary disease, the second sound may not split during inspiration. In addition, the second pulmonary sound becomes very much louder than normal. Other auscultatory signs of pulmonary hypertension are a high-pitched early systolic ejection click, which is likely due to accentuated ejection vibrations in the pulmonic area, and a presystolic gallop rhythm.

An increased pulmonary vascular resistance places a very heavy burden on the right ventricle in that it must work harder to pump blood through the pulmonary vascular bed. As a result, it frequently hypertrophies. A prominent pulsation along the left border of the sternum, along with a conspicuous retraction over the left ventricle, which gives the anterior chest a rocking motion that is synchronous with the heart beat, is suggestive of right ventricular hypertrophy.

When right-sided heart failure develops, the condition is called *cor pulmonale.* The correlation between the severity of the pulmonary hypertension and the development of right-sided heart failure is not perfect. In general, however, it has been suggested that a sustained mean pulmonary artery pressure above 40 mm. Hg is associated with a significant alteration in the electrocardiographic tracing and the radiologic evidence of an enlarged right ventricle.

EXTRAPULMONARY MANIFESTATIONS

CLUBBING OF THE DIGITS

Clubbing of the fingers and the toes is an important manifestation of certain types of intrathoracic disease, and therefore is of great diagnostic significance. Digital clubbing is most commonly associated with an intra-thoracic malignancy such as a **bronchogenic carcinoma** or a **mesothelioma**. However, it may also occur in association with suppurative diseases of the lung, such as **bronchiectasis, empyema** and **lung abscess;** in **congenital heart diseases** associated with a right-to-left shunt; and in **subacute bacterial endocarditis.** Occasionally, clubbing is seen in patients suffering from hepatic or gastrointestinal disease, particularly those characterized by chronic diar-rhea, such as **ulcerative colitis** and **steatorrhea.**

Clubbing consists of a painless, nontender enlargement of the terminal phalanges of the fingers and toes, and is usually bilateral. Initially there is hypertrophy of the soft tissues covering the root of the nail, so that the angle formed by the root of the nail and the nail bed (normally about 160 degrees) is 180 degrees or more (Fig. 71). As clubbing progresses, the skin becomes stretched and glistening. The nail gradually thickens, becomes curved and develops longitudinal ridges, and the pulp of the terminal phalanx enlarges and develops a bulbous appearance. In the advanced stages of clubbing, the nail is thickened, ridged and curved both longitudinally and laterally, and its distal end overrides the end of the finger (Fig. 72).

Clubbing of the digits usually progresses slowly, often taking months or years to develop. Occasionally it may develop acutely in the course of a

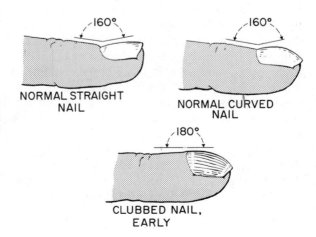

Figure 71. The "base angle" in a normal digit, a digit with a curved nail and a digit with early clubbing.

NORMAL STRAIGHT NAIL

NORMAL CURVED NAIL

CLUBBED NAIL, EARLY

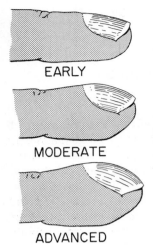

EARLY

MODERATE

ADVANCED

Figure 72. The progressive changes seen in finger clubbing. The nail thickens and becomes curved and overrides the end of the finger; the pulp of the terminal phalanx enlarges and has a bulbous appearance.

week or so if the underlying intrathoracic lesion is an acute septic process. Regression and even disappearance of digital clubbing may take place if the underlying lesion is eradicated by either medical or surgical treatment.

Pathogenesis of Clubbing

The pathologic changes in digital clubbing are the same no matter what the underlying cause. There is proliferation of the fibroelastic tissue, interstitial edema, and dilation and engorgement of the arterioles and venules. There is evidence of an increased blood flow through dilated arteriovenous anastomoses, which are very prevalent in the pulp of the terminal phalanges.

Although several theories have been advanced, the exact mechanism leading to clubbing in apparently unrelated diseases remains unexplained and is still open to conjecture. The most attractive explanation is that tissue hypoxia causes an increase in the number of arteriovenous anastomoses in the digits. This is supported by the fact that changes similar to clubbing may develop when a right-to-left shunt is produced experimentally in animals. Although tissue hypoxia may be the mechanism in pulmonary or cardiovascular disease and even in some hepatic conditions associated with right-to-left shunting, it is difficult to imagine this mechanism in patients with *steatorrhea* or *ulcerative colitis*. In addition, digital clubbing is rarely associated with chronic anemia, which can be associated with considerable tissue hypoxia.

Some investigators believe that clubbing occurs when the left ventricle delivers more blood than is necessary to meet the needs of the tissues, so that the digital blood pressure is elevated and blood flow is increased, thereby increasing the growth of the digital tissues. Chronic infection has also been proposed as a factor, since clubbing is often present in suppurative pulmonary diseases. Finally, reflex neurogenic factors have been implicated, because surgical removal of a pulmonary tumor often lessens the degree of digital clubbing. Clearly, however, such an operative procedure may also reduce venous admixture and therefore lessen the hypoxemia, so that this may explain the improvement.

HYPERTROPHIC PULMONARY OSTEOARTHROPATHY

Clubbing of the digits may progress to a condition called *hypertrophic pulmonary osteoarthropathy,* in which the gross, bulbous, enlarged terminal digital phalanges and thickened curved nails are associated with a painful, tender thickening of the wrists, ankles and long bones of the forearms and the legs. The basic pathologic process is a proliferating subperiostitis with subperiosteal new bone formation in the distal part of the long bones of the arms and legs and thickening of the connective tissue. A clear viscous effusion along with synovitis may develop in the joints of the knees, ankles and wrists. Osteoarthopathy is most frequently associated with carcinomas of the lung, particularly those in the periphery of the lung, or with central necrosis. In advanced cases the bones of the hands, feet, face and ribs may be involved, so that the individual may appear to be acromegalic.

RARE SYSTEMIC MANIFESTATIONS

When a lung tumor metastasizes to distant sites, such as the bones, liver, brain or adrenal glands, there may be manifestations that are related to the tissue or organ involved. In addition, bizarre systemic manifestations that bear no relationship to the site of metastases are occasionally seen, particularly in patients suffering from bronchogenic carcinoma, although they also occur with other primary tumors elsewhere.

Many of these systemic manifestations appear to be mediated or influenced by hormone-like polypeptides that are secreted by bronchogenic tumors of the anaplastic or *"oat-cell type."* A variety of endocrine disorders have been described, the most common being *Cushing's syndrome,* which is apparently produced by a substance similar to corticotropin. The syndrome of hyponatremia and an elevated urine osmolarity is apparently caused by excessive production of a polypeptide resembling antidiuretic hormone. The *carcinoid syndrome,* which consists of facial flushing, diarrhea and wheezing has also been reported in association with an oat cell carcinoma and is caused by the production of a substance similar to 5-hydroxytryptamine. Hypercalcemia, polyuria and weakness may be present, and even coma may rarely occur, as a result of the secretion of a parathyroid-like hormone. Finally, a number of patients with hypertrophic pulmonary osteoarthropathy have an associated *gynecomastia,* which has been attributed to abnormal estrogen metabolism.

Neuromuscular disorders may also develop in association with broncho-genic carcinoma. Cortical degeneration with a loss of Purkinje cells in the cerebellar cortex results in the rapid loss of function. In addition, peripheral neuropathy, which may be purely sensory or mixed (i.e., with both sensory and motor components) occasionally occurs.

Finally, dermatologic disorders may develop in association with a bronchogenic carcinoma. **Dermatomyositis,** in which an erythematous rash predominantly affecting the face and upper thorax is associated with weak-ness of the muscles of the shoulders and hips, occasionally develops in patients suffering from a **bronchogenic carcinoma** and often appears several months before the lung lesion is discovered. **Acanthosis nigricans,** a rare skin disease consisting of darkly pigmented verrucal lesions predominantly in the skin folds of the body, usually signifies an intra-abdominal cancer, but it also has been reported in association with lung cancer.

ASSESSMENT OF RESPIRATORY DISEASE

- CLINICAL ASSESSMENT
- RADIOLOGIC ASSESSMENT
- LABORATORY ASSESSMENT

11

CLINICAL ASSESSMENT

From the foregoing section, it is apparent that by eliciting the symptoms and signs that have resulted from a disturbance in the respiratory system, one is in a position to arrive at a tentative conclusion about the pattern and general nature of the patient's illness. A careful interview of the patient with a complete assessment of the chronologic development of a patient's symptoms, in conjunction with a thorough, systematic physical examination, usually establishes a tentative diagnosis as well as any impairment that has resulted. Confirmation and refinement of the diagnosis usually involve radiologic and laboratory investigations.

INTERVIEW OF THE PATIENT

To obtain an accurate picture of the problems that led the patient to seek medical advice, it is most important that the physician establish rapport with the patient and gain the patient's complete confidence. The patient should be treated with kindness, consideration and tact during the interview. Although specific questions may be necessary at times, it is usually a wise policy to allow patients to relate their stories in their own way, with just enough prompting and guidance to prevent irrelevancies. One should use words and phrases that the patient can understand, and avoid asking leading questions, for this may often result in an incorrect reply. On the other hand, leading questions may occasionally be necessary in order to elicit certain pertinent points, especially if the patient happens to be garrulous.

The entire historical aspect of the patient's illness should be recorded in an orderly, consecutive fashion. The following sequence is recommended: present complaints; personal and family history; previous illnesses and medical examinations; review of the nonrespiratory systems; medications taken in the past or currently being taken; and finally, a detailed history of the current illness.

PRESENTING COMPLAINTS

The complaints that led the patient to seek medical advice are, in effect, a capsule account of the patient's illness. These symptoms should be enumerated in a chronologic order and recorded with their approximate dates of development. It is best to begin by asking patients when they last felt well and then noting each symptom in the order its onset. With this information, the examiner can determine whether one is dealing with a chronic, a subacute or an acute illness and whether it has remained stationary, progressed in severity or been complicated by subacute or acute exacerbations.

PERSONAL HISTORY

The patient's background, living habits, hobbies and environment may have some bearing and may even play an important role in the development of the illness.

Background

The date of birth, birthplace, racial origin and economic status of the patient's parents should be recorded. An early life of extreme poverty, with malnourishment and poor hygienic standards, may have predisposed the patient to the development of various diseases, such as *tuberculosis* in childhood. Certain ethnic groups, such as the native Indian and Eskimo, are especially susceptible to tuberculosis. The level of education and the age at which the patient left school often provide considerable information about the extent of insight into the complaints.

Personal Habits

Susceptibility to disease may be increased because of an inadequate protein intake, which may occur in individuals who diet injudiciously to lose weight or in chronic *alcoholism,* when alcohol may be sacrificed for food. In contrast, gross overeating and *obesity* may in themselves lead to respiratory insufficiency or cardiac failure.

A history of the patient's smoking habits is clearly essential and should include the age at which smoking began; the current daily consumption of cigarettes, cigars or pipe tobacco; and the average cigarette consumption to date. If the patient has stopped smoking, the date of smoking cessation should be recorded along with the reasons for stopping, for it may have been because of cough, breathlessness or wheezing. Cigarette smoking is associated with the development of *bronchogenic carcinoma* and is particularly important in the pathogenesis and perpetuation of *chronic bronchitis and emphysema.* For reasons that are as yet not fully understood, the prevalence of chronic bronchitis or bronchogenic carcinoma among pipe and cigar smokers is only slightly higher than that of nonsmokers.

Hobbies and Pets

Close contact with pets or flowering plants may be important. Diseased pigeons or budgerigars or the mere repeated contact with a number of birds (or their droppings) may be the cause of an *acute hypersensitivity pneumonitis.* Attacks of *asthma* may be precipitated by exposure to the dander of dogs, cats or horses, as well as to the pollen of flowering plants. It is important to emphasize that individuals who have become allergic to their house pets have a tendency to deny any association between their symptoms and exposure to the pets.

Residence

A detailed chronologic account of the specific areas of residence or those visited in the past should be obtained. Certain countries are notorious for the prevalence of endemic diseases, especially those that are fungal in origin. *Histoplasmosis* is endemic in the valleys of the great rivers of North America, such as the Mississippi, the Ohio and the St. Lawrence. *Coccidioidomycosis* is common in the deserts of California, Arizona, and northern Mexico, and *schistosomiasis* is prevalent in Puerto Rico, Central America, and Egypt.

An area may be particularly polluted or have a high concentration of pollens or molds. The types of atmospheric pollens and saprophytic mold spores vary from one geographic area to another. Since patients with *rhinitis* or *asthma* caused by pollen allergies have increased symptoms at particular times of the year, it is important to know the time and duration of the seasons for tree, grass and weed pollens and for saprophytic mold spores in the patient's locale. In addition, the importance of mites as a major component of the house dust allergens varies a great deal from one geographic area to another, depending on the climatic condition and home environment. A moist, warm climate and suboptimal cleanliness in the home presumably present favorable conditions for mite growth.

Occupation

A detailed and complete occupational history, beginning with the patient's first employment and including the duration of each job, may point to the pattern of the disease that is present. For instance, underground work in a mine, even 20 to 30 years previously, may be responsible for the development of *silicosis.* Occupational exposure to a high level of irritants such as smoke, dust, or fumes may lead to the development of *chronic bronchitis and emphysema;* the manufacturing of fluorescent light bulbs to *berylliosis;* the cotton industry to *byssinosis;* and meat wrapping to *asthma;* the inhalation of asbestos fibers predisposes one to *asbestosis, mesothelioma* or a *bronchogenic carcinoma.*

Farming may be associated with the development of variety of respiratory diseases. Acute *interstitial pneumonitis* or *obliterative bronchiolitis* may follow the inhalation of nitrogen dioxide fumes in a silo; a *hypersensitivity pneumonitis* may be induced by fungal spores in moldy hay *(farmer's lung); histoplasmosis* may develop in chicken farmers; and *asthma* may result from the inhalation of grain dust. Although there may be no obvious work-related exposure, one should inquire about surrounding industries, because the air intake of a heating or air conditioning system may be near a source of a particular antigen.

Finally, exhausting labor in poorly ventilated surroundings, as well as insufficient rest, may contribute to a reduced resistance to disease. Worries over financial difficulties or the anxiety associated with the pressure of employment may also contribute to mental fatigue.

FAMILY HISTORY

All serious illnesses, whether acute or chronic, that may have affected any member of the patient's immediate family should be recorded, together with the cause of death of any deceased relative. This is important because it may direct attention to a possible hereditary predisposition to certain diseases, such as *cystic fibrosis, atopy* or *alpha-1-antitrypsin deficiency,* or it may indicate contact with an infectious disease, such as *tuberculosis,* during some period in the patient's life.

PREVIOUS ILLNESSES AND MEDICAL EXAMINATIONS

All illnesses or injuries suffered by the patient in the past, including the infectious diseases of childhood, should be elicited. In the case of *asthma,* there may have been a previous episode of *infantile eczema, atopic dermatitis* or *allergic rhinitis. Measles* or *pertussis* in childhood, especially if prolonged or complicated by pneumonia, may have led to the development of *bronchiectasis,* which should be suspected if there is a history of repeated episodes of pneumonia affecting the same area of the lungs. A *bronchogenic carcinoma* should be suspected when repeated episodes of pneumonia involving the same area occur in a middle-aged or elderly individual. Chronic sinus infection or postnasal discharge may be the source of attacks of recurrent bronchitis. A *lung abscess* should be suspected if the illness followed either a dental extraction or an operation on the upper respiratory tract. *Sarcoidosis* should be suspected if there is a past history of either enlarged, painless lymph nodes, dimness of vision in one or both eyes, a chronic skin eruption or *erythema nodosum,* especially if these episodes disappeared spontaneously. *Tuberculosis* should be suspected if the patient has suffered from a draining abscess in a lymph node or if there is a history of a *pleural effusion.*

REVIEW OF THE NONRESPIRATORY SYSTEMS

A functional enquiry into the nonrespiratory systems is important because certain respiratory illnesses may be the consequence of disease processes that primarily affect other organs. For example, a *renal carcinoma* may have metastasized to the lung, or a pneumonitis may be due to aspiration of gastric juices because of *esophageal reflux.*

Nervous System

A cerebral metastasis from a *bronchogenic carcinoma,* a cerebral abscess secondary to *bronchiectasis,* or *tuberculous meningitis,* may cause a severe intractable throbbing headache, vertigo, diplopia, drowsiness, confusion, disorientation, syncopal attacks and convulsions. On the other hand, many of these symptoms may also be due to hypoxemia and carbon dioxide retention. Paresthesias, muscular wasting and limb weakness may be due to a *peripheral neuropathy,* which occasionally complicates a *bronchogenic carcinoma.*

Emotional disturbances may be responsible for many of the patient's complaints. The thought that respiratory symptoms may be due to some incurable organic disease may engender symptoms of anxiety and apprehension in any patient, and as a result, the patient may experience irritability, depression and emotional upsets, as well as difficulty in sleeping. Occasionally, the emotional disturbances may lead to numbness and tingling in the extremities as well as faintness, as a result of chronic hyperventilation.

Cardiovascular System

Cough and dyspnea are also cardinal symptoms of cardiovascular disease. The development of orthopnea and the need for more pillows when lying down suggests the onset of left ventricular failure. A recent attack of severe substernal pain followed by dyspnea suggests the possibility of a *myocardial infarction* with consequent pulmonary congestion. An increase in exertional dyspnea, and the development of ankle swelling in a patient suffering from a respiratory disease may herald the development of *cor pulmonale.* Pleuritic chest pain in a patient who is suffering from heart failure, or a swollen, painful and tender limb suggests the possibility of *pulmonary embolism.*

Gastrointestinal System

Aspiration of esophageal contents into the tracheobronchial tree may occur if there is difficulty in swallowing because of a stricture or malignant involvement of the esophagus. Aspiration may also occur as a result of *esophageal reflux,* with or without a hiatus hernia, particularly in patients receiving aminophylline or beta-2 agonists. Anorexia and vague dyspeptic complaints may be associated with active pulmonary *tuberculosis* or any other chronic infective bronchopulmonary disease, such as *bronchiectasis.* Postprandial epigastric pain that is relieved by food or alkalies suggests *peptic ulceration,* which is occasionally seen in patients suffering from *emphysema* or other chronic diseases. Chronic diarrhea may indicate a *carcinoid tumor of the bowel, tuberculous enteritis, adrenal insufficiency* resulting from **tuberculosis** or malignant metastases. It may also be due to **amyloidosis** in a patient suffering from a suppurative pulmonary disease.

Genitourinary System

Frequency, dysuria and hematuria may be due to **renal tuberculosis.** Hematuria may also be due to a **renal carcinoma.** A painful or swollen testicle may be due to tuberculous or malignant involvement. Amenorrhea often accompanies pulmonary tuberculosis as well as many other wasting diseases.

Metabolic System

Fatigue, weakness, and weight loss occur frequently in patients suffering from chronic respiratory diseases. Considerable weight loss can occur fairly rapidly in active pulmonary tuberculosis or malignancy. Conversely, excessive weight may lead to alveolar hypoventilation and symptoms of hypoxemia and carbon dioxide retention.

Locomotor System

If clubbing of the fingers has been noted by the patient, the date it was first detected should be established, if possible. A recent onset suggests a malignant process. *"Familial clubbing,"* a hereditary form of bilateral digital clubbing that is present at birth but is slowly progressive and only becomes evident at puberty, is not associated with any organic disease. Pain and tenderness in the lower parts of the patient's forearms and legs may be due to **hypertrophic pulmonary osteoarthropathy.** A fine tremor may implicate **hyperthyroidism** as the cause of dyspnea. On the other hand, a flapping tremor such as that which occurs with hepatic coma, is seen in association with severe carbon dioxide retention and acidemia. Painful, tender, discolored areas of **erythema nodosum** commonly develop over the extensor surfaces of the legs and may be due to tuberculosis, sarcoidosis or coccidioidomycosis. Weakness in specific groups of muscles may suggest **poliomyelitis, infectious polyneuritis** or a myopathy caused by a pulmonary malignancy.

MEDICATIONS

Current medications as well as those taken in the past should be itemized. Some or all of the patient's symptoms may be related to the side effects of these drugs. For instance, the development of wheezing and shortness of breath may be related to the administration of a beta-blocking agent, aspirin or acetylsalicylic acid (ASA), which is present in the great majority of pain remedies, and interstitial lung disease may be a complication of the administration of furadantoin or other drugs.

HISTORY OF THE PRESENT ILLNESS

With the background information obtained by the judicious questioning, as suggested above, one is equipped to tackle the important aspect of the history of the respiratory illness itself.

A chronologic description of the respiratory illness should be obtained, beginning from the time the patient last felt "completely well." The evolution of the illness and the symptomatology, as well as their course, should be carefully noted. Precipitating factors should be painstakingly searched for. If it is an acute illness, a description of its day-by-day or even hour-by-hour manifestations should be elicited. If it is a chronic illness, the progression of events from month to month or year to year is important.

Having obtained this general picture of the illness, the physician should now obtain a more detailed description of each symptom. The date and mode of onset of each symptom, whether acute or gradual; its progress, whether continuous or recurrent; and its development, whether progressive or stationary, should all be carefully elucidated.

The mechanism of development and the significance of the symptoms associated with respiratory disorders have already been discussed in a previous section. The following discussion indicates the type of the questions that should be asked in order to obtain a complete description of each symptom.

Cough

If cough is present, its approximate time of onset and its progress should be recorded. If there are acute exacerbations of cough, the frequency and duration of the attacks and whether they are becoming more frequent, more prolonged or more severe, as well as any known precipitating factors, should be determined. If the cough is fairly constant, one should note the effect of smoking, seasonal weather changes, dust, irritating fumes or other precipitating factors. A cough that is aggravated by a change in posture suggests **bronchiectasis.**

A harassing cough of recent onset suggests an acute infection. Repeated episodes of coughing with free intervals between the attacks is a feature of recurrent bronchitis as well as hyperreactive airways. Indeed, chest tightness and cough, which may or may not be associated with wheezing, are the commonest complaints of a patient with **asthma.** A chronic recurring cough that persists for approximately three months during each year for at least two successive years and is not associated with any localized bronchopulmonary disease is a feature of **chronic bronchitis.**

Expectoration

A cough may be nonproductive initially and then may become productive with the expectoration of sputum. If this occurs, the approximate time of this change should be recorded. Both children and the occasional adult habitually swallow their sputum and therefore may not recognize or admit that they ever produce any sputum.

Although it may be difficult to be accurate, an approximate estimate of the amount of sputum that is currently being expectorated during a 24-hour period, as well as the amount previously expectorated, should be obtained. One can generally obtain a rough estimate of the amount of expectoration if the patient is asked to relate the amount to a common measure such as a cup, half-cup, tablespoon or teaspoon.

Pinkish, frothy, watery sputum is characteristic of acute pulmonary edema. The mucoid sputum of *chronic bronchitis* is usually white or gray, and, because it is quite viscous, it may be difficult to expectorate. In septic lesions of the lungs, such as bronchiectasis or a lung abscess, the sputum is usually thick and yellow, may have an unpleasant taste and occasionally an offensive odor. This purulent sputum is generally less viscous than mucoid sputum and is therefore easier to cough up. The sudden expectoration of a very large quantity of purulent sputum suggests that a *lung abscess* may have erupted into a major bronchus.

The presence or absence of a *postnasal discharge* should be noted, and its duration ascertained. The patient will recognize this as "phlegm" in the back of the throat, and if present, its color and consistency should be noted. Generally, the patient attempts to expectorate this material by "hawking" and clearing his throat rather than by coughing. Such a discharge may, of itself, induce a chronic cough by irritation of the posterior pharyngeal wall, or it may increase the amount of sputum expectorated, particularly in the morning.

Hemoptysis

The expectoration of blood is an alarming symptom that frequently prompts the patient to seek medical advice. In discussing the blood spitting with the patient, it is important to determine whether the expectorated material was pure blood or whether the sputum was stained, streaked, or spotted with blood. When frank blood is expectorated, it is generally bright red initially, and then it gradually darkens and decreases in amount over the next few days. The amount of blood that was expectorated should be ascertained, although this is often exaggerated by the patient.

Hemoptysis may occur in *pulmonary tuberculosis, bronchiectasis, bronchogenic carcinoma, pulmonary infarction* and *mitral stenosis*. A recent painful tender swelling in a lower extremity may point to a *thrombophlebitis* that has been followed by a *pulmonary embolus*. This may be encountered in individuals who have been confined to bed for long periods of time because of either *congestive heart failure, multiple fractures* or extensive surgery.

Blood-stained sputum may be caused by a *bronchogenic carcinoma*. Streaks or spots of blood in the sputum may be of less consequence and may be due to a hyperemic bronchial mucosa, which develops during an acute infection of the tracheobronchial tree.

The upper respiratory tract may be the source of expectorated blood, and if the patient had an epistaxis, the blood may have been aspirated into the trachea and then expectorated. The expectoration of blood may also occur in patients suffering from certain blood dyscrasias, such as *hemophilia* and *leukemia,* or those taking maintenance anticoagulant therapy for the treatment of a *myocardial infarction.* For this reason, it is necessary to determine whether there is or has been bleeding from other orifices, the gums, or the skin.

Occasionally, a patient may not be sure whether the blood was coughed up or vomited. The distinguished feature of hemoptysis is that the expectorated blood is generally bright red and frothy, whereas in a hematemesis, the blood is generally dark red without froth and often contains food particles. In addition, blood that originates in the stomach is usually associated with the passage of black, tarry stools.

Breathlessness

If breathlessness on exertion is present, its time of development and its progress should be noted. It may have remained fairly stationary over the course of the illness, gradually increased in severity, or increased episodically during acute exacerbations of the illness. It may occur spontaneously in the absence of any exertion, as in *asthma,* and the patient may be completely free of dyspnea between attacks.

An accurate assessment of the severity of the breathlessness is generally fairly difficult to obtain, because the degree of exercise tolerance is related to the amount of the physical activity habitually undertaken as well as the level of physical fitness. One can obtain a rough estimate by determining whether the patient was previously able to perform this level of exertion without any difficulty. As indicated earlier, the severity of the dyspnea should be semiquantitated by determining whether the breathlessness occurs while walking up a slight incline or a flight of stairs; while walking with others at a normal pace on level ground; while performing ordinary activities, such as dressing and shaving; or while sitting quietly at rest.

If the patient is breathless while lying down *(orthopnea)* and requires several pillows in order to be comfortable, pulmonary congestion secondary to left-sided heart failure must be considered. However, patients suffering from chronic airflow limitation may also be more comfortable in an upright position. Breathlessness that awakens the patient may be either cardiac or bronchial in origin. If due to left ventricular failure, it may be relieved by sitting up; if due to accumulated secretions, by the expectoration of sputum; and if due to bronchospasm, by inhalation of a bronchodilating agent.

Chest Pain

If chest pain is present, the time and the mode of onset, as well as its relationship to the other respiratory symptoms, should be ascertained. The anatomic site of the pain, its radiation, and its characteristics are most helpful in determining its cause. If the diaphragmatic pleura is involved, the pain will be felt along the superior ridge of the trapezius muscle of the affected side and along the costal margin. The squeezing anterior chest pain of myocardial ischemia, which may radiate into the neck and down one or both arms, is usually induced by exertion and relieved by rest. The raw, burning discomfort of *acute tracheitis* is usually situated over the upper anterior chest wall, and that due to *esophageal reflux* is over the lower sternum or upper abdomen and may simulate that of myocardial ischemia. An acute onset of chest pain may be due to a fractured rib or costal cartilage, a fibrinous pleurisy secondary to pneumonia, or a *pulmonary infarct*. Pain due to pleuritic involvement is usually sharp and knifelike, and is aggravated by deep breathing or coughing. On the other hand, pain due to *fibrositis* of the intercostal muscles is also aggravated by deep breathing and coughing.

Upper Respiratory Symptoms

The upper respiratory tract is often the cause of an aggravating factor in a patient's lower respiratory tract illness. Drainage from the upper respiratory tract may enter the tracheobronchial tree, particularly during sleep, and aggravate chronic airway disease. A purulent *postnasal discharge* indicates an infective process. Episodic attacks of profuse watery nasal discharge, nasal obstruction, paroxysmal sneezing spells, irritation of the eyes or marked tearing suggest *hay fever*. Attacks of *acute sinusitis* are often associated with pain and tenderness over the area overlying the affected sinus. A deviated nasal septum or polyps may cause constant nasal obstruction.

Hoarseness that develops immediately after a thyroidectomy suggests injury to one of the recurrent laryngeal nerves. It may also be due to ulceration of the larynx, which occasionally complicates an active *tuberculous cavity,* or to a localized growth on one of the vocal cords, whether benign or malignant.

Constitutional Symptoms

Feverishness, chilly sensations, excessive sweating, anorexia, weakness, easy fatiguability and weight loss may be associated with any chronic pulmonary disease and are especially common in *tuberculosis, bronchiectasis, pulmonary abscess* and *bronchogenic carcinoma*. *"Night sweats,"* necessitating a complete change of night clothes, may also occur in these diseases. Severe chills, associated with chattering of the teeth and involuntary shaking of the limbs, may occur with bacterial infections, particularly a *pneumococcal pneumonia.*

EXAMINATION OF THE PATIENT

After obtaining a detailed history of the patient's illness, the physician is able to put the pertinent aspects together into patterns that suggest several possible diagnoses. These various possibilities may now be strengthened and perhaps confirmed by abnormalities detected during the physical examination. While carrying out the examination, the examiner should be courteous and considerate and avoid unnecessary physical discomfort for the patient. In addition, the room temperature should be comfortable, and the lighting adequate.

Proficiency in the physical examination can be attained only by repeated examination of healthy individuals, as this will facilitate recognition of even a minimal abnormality. Just as a functional inquiry into the nonrespiratory systems is important in eliciting the history of the respiratory illness, a thorough and complete physical examination should be carried out in an orderly, systematic and consistent manner so that no abnormal physical signs will be missed. It is through errors of omission that failure to arrive at the correct diagnosis occurs.

Although it is not within the scope of this discussion to describe the technique of performing a complete physical examination, it is clear that respiratory disturbances may produce signs and symptoms referable to other systems. Indeed, abnormal physical findings in other organs frequently yield valuable clues about the nature of the respiratory illness. However, only those findings that may be helpful in the assessment of findings in the respiratory system will be referred to, and the majority of the discussion will deal with the examination of the respiratory system.

GENERAL OBSERVATION

Inspection of the patient, the initial phase of the physical examination, should be conducted conscientiously and very carefully. Much that is learned from observation is acquired automatically and unconsciously. For example, most individuals are able to guess the age of a casual acquaintance fairly accurately but are quite unable to describe the physical evidence upon which the judgment is based. Even lay individuals will habitually scrutinize someone and decide that the individual "looks well" or "does not look well." In a similar manner, experienced clinicians unconsciously gather valuable impressions, an occult faculty that largely accounts for what is termed "clinical intuition."

In the discussion that follows, some of the more common abnormalities that may be observed are enumerated and briefly discussed. Any single observation may be of little significance, but in combination with other signs, it may be of considerable value in arriving at a final assessment of the underlying respiratory disease.

The Head

It is impossible to enumerate all the factors that may be detected from even a casual glance at a patient's face, but one can usually determine whether the patient is in distress, and often one can estimate the mental capacity, temperament and mood of the patient.

The presence or absence of respiratory distress is particularly important, and one should attempt to ascertain whether there is inspiratory or expiratory difficulty. The respirations may be rapid, shallow and gasping in nature, or the lips may be pursed during expiration. The patient may be using the sternomastoid muscles and the other accessory muscles of respiration, and the alae nasae may widen during inspiration. Some patients attempt to relieve the respiratory difficulty by assuming a characteristic forward-leaning posture with both hands pressed on the thighs, if in the sitting position, or pressed against a chair or a desk if standing. Noisy breathing or wheezing suggests widespread airflow obstruction, and stridor indicates upper airway obstruction.

Other specific signs, such as the presence of respiratory distress, pallor, plethora, cyanosis, pigmentation or a rash, jaundice, edema, venous dilatation, emaciation, or obesity, should also be noted. Facial neurologic signs may suggest a localized lesion such as a *cerebral abscess* secondary to a *lung abscess* or *bronchiectasis* or a metastasis from a *bronchogenic carcinoma*. Confusion, irrational behavior and even hallucinations may be caused by severe respiratory insufficiency.

The Eyes

Exophthalmos may be due to *hyperthyroidism* or compression of the trachea by a substernal toxic thyroid gland. Examination of the fundi with the aid of an ophthalmoscope may reveal engorged retinal veins and swelling of the optic discs, which indicate increased cerebrospinal fluid pressure that is most often due to a cerebral lesion, although it is occasionally seen during acute respiratory failure. Small, yellowish, round miliary lesions in the choroid are diagnostic of *miliary tuberculosis.*

The pupils may be affected by respiratory disease. Irritation of the cervical sympathetic ganglia by a *bronchogenic carcinoma* in the apex of the lung, the so-called *thoracic inlet tumor,* or by the pressure of enlarged metastatic lymph nodes may cause dilatation of the pupil of that side. As the condition progresses, the sympathetic ganglia become paralyzed; this results in constriction of the affected pupil, narrowing of the palpebral fissure, and absence of sweating on the same side of the face, the so-called *Horner's syndrome.*

The Upper Respiratory Tract

As had been described earlier, diseases that affect the upper respiratory tract may be a cause of respiratory symptoms, or they may play a contributing role. Whether this particular portion of the respiratory tract is healthy or diseased can largely be determined by inspection. A searching examination of the mucous membranes of the nose, mouth, tongue, pharynx and larynx should therefore precede the examination of the lungs.

The Nose. The patency of each nasal passage should be tested by having the patient sniff through one passage while the other is obstructed. In addition, the interior of each nasal passage should be examined with either an otoscope or a nasal speculum, using a head mirror to reflect light into the passage. The appearance of the nasal mucosa as well as the character of any nasal discharge should be noted. Healthy nasal mucosa is smooth, pink and glistening in appearance, whereas an inflamed mucous membrane is dull and red. An allergic nasal mucosa appears swollen and pale and is associated with a thin, watery and clear nasal discharge. *Nasal polyps* have a glistening, grapelike appearance and are frequently associated with an allergic diathesis.

A deviated septum may be the cause of nasal obstruction. A thick yellow or green exudate in one or both passages or a purulent postnasal discharge points to a purulent infection. Fresh blood in one of the nasal passages may indicate the source of a recent episode of hemoptysis.

The Mouth. The buccal mucosa should be carefully examined for eruptions, petechiae, pigmentation, cyanosis or the reddish purple color associated with polycythemia. It is important to note the presence or absence of a *postnasal discharge* in the posterior pharynx and, if present, whether it is mucoid or purulent in appearance. The condition of the gums and the teeth should be checked, because poor dental care and pyorrhea may be factors in the development of bronchopulmonary diseases. A malodorous breath may be due to either improper oral hygiene and pyorrhea or a chronic infection of the tonsils, adenoids or nasal mucosa. In addition, any septic diseases of the lungs, such as *bronchiectasis* or a *lung abscess,* as well as pyloric obstruction may make the breath malodorous.

The Larynx. The larynx is usually not inspected routinely. However, it must be examined if the patient complains of hoarseness or a croupy cough or if stridor is evident. Indirect examination of the larynx provides a functional assessment of the vocal cords and causes very little discomfort to the patient. The patient's tongue is held out with some gauze, and a warmed laryngeal mirror is placed against the soft palate in front of the uvula. With the reflected light from a head mirror, the epiglottis, the arytenoid regions and the vocal cords can be viewed. Laryngoscopic examination of the larynx is more uncomfortable but is necessary if a biopsy of one of the vocal cords is contemplated.

Aphonia associated with a cough that seems to have lost its explosive character suggests paralysis of one of the vocal cords. This, in turn, is caused by pressure or injury of a recurrent laryngeal nerve, as can occur with a *bronchogenic carcinoma.* In this condition, the affected vocal cord sits midway between adduction and abduction during quiet respiration and fails to move toward the midline during phonation.

The Neck

A painful stiff neck caused by cervical disc degeneration may be associated with irritation of a cervical nerve root. Scars on the neck may be due to either previous draining sinuses or excision of tuberculous lymph nodes. Enlargement of the cervical nodes or the thyroid gland may be evident. Cervical lymphadenopathy may be due to either *tuberculosis, malignancy, sarcoidosis, infectious mononucleosis,* or a *lymphoma.* An enlarged, hard, fixed thyroid gland may be the source of pulmonary metastases.

The position, consistency, size and anatomic relations of any masses that are obvious on inspection should be determined in order to differentiate between lymph nodes, the thyroid gland or a soft tissue mass that may be of no significance. Palpation of the neck in the search for enlarged lymph nodes should be carried out with the fingertips, using gentle pressure and a rotary movement, in the posterior and the anterior triangles of the neck, the submental region, the supraclavicular areas and the area directly behind the clavicular insertion of the sternomastoid muscle.

Engorgement of the external jugular veins, as well as visible pulsation in them, in a patient who is lying propped up at an angle of 45 degrees (i.e., the veins are at a higher level than the right atrium) indicates that the central venous pressure is elevated. Bilateral distension of the jugular veins is usually due to **congestive heart failure,** although this may also be produced by **superior vena caval** obstruction, in which case collateral veins are visible over the neck and the anterior chest wall. Distension of both jugular veins during expiration, and their collapse during inspiration, are often seen in patients who are suffering from severe obstruction to airflow.

The Extremities

Inspection of the hands may reveal an intensely brown-stained thumb and index finger resulting from cigarette smoking. Pigmentation of the creases in the skin is suggestive of **Addison's disease.** Pallor in the palms, the nailbeds and finger pulps of the hands suggests anemia. For many reasons, this is a much safer reflection of the hemoglobin content than is the color of the face, which may be weather-beaten or disguised by cosmetics. The nail beds should also be examined for the presence or absence of **cyanosis** and **digital clubbing.**

The axillae, epitrochlear and inguinal regions should be examined to determine whether there are any enlarged lymph nodes. A painful, tender, thrombosed vein due to **thrombophlebitis** may account for the source of a **pulmonary embolus.** Bilateral edema of the extremities is caused by **congestive heart failure, renal failure, hypoproteinemia** or **inferior vena cava obstruction.** The typical deformed joints of **rheumatoid arthritis** may be associated with **diffuse pulmonary fibrosis.**

Atopic dermatitis or **urticaria** may be present in an allergic state. **Erythema nodosum** may occur in association with either **streptococcal sore throat, tuberculosis, sarcoidosis,** or **coccidioidomycosis.** Metastases from a **bronchogenic carcinoma** may develop in the subcutaneous tissues, where they may be felt as firm, nontender nodules. Chronic infiltrations in the skin may occur with either **sarcoidosis,** fungal infections or **histiocytosis "X."** Icterus is occasionally associated with a **pulmonary infarct.**

The Abdomen

The abdomen should be palpated to determine whether the liver or spleen is enlarged or if any abnormal masses are present. An enlarged liver may be due to **congestive heart failure,** metastatic infiltration from a **bronchogenic carcinoma,** a **lymphoma,** or an **amebic abscess.** A palpable spleen is found in association with a **lymphoma, sarcoidosis, septicemia,** or **subacute bacterial endocarditis.** A tumor involving the stomach, bowel, kidney or one of the ovaries may produce a palpable mass. A benign tumor of the ovary may be the cause of *Meig's syndrome,* a condition in which ascites and hydrothorax develop. A hard, fixed, nodular prostate suggests a malignant process that may be the source of pulmonary metastases. A *rectal carcinoma* is easily accessible to the examining finger. A *fistula-in-ano* should make one suspect a tuberculous etiology, especially if a pulmonary lesion is present.

External Genitalia

The scar of an old primary chancre from a syphilitic infection or an enlarged nontender *syphilitic orchitis* might explain the presence of an *aortic aneurysm.* A *tuberculous epididymitis* should make one suspect the possibility of active pulmonary *tuberculosis.*

EXAMINATION OF THE CHEST

Although abnormal findings elicited during the clinical examination of the chest reflect only certain patterns of disease and their approximate location, a presumptive clinical diagnosis often may be made when taken in conjunction with the systemic inquiry into the development of symptoms. The physical examination of the chest is directed at answering the following questions:

1. Is there an abnormality in the chest?
2. Does the disease process affect one or both lungs?
3. If the disease is present in both lungs, is it predominant in one lung or are both lungs equally affected?
4. Is the volume of the affected lung or lungs altered?
5. Is the density of the affected lung or lungs altered?
6. Is the transmission of sound altered?
7. Is pulmonary hypertension present?
8. Is ventilatory function impaired?
9. What is the extent of disability present?

Before proceeding with the physical examination of the chest, one must be thoroughly acquainted with the boundaries of the thoracic contents. With this knowledge, it is possible to have a mental picture of the anatomic location of any signs that are found. With this in mind, the landmarks, topographic lines and surface markings of the fissures, lobes and bronchopulmonary segments, and the pleurae will be reviewed.

Landmarks

The spinous processes of the thoracic vertebrae and the sternal angle serve as important landmarks that orient the examiner with regard to the position of the underlying thoracic contents. In the erect position with the head bent slightly forward, the first thoracic spinous process is the lower of two prominent projections at the junction of the neck and the thorax; the upper projection is the spinous process of the seventh cervical vertebra. The projection due to the third thoracic spinous process is at the level of the root of the spine of the scapula, and the seventh thoracic spinous process lies at the level of the inferior angle of the scapula. The kidney angle, which is at the junction of the posterior end of the costal margin and the sacrospinalis muscle, is situated at the level of the twelfth thoracic spinous process.

The sternal angle, which is also known as the angle of Louis, marks the attachment of the second costal cartilage, so that it serves as a landmark for the identification of the costal cartilage and the ribs. It is at the same level as the bifurcation of the trachea, and indicates the approximate upper level at which the lungs meet anteriorly and the upper borders of the atria of the heart. To determine if the venous pressure is abnormal, therefore, the arms must be elevated above the level of the sternal angle. If the pressure is normal, the veins will collapse when the arms are raised above this level.

Topographic Lines

Certain conventional topographic lines are used to demarcate various areas of the chest wall. The *midclavicular line* runs vertically downward over the anterior chest wall from the middle of the clavicle to the lower costal margin. The *anterior axillary line* runs vertically downward from the origin of the anterior axillary fold, and the *posterior axillary line* runs downward from the orgin of the termination of the posterior fold. The *midaxillary line* runs vertically downward over the lateral aspect of the chest wall from the middle of the apex of the axilla to the lower costal margin, midway between the anterior and the posterior axillary lines. The *midscapular line* runs vertically downward from the middle of the inferior angle of the scapula to the kidney angle.

Surface Markings

The apices of both lungs lie in the root of the neck, occupying an area that starts at the lower end of the sternoclavicular junction, curves upwards to about 2.5 cm. above the upper border of the clavicle, and then descends to the lower border of the clavicle at the junction of its lateral and middle thirds. The hilum of the lung, which is situated posteriorly within the chest, corresponds to a rectangular area that lies between the fourth, fifth and sixth thoracic vertebrae and is bordered laterally by the vertebral borders of both scapulae.

Pleural and Lung Borders. The anterior border of the right pleural space (and that of the right lung) runs from the sternoclavicular joint to the center of the angle of Louis and then down the sternum as far as the xiphisternal joint. The anterior border of the left pleural space runs from the left sternoclavicular joint to the center of the angle of Louis and then downward to the level of the fourth costal cartilage, where it turns laterally to the left border of the sternum. It then runs downward to the level of the seventh costal cartilage. The anterior border of the left lung runs just inside the pleural border until it reaches the fourth left costal cartilage; it then turns laterally, until it is about 3 cm. from the left sternal border, and then downward to the sixth costal cartilage, about 2.5 cm. from the border of the sternum.

The inferior borders of both pleural spaces and lungs run backward from the lower anterior margins, crossing the sixth ribs at the midclavicular line and the eighth ribs at the midaxillary lines. The lungs cross the midscapular lines at the tenth rib, and the pleurae cross at the twelfth rib. The posterior borders of both the pleurae and the lungs lie parallel to one another, that of the lungs being just lateral to the pleural borders, which lie about 2.5 cm. lateral to the thoracic spinous processes.

Fissures. The situation of the various lobes of both lungs is illustrated in Figures 73 to 75. The major, or *oblique, fissures* which separate the upper and lower lobes, run identical courses in both lungs. Their projections on the surface of the chest wall run obliquely downward from the second thoracic spinous process, curve around the chest over its posterior, lateral and anterior aspects, crossing the midaxillary line at the fifth rib, and end anteriorly at the inferior border of the sixth costal cartilage, midway between the midsternal and the midclavicular lines. When the patient is standing erect, with both hands behind the neck, the vertebral borders of both scapulae correspond to the posterior portions of both oblique fissures.

The minor, or *transverse, fissure* separates the upper and middle lobes of the right lung. The lingular segment of the left upper lobe corresponds to

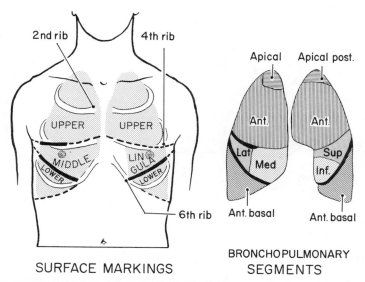

Figure 73. Surface markings of the lungs (anterior aspect). The underlying bronchopulmonary segments are also shown.

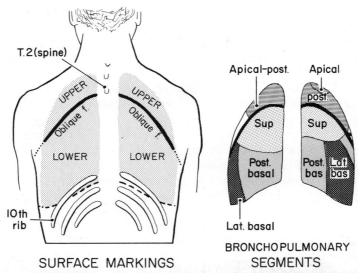

SURFACE MARKINGS

BRONCHOPULMONARY SEGMENTS

Figure 74. Surface markings of the lungs (posterior aspect). The underlying bronchopulmonary segments are also shown.

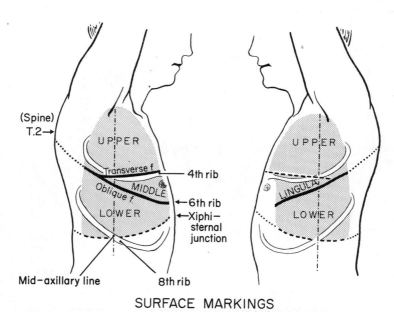

SURFACE MARKINGS

Figure 75. Surface markings of the lungs (lateral aspect).

the right middle lobe, although a true fissure is generally absent. The transverse fissure can be outlined on the chest wall by a line that starts anteriorly at the level of the third or fourth intercostal space on the right and passes laterally, in a slightly upward direction, ending at the point where the oblique fissure crosses the midaxillary line.

Bronchopulmonary Segments. The lobes of the lungs can be further subdivided into bronchopulmonary segments (Fig. 73–74). The surface markings of the *anterior segments* of both upper lobes lie anteriorly between the levels of the clavicle and the transverse fissure. The *apical segment* of the right lung lies predominantly anteriorly above the clavicle, and to a small extent posteriorly in the apex of the lung. The *posterior segment* occupies the remainder of the posterior aspect of the right upper lobe. The *apical-posterior segment* of the left upper lobe occupies an area on the left side that is equivalent to that occupied by the apical and the posterior segments of the right upper lobe.

The right middle lobe is divided into a *medial segment,* which occupies the anterior surface of the chest wall, and a *lateral segment,* which occupies the remaining area overlying the anterior portion of the axilla. The lingular segment of the left upper lobe lies under an area of the left anterior chest wall that is identical to that of the right middle lobe. The lingula is also divided into two bronchopulmonary segments: a *superior segment,* which occupies approximately the upper half of the area, and an *inferior segment,* which occupies the lower half.

The surface markings of the two lower lobes are very similar. The superior, or *apical, segment,* occupies the upper part of the posterior aspect of the lower lobe; its upper boundary is the oblique fissure, and its lower border corresponds approximately to the spinous process of the seventh thoracic vertebra. The remainder of the posterior aspect of the lower lobe is occupied by the *posterior basal segment.* The *lateral basal segment* occupies the axillary aspect of the lower lobe, whereas the *anterior basal segment* occupies that part of the lower lobe which lies under the anterior chest wall. The *medial basal segment* of the right lower lobe lies next to the mediastinum and so has no comparable area over the surface of the chest wall.

The Heart. The apex beat of the heart, which corresponds to the apex of the left ventricle, can often be seen as well as felt in the fifth left intercostal space, about 8 to 9 cm. from the midline of the sternum. The left border of the heart, which is formed by the left atrial appendage superiorly and by the left ventricle, starts 2.5 cm. from the left sternal border at the level of the second costal cartilage and runs laterally to the apex of the heart. The right border of the heart, which is formed entirely by the right atrium, corresponds to a line that is slightly convex to the right, running between the third and sixth costal cartilages, about 1 cm. from the right sternal border. The superior border of the heart, which is formed by the right and left atria, corresponds to a line drawn between the upper ends of the right and left borders. The inferior border of the heart, which is formed predominantly by the right ventricle, is located by a line that joins the lower ends of the right and left borders and passes over the xiphisternal joint. Normally, the borders of the pericardial sac correspond to those of the heart.

Inspection

There are wide variations in the contour of the normal chest cage, but its bony structure is generally symmetrical, largely because the thoracic spine is normally straight. Consequently, alterations in the contour of the thoracic cage are produced by deformities of the spine. These may be easily overlooked unless the thoracic spine is routinely examined by both inspection and palpation of the spinous processes. In *scoliosis,* the lateral margins of the thoracic vertebrae are widely spaced on the convex side, and converged on the concave side. In *kyphosis* the convexity of the curvature of the thoracic spine is directly backward; so that the ribs are crowded and the chest and sternum bulge forward anteriorly, producing a pigeon-breast type of deformity. *Angular kyphosis,* which is less common and which results from a destructive lesion of one or more vertebral bodies by *tuberculous osteomyelitis,* can also produce this type of deformity. **Kyphoscoliosis,** a combination of kyphosis and scoliosis, is most often due to postural abnormalities, and the underlying lungs are not usually affected. A severe form of kyphoscoliosis follows *poliomyelitis*, which affects the spinal muscles; here, one side of the chest may be very retracted and the opposite side may protrude markedly.

The *funnel-chest deformity,* an abnormal depression of the lower end of the sternum and its attached costal cartilages, and the *pigeon-breast deformity,* a protrusion of the lower end of the sternum with its attached cartilages, are generally of no serious significance. However, a severe funnel-chest deformity may so distort and compress the mediastinum that cardiac, as well as respiratory, embarrassment may develop in later years.

Unequal movement of the two sides of the chest suggests that there is an underlying condition on the side whose movement is decreased. In diffuse obstructive disease, the chest may move up and down "as a whole" during breathing. Paradoxical movement of the costal margin (i.e., inward during inspiration and outward during expiration) suggests depression of the diaphragm. In addition, inspiratory "in-drawing" of the intercostal spaces may be seen in the lower lateral areas of the chest cage in *interstitial fibrosis* and *emphysema.*

If the cardiac impulse is visible, its exact position, character and intensity should be noted. A shift away from the normal position may indicate an underlying pulmonary problem, and the character of the impulse may suggest either right or left ventricular enlargement. Engorged superficial veins over the chest wall suggest either a partial or complete obstruction of the superior vena cava. If the vena azygos is still patent, the veins will be dilated only over the upper half of the anterior chest wall; if it is obstructed, the veins will be dilated over the entire anterior chest wall.

Palpation

An alteration in volume of the chest cage on one side is reflected by a shift of the mediastinum from its normal midline position. This is assessed by palpation of the position of the trachea and the apex beat of the heart. Of the two, the trachea is a more sensitive index of the position of the mediastinum, because the heart does not shift as easily. The trachea should be palpated at the level of the suprasternal notch, because minor deviations of the mediastinal position are not obvious at higher levels. As is shown in Figure 76, the tip of the fully extended index finger is inserted into the patient's suprasternal notch, just medial to one sternoclavicular joint, and then gently pressed backward toward the cervical spine, first on one side and then on the other. If the trachea is in its normal midline position, the resistance felt by the examining finger will be equal on both sides. If it is deviated to one side, the examining finger will encounter the cartilaginous rings of the trachea on the side to which the trachea is deviated and only soft tissue on the other side. It is important to note that in many elderly individuals, the trachea may normally be shifted to the right, because of the pressure of an elongated atherosclerotic arch of the aorta.

The most lateral point at which a definite localized systolic thrust is felt when the tip of the index finger explores the third to the sixth intercostal spaces from the left midaxillary line to the middle of the sternum defines the position of the apex beat of the heart. It is normally felt in the fifth left interspace about 9 cm. from the midsternum, but it may be difficult to palpate, especially in sthenic or obese subjects or in patients who are hyperinflated because of chronic airflow limitation. In these individuals, the action of the heart may be seen and felt in the epigastrium.

If the apex beat of the heart is displaced to the left but the trachea is situated centrally, then left ventricular hypertrophy is the likely cause. Both

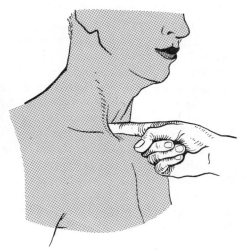

Figure 76. Palpation for the position of the trachea. The tip of the fully extended finger is inserted just medial to the sternoclavicular joint; the part of the trachea just before entrance to the thoracic inlet is the most mobile and reflects shifts of the mediastinum.

the trachea and apex beat may be shifted by an abnormality of the thoracic cage, a lung lesion or a disorder of the pleural space. In a thoracic cage deformity, they are displaced to the side of the compressed underlying lung. In atelectasis or a localized fibrosis, they are displaced to the side of the diseased lung, and in a pleural effusion or pneumothorax, they are shifted to the opposite side. The mediastinum may also be shifted to the opposite side when abdominal contents herniate into the thorax.

The intensity of the cardiac impulse should be determined by firmly placing the palm of the hand over the patient's left inframammary region. Normally a localized systolic thrust is felt, but if left ventricular hypertrophy is present, a systolic heave may be imparted to the ribs. If right ventricular hypertrophy is present, there may be a systolic thrust close to the left sternal border and a simultaneous retraction over the left ventricle, resulting in a rocking motion.

Source of Chest Pain. If the patient complains of chest pain, one should search carefully and systematically for tender areas in the chest wall. The patient should first outline the borders of the painful area on the chest wall. Then, starting well away from this area, the tip of the thumb should be pressed firmly along the course of the ribs and the intercostal spaces.

A localized area of exquisite tenderness and a grating sensation may be felt at the site of a fractured rib cartilage. A localized area of tenderness in an intercostal space may also indicate fibrositis of an intercostal muscle. With subluxation of a costal cartilage, the pain will be reproduced by squeezing the ribs on either side of th dislocated cartilage.

Chest pain suggestive of nerve root irritation can be confirmed by demonstration of a zone of hyperalgesia at the site of the pain by drawing the point of a needle or pin across the skin from above and below the painful area.

Movement. Diminished movement of a part of the chest is the earliest evidence of reduced distensibility of a portion of the lung, often developing before any other clinical abnormality can be detected.

Movement of the upper lobes is checked anteriorly over the first four ribs (Fig. 77) while the patient is sitting or lying and facing the examiner. The palms of both hands are placed firmly over the upper anterior chest wall with the fingers extended over the trapezius muscles. The palms of the hands are dragged downward, until they lie firmly over the infraclavicular areas, the extended fingers remaining over the supraclavicular regions. With the thumbs kept fully extended, the skin is pulled medially toward the sternum by the hands until the tips of both thumbs meet at the midsternal line. The examiner's elbows and shoulders should be maintained in a relaxed state with only the wrists applying pressure to the chest wall. In this way, the shoulders can act as a fulcrum that helps to exaggerate the movement of the hands. If both lungs are healthy, the hand will move an equal distance from each other when the patient inspires deeply. It is the comparison of the two sides that is important. If one side is diseased, then its

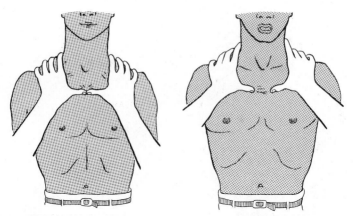

Figure 77. Examination of the movement of the upper lobes. Both hands move an equal distance with inspiration.

movement will be diminished, or if the disease process is minimal, there may be a lag in movement at the beginning of the inspiration.

Movement of the right middle lobe and the lingular segment of the left upper lobe is assessed by placing the widely outstretched fingers of both hands over the posterior axillary folds high up in the axillae, with the palms lying flat against the chest wall. The underlying skin is then pulled medially until the outstretched thumbs meet at the midsternal line, and the hands are allowed to follow the chest movement (Fig. 78).

Movement of the lower lobes is assessed while the patient sits with his back to the examiner. As is shown in Figure 79, the examiner places both hands high up in the axilla with the outstretched fingers overlying the anterior

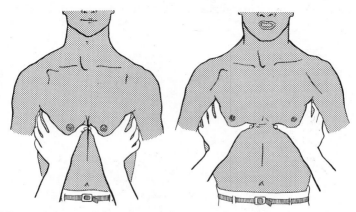

Figure 78. Examination of the movement of the middle lobe and lingula. Both hands move an equal distance with inspiration.

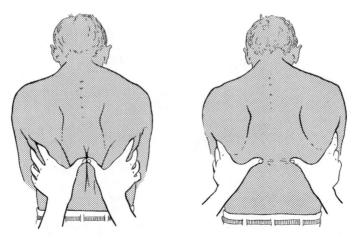

Figure 79. Examination of the movement of the lower lobes. Both hands move an equal distance with inspiration.

axillary folds. Both hands are then drawn medially, pulling the underlying skin with them until the outstretched thumbs meet in the midline over the vertebral spinous processes. They are then allowed to follow the movement of the chest.

Because of its dome shape, the diaphragm also causes inspiratory elevation of the lower ribs. To determine the diaphragmatic movement, the examiner stands beside the supine patient and places both hands lightly over the lower anterior chest wall, with the thumbs overlying the respective costal margins and almost meeting in the midline over the xiphoid process. As is shown in Figure 80, the examiner's thumbs normally move apart equally when the patient inspires deeply. If the diaphragm is no longer dome shaped, as occurs when the lungs are hyperinflated or there is fluid or air in the pleural space, the costal margins may move inward on inspiration.

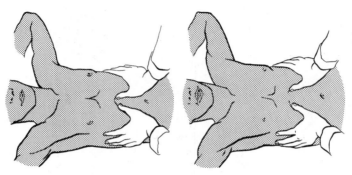

Figure 80. Examination of the action of the diaphragm on the costal margins. Both hands move an equal distance with inspiration.

Fremitus. Palpation of the vibrations produced over the thoracic wall by the conduction of vocal sounds through the tracheobronchial tree and the lung parenchyma is known as *tactile fremitus.* The side of the hand is applied to the chest wall at different locations while the patient slowly repeats a combination of words such as "one, two, three" or "ninety-nine." The intensity of tactile fremitus is normally uniform over healthy lungs, although it is often increased over the apex of the right lung because the bronchi are closer to the chest wall.

All areas of both sides of the chest should be compared with one another in order to detect any abnormality. Often there is a striking change from normal fremitus to an increase or decrease when the side of the hand reaches a diseased area. The intensity of the fremitus is greater when the density of the underlying lung parenchyma is increased, as in consolidation, provided that the bronchi are patent. Fremitus is diminished or absent when there is fluid or air in the pleural space or when there is an atelectasis due to bronchial obstruction.

Percussion

Two methods of percussion may be used to determine whether there is an alteration in the density of the underlying lung or the pleural space. *Indirect,* or *mediate, percussion,* which is the method most commonly in use, is effected by placing the third finger of the left hand (the pleximeter) on the surface of the chest and tapping it with the third finger of the right hand (the plexor). *Direct,* or *immediate, percussion* is effected without the interposition of a pleximeter, the chest wall being struck directly with the pads of one or two fingers. This latter technique is occasionally used to detect an abnormality in an upper lobe by tapping the central portion of the clavicles with the tips of one or two fingers.

The position of the fingers during the act of indirect percussion is shown in Figure 81. The terminal phalanx and the interphalangeal joint of the pleximeter finger are applied to the chest wall with very little pressure, while the rest of the finger and the other four fingers are raised away from the

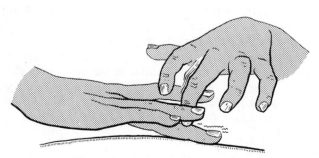

Figure 81. Percussion of the chest.

chest wall to avoid dampening of the percussion note. Using the wrist as a fulcrum, with the elbow fixed in a semiflexed position, the plexor finger taps the terminal phalanx of the pleximeter finger in a rapid staccato manner. The blows should be short, sharp and light with instantaneous recoil of the finger; if the recoil is slow, the sound may be dampened. Too forceful percussion may cause large areas of the chest wall to vibrate, so that small pulmonary lesions may be overlooked. Conversely, if the lesion is very small and is more than 5 cm. beneath the chest wall, it may not be detected by percussion.

The pitch of the sound produced by percussion is determined by the ratio of air-containing tissue to solid tissue in the area directly beneath the percussing finger. Well-aerated lung parenchyma produces a low-pitched resonant sound that is similar to that of a muffled drum. A sound that is higher in pitch, with a dull-to-flat note, implies that there is an increased amount of solid tissue beneath the percussing finger. This may be due to *atelectasis, consolidation,* or a *pleural effusion.* The percussion note over a *pneumothorax* is hyperresonant, the degree of resonance depending on the amount of air present.

In most cases, the detection of diminished movement will already have alerted the examiner to the particular area that may be affected. It is a good plan to percuss over the supposedly healthy lung first. The pleximeter finger is moved slowly and continuously from the apex down to the base anteriorly, in the axilla, and posteriorly, with the plexor finger tapping continuously, rapidly and lightly. A practically continuous sound that has the same pitch throughout will be elicited over a healthy lung. The same procedure is then carried out on the side of the chest that is suspected to be abnormal. If a disease process is suspected in the lower part of the chest, then percussion should begin over the apex, proceeding downward toward the abnormal area. If an abnormality is suspected in the upper part of the chest, then percussion should begin over the base of the lung and proceed upward. To be certain that the pitch is truly altered, it should be compared with the corresponding area of the opposite side.

One can also assess the inspiratory descent of the diaphragm by percussion over the lower posterior surface of the chest wall while the patient is sitting. The pleximeter finger should be placed in a horizontal position so that it lies parallel with the plane of the diaphragmatic dullness. It is easier to detect a change in the note if percussion is carried out from the area of resonance to that of dullness, starting over the lower lobes and then moving downward until an abrupt flat note indicative of the position of the diaphragm is reached. This is carried out while the patient holds his breath at full inspiration and again at full expiration. If the diaphragm is paralyzed on one side, it will move paradoxically, rising above its resting level when a deep inspiration is made.

Auscultation

Auscultation, derived from the Latin meaning the act of listening, is carried out with a stethoscope.

Breath Sounds. One can best appreciate the soft rustling quality of normal breath sounds by listening with the stethoscope over the axillary region of one's own chest wall. The inspiratory phase is easily heard, but the expiratory phase is considerably fainter, and its length is approximately one-third of the inspiratory phase. An appreciation of bronchial breath sounds can be gained by listening over the trachea, where the inspiratory and the expiratory notes are equal in pitch, intensity and duration and are separated by a silent interval. These sounds are normally heard over the trachea, the upper anterior chest wall and the posterior chest wall in the midscapular region. If bronchial breath sounds are detected over other areas of the chest wall, it implies that a disease process has led to a reduction of air-containing alveoli and that patent bronchi are surrounded by solid lung tissue. Conversely, if, for some reason, the bronchus is completely occluded so that there is no airflow, the breath sounds may be faint or even absent.

Vocal Sounds. Auscultation while the patient whispers a combination of words, such as "one, two, three," may confirm the suspicion of consolidation. By whispering, vibrations with a very high frequency are deliberately created in the tracheobronchial tree, and as long as the underlying lung parenchyma is healthy, these vibrations will be poorly transmitted to the chest wall because of the low-pass filter property of the lung parenchyma. However if the underlying lung tissue is consolidated, the high frequencies of the whispered sound are transmitted to the chest wall with great clarity. Thus, *whispering pectoriloquy* is a helpful physical sign, particularly when the areas of consolidation are small and patchy, as in lobular pneumonia.

Adventitious Sounds. Abnormal vibrations produced by a pathologic process in the lung are called adventitious sounds.

WHEEZES. Wheezes may be high or low pitched, inspiratory or expiratory, short or long, and single or multiple. Wheezes that are heard at a distance may sound different from those that are heard over the chest wall, but this difference is due to filtration of the sound as it passes through the lung. If one listens over the mouth as well as the chest wall while the patient expires forcibly, it may be possible to determine the site of origin. A wheeze that is audible over the open mouth, implies that the large central airways are involved, because wheezes produced by narrowed peripheral airways are generally not transmitted to the mouth.

A persistent wheeze that is localized to one area is very important, for it signifies a localized narrowing which may be due to a new growth, bronchostenosis, an aspirated foreign body or secretions.

Stridor is a very loud, fixed, high-pitched inspiratory muscial sound similar to that of a wheeze, but it occurs during inspiration and expiration and can easily be heard at a distance from the chest. It can be caused by laryngeal spasm, as in whooping cough, tracheal stenosis, or edema of the vocal cords.

CRACKLES. These sounds, which have also been called rales, are short, explosive nonmusical sounds that occur in brief bursts and resemble the crackling sounds of a fire. They may be high or low pitched, scanty or profuse, and loud or faint, and they may occur early or late during either inspiration, expiration, or both phases of respiration.

Crackles may be present in severe chronic airflow limitation such as *chronic bronchitis* or *asthma*, and in restrictive lung disorders, such as *interstitial pulmonary fibrosis* or *pulmonary edema.* The distinguishing feature between the crackles in the two groups of conditions is the time of occurrence during inspiration. Because the proximal and larger airways are affected primarily in bronchitis or asthma, crackles are more manifest near the beginning of inspiration and may extend to midinspiration before disappearing. They are generally scanty in number, may be heard over one or both lung bases as well as at the open mouth, and are unaffected by a change in posture. Secretions in the proximal larger airways can cause crackles that have no orderly sequence. These rales can occur randomly during either inspiration or expiration, and are frequently reduced or disappear following a cough.

In *interstitial pulmonary fibrosis* the crackles are due to the opening of small peripheral airways that closed during expiration. The abrupt opening of the airways results in "Velcro-like" crackles at the lung bases, which are manifest during the latter part of inspiration. They are usually profuse and are rarely transmitted to the open mouth. Coughing does not change their character, but they may be altered by a change in posture.

RUBS. A pleural crackle is also commonly called a "pleural rub." Roughening of the pleural surfaces by inflammation, fibrin or neoplastic deposits probably produces the low-pitched, crackling, leathery sounds that are characteristically audible at the end of inspiration and the beginning of expiration. They are most frequently detected over the lower areas of the chest, presumably because the excursion of the pleural layers is greatest over the lower lobes.

PATTERNS OF DISTURBANCES

It must be emphasized that abnormal physical signs, of themselves, do not yield information about the exact etiology or nature of the disease. However, these signs frequently form patterns that indicate the anatomic disturbance present. A summary of the altered physical characteristics and the clinical findings in the various patterns of respiratory disorders that affect one hemothorax is presented in Table 12. This table shows the signs found when a right-sided lesion is present.

TABLE 12. Physical Signs in Various Patterns of Diseases*

	Consolidation†	Atelectasis†	Localized† Fibrosis	Pneumothorax†	Pleural† Effusion	Obstructive Lung Disease**
Size						
Trachea position	↕	→(R)	→(R)	→(L)	→(L)	↕
Apex position	↕	→(R)	→(R)	→(L)	→(L)	↕
Distensibility						
Movement	↓ (R)	↓ (R)	↓ (R)	↓ (R)	↓ (R)	→ Bilateral
Sound transmission						
Percussion	↓ (R)	↓ (R)	↓ (R)	↑ (R)	↓ (R)	↑ Bilateral
Tactile fremitus	↑ (R)	↓ (R)	↑ (R)	↓ (R)	↓ (R)	↓ Bilateral
Breath sounds	Bronchial (R)	Diminished or absent (R)	Bronchovesicular (R)	Absent (R)	Absent (R)	Prolonged expiration
Adventitious sounds	Whispering pectoriloquy Crackles (R)		Crackles (R)		? Rub (R)	Wheezes

*Note that there is usually only one sign that is significant in establishing the correct diagnosis.

**The signs are bilateral.

†The signs are those found when a right-sided lesion is present. If the lesion is left-sided, L should be substituted for R and R for L.

CONSOLIDATION

In this condition, the alveolar air is replaced by fluid and inflammatory cells and the volume of the affected area of lung remains unchanged. Characteristically, therefore, the mediastinum continues to occupy a central position, so that the trachea is centrally located and the apex beat is in its normal position. The distensibility of the lung is reduced, so that movement is diminished. The ratio of air to tissue (i.e., the density) is increased, so that the percussion note is impaired and tactile fremitus is increased while bronchial breath sounds and whispering pectoriloquy are heard over the affected area. In addition, inspiratory crackles may be present during the latter part of inspiration over the affected area.

ATELECTASIS

When a portion of the lung is collapsed and airless (because of a complete obstruction), the volume is reduced, so that the trachea and apex beat are deviated to the affected side. The distensibility of the lung is reduced, so that movement is diminished. The density is increased, so the percussion note is impaired. Because there is no airflow in the underlying bronchus, the transmission of sound is reduced, so that tactile fremitus and breath sounds are diminished or absent over the affected area.

LOCALIZED PULMONARY FIBROSIS

Fibrosis confined to a large enough area of a lung also results in a reduced volume in the affected lung, diminished distensibility, an increased density and a variable alteration in the ability to transmit sound. Again, the mediastinum is deviated to the affected side, movement is diminished, and the percussion note is impaired. Tactile fremitus and the breath sounds are frequently diminished over the affected area, and Velcro-like crackles may occur late in inspiration.

PNEUMOTHORAX

When there is air in a pleural cavity, the size of the affected side is increased and the trachea and apex beat are deviated to the opposite side. The distensibility of the affected hemithorax is reduced, so that movement is diminished. The ratio of air to tissue is markedly increased, leading to hyperresonance on percussion. Because there is air in the pleural space, there are an increased number of surfaces available for reflection of the sound waves. As a result, tactile fremitus and the breath sounds are distant or absent over the affected area.

PLEURAL EFFUSION

When there is fluid in a pleural cavity, the trachea and apex beat are usually deviated away from the diseased side, because the size of the affected side is increased. The distensibility of the hemithorax is reduced, so that movement is diminished, while the ratio of air to tissue (fluid) is reduced, so that there is a flat note on percussion. Since the fluid separates the pleural surfaces, there is increased reflection of sound waves, and tactile fremitus and breath sounds are absent over the involved area. Bronchial breath sounds may occasionally be heard at the upper limit of the fluid, because the underlying lung is compressed and the bronchi are patent. Pleural crackles may also occasionally be present at this level.

EXAMINATION OF THE HEART

The presence of cardiac murmurs or abnormalities of cardiac rhythm may reveal the source of respiratory symptoms. The typical apical diastolic murmur of mitral stenosis may indicate the origin of a recent hemoptysis, and atrial fibrillation may explain the onset of shortness of breath.

Respiratory disease may lead to an increase in the pulmonary vascular resistance, pulmonary hypertension and the consequent development of right ventricular hypertrophy. There are no physical findings in the lungs that are indicative of an increased pulmonary vascular resistance; this is elicited only during the cardiac examination. In the following discussion, only those abnormalities that are indicative of an increased pulmonary vascular resistance will be presented.

Cardiac Impulse

If the cardiac impulse, or apex beat, is visible, its position and character should be noted. The character of the cardiac impulse is an important as its location. One can frequently feel a heave just to the left of the lower sternum along with a conspicuous retraction of the chest lateral to it, producing a characteristic rocking motion of the precordium, when there is right ventricular hypertrophy associated with pulmonary hypertension. In addition, dilation of the pulmonary artery may produce a visible systolic pulsation in the pulmonic area just to the right of the upper sternum.

Heart Sounds

The presence of palpable vibrations and an accentuated pulmonic sound over the pulmonic area, as well as a systolic ejection click, is indicative of pulmonary hypertension. The high-pitched systolic click in the pulmonic area occurs during systole just after the opening of the pulmonic valve, at the end of the period of isometric contraction. The click is probably caused by accentuated ejection vibrations and is almost invariably found in patients with large left-to-right shunts, mild pulmonary stenosis or dilation of the pulmonary artery.

Failure of the second pulmonic sound to split during inspiration further suggests the presence of pulmonary hypertension. Conversely, a prolonged widening of the inspiratory split of the pulmonic second sound is probably caused by a delay in closure of the pulmonic valve, which is usually due to a bundle branch block or a mild pulmonary stenosis.

Pulsus Paradoxus

In many healthy individuals, systolic blood pressure drops by up to 5 mm. Hg during inspiration, and the magnitude of the pulse decreases slightly. In *pulsus paradoxus*, the systolic blood pressure falls by 10 mm. Hg or more during inspiration, and the decrease in the magnitude of the pulse becomes very evident. This physical sign is particularly important when assessing patients with **asthma**. It is present when airflow limitation is severe, and marked hyperinflation and great swings in transpulmonary pressure are also present. This combination effectively traps the heart in a manner analogous to constrictive pericarditis, so that there is restriction of cardiac filling and emptying.

ASSESSMENT OF IMPAIRMENT AND DISABILITY

Just as estimation of the systolic and diastolic blood pressure and, in some cases, the electrocardiogram, are an essential component of the examination of the cardiovascular system, assessment of the distensibility of the respiratory system and air flow resistance are integral components of the examination of the respiratory system. An index of the distensibility of the lungs and chest wall can be obtained with a simple spirometer by recording a forced expiratory vital capacity (FVC). Similarly, the amount of air expired in the first second (FEV_1) or the mean flow during the middle half of the forced expiration (FE_{25-75}) provides an index of the degree of expiratory airflow limitation present. In a **restrictive disorder**, such as pulmonary fibrosis, the FVC and the FEV_1 are low, but the FEV_1/FVC ratio is greater than 70 per cent. In an **obstructive disorder,** the FVC is also usually less than expected, but the FEV_1 is markedly reduced, so that the FEV_1/FVC ratio is lower than normal.

In addition to determining the extent of impairment produced by pulmonary disease, one can also evaluate the extent of disability present during the clinical examination. This entails having patients undergo a form or walking on the level at a brisk pace, and noting when breathlessness and tachycardia develop.

These simple assessments of function and respiratory difficulty provide a rough index of the functional disturbances produced by respiratory disease. In some cases, more specific studies of pulmonary function may be required, and their interpretation has been discussed earlier.

ASSESSMENT OF THE INFANT AND CHILD

Much of the previous discussion about the examination of the respiratory system and the patterns of pulmonary disturbances is applicable to the assessment of respiratory disorders in infants and children. However, there are a number of diseases that are peculiar to this age group and that require historical information of a different nature. The history must be obtained in large part from the parents, and since considerable probing may be necessary, the questioning requires much tact and consideration of personal feelings. In addition, although the approach to the physical examination is essentially the same as in the adult, examination of the child requires a greater degree of gentleness and patience in order to obtain optimal information.

HISTORY

The Newborn Infant

When approaching the problem of a newborn infant with respiratory distress, one must obtain detailed information about previous pregnancies and their outcome, as well as the present pregnancy and delivery. The gestational age of the infant is important, since the preterm infant (born before 37 completed weeks of gestation) has a 10 per cent chance of developing *hyaline membrane disease.*

The quality and quantity of amniotic fluid must be ascertained; foul-smelling, murky amniotic fluid suggests infection, and meconium staining of the amniotic fluid suggests meconium aspiration. Excessive amniotic fluid *(hydramnios)* is often associated with a tracheo-esophageal fistula. Rupture of the amniotic sac with leakage of fluid for longer than 24 hours is associated with an increased incidence of infection and is a likely cause of pneumonia in the newborn infant. There is an unusually high incidence of aspiration pneumonia and spontaneous pneumothorax in postterm infants (born after 42 completed weeks of gestation), presumably because of the *in utero* aspiration of amniotic fluid, which, at this time, contains a large number of squamous epithelial cells.

The type of presentation and delivery is important, since a traumatic delivery or a breech presentation may be associated with cerebral hemorrhage and subsequent respiratory distress. Conditions such as placenta previa, a prolapsed or entangled umbilical cord, or fetal bradycardia are often associated with asphyxia before birth and a flaccid, apneic and cyanotic infant. Similarly, excessive administration of narcotic medications to the mother immediately before delivery of the infant may cause respiratory depression. The Apgar score (Table 13), determined one minute following delivery, is useful in assessing the condition of the infant immediately postpartum. Each of the five signs indicated in the table is rated from 0 to 2, so that the total score calculated (i.e., the Apgar score) for a newborn infant is rated out of a maximum of 10.

The Child

Assessment of older children involves careful evaluation of growth and development as well as knowledge of the previous and the current state of immunizations. Children are now routinely immunized against diphtheria, whooping cough, tetanus, polio, measles and mumps within the first year or two of life. The birth weight and the pattern of growth (both height and weight) should be compared with those of other children of the same age

TABLE 13. The Apgar Method of Scoring Newborn Infants*

Sign	Score		
	0	1	2
Heart rate	Absent	Slow (below 100)	Over 100
Respiratory rate	Absent	Slow, irregular	Good, crying
Muscle tone	Limp	Some flexion of extremities	Active motion
Reflex irritability (response to catheter in nostril)	No response	Grimace	Cough or sneeze
Color	Blue, pale	Body pink, extremities blue	Completely pink

*The score is taken first 60 seconds after the complete delivery of the infant and may be repeated at 1- to 5-minute intervals until the total score reaches at least 8.
Score: >7 Normal
4–7 Suspicious
<4 Marked abnormality

and sex. Developmental milestones, such as when the child first smiled, sat, walked, spoke words and spoke phrases, should be noted. The first sign of any illness in childhood is often anorexia, so careful attention should be paid to recording the food and water intake of the patient. Since vitamin supplements are necessary in the first year of life, it is important to assess the adequacy of vitamin intake.

PHYSICAL EXAMINATION

As has been pointed out, examination of the child requires both patience and gentleness, particularly in the uncooperative age group from one to three years old. Unlike the examination of the adult, it is the child who dictates the order in which the physical examination is conducted. Often most of the examination is best conducted while the child is being held by the mother, either sitting on her lap or held over her shoulder. Even so, any use of instruments should usually be left to the end of the examination, since such utensils as the stethoscope, otoscope and tongue blades often frighten the child.

In the newborn, inspection is the most important part of the physical examination. The frequency of breathing may normally vary from 30 to 60 breaths per minute in the first few days of life; a greater respiratory rate is definitely abnormal. Preterm infants often have Cheyne-Stokes respiration with periods of apnea lasting from 10 to 15 seconds. Apnea lasting longer than 15 seconds is abnormal and is usually associated with bradycardia.

Frothy blood in the mouth suggests pulmonary hemorrhage. Newborn infants commonly demonstrate peripheral cyanosis, but cyanosis due to hypoxemia is as difficult to judge as in the adult. Cyanosis and tachypnea in the absence of pulmonary disease suggest the presence of a cyanotic congenital heart disease. The presence of a scaphoid abdomen suggests the possibility of a diaphragmatic hernia.

Inability to breathe without an oral airway is suggestive of atresia of the posterior nares *(choanal atresia)*. A routine part of the physical examination on admission to the nursery should be passage of a #8 French catheter through each nares. It should be noted that the newborn infant is an obligate nose breather, and it may take several weeks before he learns to breathe through his mouth.

The anteroposterior and transverse diameters of the thorax are nearly equal in the newborn. With time there is a greater increase in the transverse diameter, and the chest contour has the proportions of an adult at the time of puberty. Because the infant's chest wall is very compliant, it is often easier to judge the degree of respiratory difficulty. Retraction in the suprasternal, intercostal, and subcostal areas and even of the entire sternum may occur in association with respiratory difficulty. Flaring of the alae nasae is also common. A typical sign of severe respiratory distress is the expiratory grunt, which may or may not be heard without the aid of a stethoscope. The expiratory obstruction that is produced by closure of the glottis is probably beneficial, because it prolongs the time for gas exchange in the lung and also may prevent collapse of alveoli and airways during expiration. The presence of a laryngeal web or a congenital vascular ring that is compressing the trachea should be suspected if a baby tends to keep his head extended or has stridor.

Percussion is very difficult to interpret in the small infant, since the percussion note is easily transmitted by the small thorax. The percussion note tends to be more hyperresonant in infants than in adults, and it is only after the first few months of life that percussion becomes a reliable clinical sign. However, the rest of the examination of the chest can be very informative. A shift of the apical impulse, with or without a similar shift of the trachea, is highly suggestive of a pneumothorax. In children, the high-pitched voice sounds penetrate the chest wall poorly, so that vocal fremitus is not a reliable part of the examination. However, fremitus can be picked up through the chest wall during crying, but this makes auscultation difficult.

Since auscultation is extremely difficult or impossible if the infant is crying, this part of the physical examination should always be carried out first if the child is quiet. However, as indicated earlier, the sight of the stethoscope may induce a crying episode, so that the approach to each child must be individualized. The mother may have to gently restrain the hands of the curious infant who reaches for the stethoscope tubing, or alternatively, he may be induced to play with another object such as a reflex hammer or a tongue blade. The child's head should be in a central position, since the mere turning of the head often reduces breath sounds on one side of the chest, even in the absence of pulmonary disease. Breath sounds in small children and infants are harsher and louder and appear closer to the ear than those of adults, because the chest wall is thin and the airways are in close proximity to the chest wall. The breath sounds radiate widely in the small chest, so that they may not be decreased even when there is a loss of lung volume or even a pneumothorax. In premature infants with *hyaline membrane disease,* breath sounds are often completely absent. An audible expiratory grunt may be picked up by holding the stethoscope in front of the infant's nares. Fine inspiratory crackles are common immediately after birth and presumably represent the opening of the unexpanded airways and alveoli.

SUMMARY

When abnormal physical findings are taken in conjunction with a thorough inquiry into the chronologic development of the symptoms, the duration of the illness and the nature of its progress, it is frequently possible to arrive at a presumptive clinical diagnosis of a disease process and the resultant impairment in function. This, in turn, should now be supplemented by appropriate radiologic and laboratory investigation to establish the etiology of the disorder, and when necessary, additional physiologic assessment to quantitate the degree of impaired function.

12

RADIOLOGIC ASSESSMENT

After taking a complete history and performing a thorough physical examination, one is usually able to arrive at a conclusion about the anatomic location of a pulmonary lesion and a tentative diagnosis. Further valuable information leading to a more definitive diagnosis may be obtained by radiologic assessment of the patient's chest. Although there are many bronchopulmonary diseases in which the x-ray examination of the chest is entirely noncontributory, many pulmonary lesions can be demonstrated on a chest roentgenogram before they can be detected by clinical examination. In addition, in many pulmonary conditions, roentgenograms and special radiographic techniques are often extremely useful in following the course of disease and its response to therapy. The standard radiologic examination of the chest should consist of roentgenograms taken in the posteroanterior and lateral positions and then, when indicated, more detailed and specialized techniques.

THE ROENTGENOLOGIC APPEARANCE OF
THE NORMAL CHEST

The thorax is an ideal region for a radiologic examination. The aerated lung parenchyma offers very little resistance to the passage of the roentgen rays, and it therefore produces very radiant shadows. On the other hand, the rays are not transmitted as well by the soft tissues of the thoracic wall, the mediastinum, the heart, the great vessels and the diaphragm, so that they appear as denser opacities on the roentgenogram. The bony structures of the thorax—the ribs, vertebrae and sternum—are even less readily penetrated, and their shadows are even more dense. To determine whether an abnormality is present, one must clearly understand the normal appearance of the heart and lungs on the chest roentgenogram, since normal findings vary considerably with age, sex and habitus.

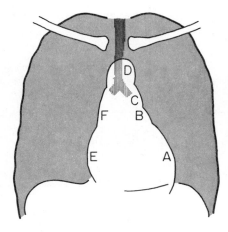

Figure 82. The roentgenologic appearance of the heart. *A*, Left ventricle; *B*, left atrial appendage; *C*, pulmonary artery; *D*, aortic knob and margin of descending aorta; *E*, right atrium; and *F*, superior vena cava.

THE HEART

In the posteroanterior roentgenogram (Fig. 82) the right heart border is formed entirely by the right atrium. The inferior vena cava may be seen entering the right atrium, and the ascending arch of the aorta and the superior vena cava often overlap and form the border superior to the right atrium. The left heart border, beginning at the level of the diaphragm, is composed of the border of the left ventricle, the left atrial appendage, the undivided segment of the pulmonary artery and the aortic knob, which is produced primarily by the transverse arch of the aorta.

On the lateral chest roentgenogram, the posterior mediastinum is visualized as an area of radiolucency between the posterior border of the heart and the anterior aspect of the spine. The descending aorta is outlined in this space.

In the right anterior oblique position, the posterior border of the heart shadow is made up of the left and right atria, with the superior vena cava above. The anterior border of the heart shadow is formed by the right ventricle.

The left anterior oblique position is particularly valuable for the visualization of the right ventricle, which lies along the diaphragmatic and the inferoanterior portion of the cardiac outline. The left atrium and the left ventricle form the posterior portion of the silhouette.

THE LUNGS

In the posteroanterior view of the chest, the trachea is a vertical translucent shadow situated in the midline and overlying the cervical vertebrae. The hila, or lung roots, are poorly defined areas of increased density in the medial part of the central portion of the lung fields and consist of the pulmonary blood vessels, the bronchi and a group of lymph nodes. The left hilum is partially obscured by the overlying shadow of the heart and great vessels, and it lies at a slightly higher level than the right hilum. In the middle third of the lung fields there is a series of linear reticular shadows formed principally by arteries, veins and lymphatics. A bronchus seen end-on forms a ringlike area of increased density with a central translucency, whereas a blood vessel seen end-on forms a round solid shadow. In the peripheral portions of the lung these linear markings are much less obvious.

The lobes of the lungs cannot normally be distinguished on the chest roentgenogram. The major, or oblique, fissures of both lungs are usually seen only in the lateral view as a very thin dense line. The minor, or transverse, fissure on the right side is normally seen on the posteroanterior film as a fine hairlike line running transversely in either the third or fourth intercostal space; on the lateral view it runs horizontally from the hilum to the anterior margin of the chest cage. The position of this fissure is frequently of diagnostic value. For instance, if the right upper lobe is contracted or atelectatic, the fissure is drawn upward; if the middle lobe is atelectatic, it is drawn downward. Similarly, when the lower lobe is collapsed, the major fissure is drawn downward and posteriorly.

Just as it was important to understand the surface anatomy of the chest in carrying out the physical examination, so it is necessary to have clearly in one's mind the anatomic location of each of the lobes and the various bronchopulmonary segments when the chest roentgenogram is examined.

Bronchopulmonary Anatomy

The trachea extends anteriorly from the lower edge of the cricoid cartilage to the level of the second costal cartilage, and this corresponds posteriorly to the lower border of the body of the fourth thoracic vertebra. Here the trachea divides into the right and left major bronchi, which serve each lung.

The right major bronchus divides into three main branches: a bronchus to the upper lobe, one to the middle lobe and one to the lower lobe. The lobar bronchi divide into smaller branches, which are known as *segmental bronchi,* each supplying a portion of a lobe called a *bronchopulmonary segment.* These are illustrated in Figures 83 and 84. A given segment has its own bronchus and its own artery, vein and lymphatics.

The Right Lung. The upper lobe bronchus of the right lung arises about 2.5 cm. beyond the bifurcation of the trachea and almost immediately divides into three branches, each supplying a segment. The anterior segment of the right upper lobe is situated anteriorly between the levels of the clavicle and the fourth rib. The apical segment lies in the area above the level of the clavicle, and the posterior segment lies posterior to the other segments of the right upper lobe.

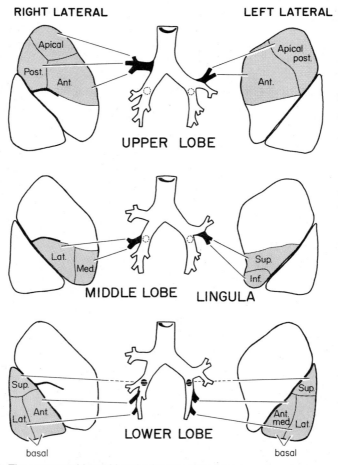

Figure 83. The segmental bronchi and a lateral view of the bronchopulmonary segments.

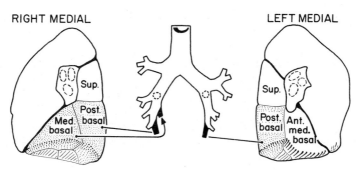

Figure 84. The bronchopulmonary segments of the lower lobes (medial aspect).

The middle lobe bronchus of the right lung arises from the anterior aspect of the right major bronchus about 2 cm. below the opening of the upper lobe bronchus. It runs in a downward and forward direction, finally dividing into two branches that supply the medial and the lateral segments of the middle lobe.

After giving off its branch to the middle lobe, the right main bronchus gives off the superior, or apical, branch posteriorly, then continues its downward course, and finally divides into four branches, each supplying a particular segment of the lower lobe. These are the anterior basal, the medial basal, the lateral basal and the posterior basal segments of the right lower lobe.

The Left Lung. The bronchus of the upper lobe of the left lung arises from the anterolateral aspect of the left major bronchus about 5 cm. from the bifurcation of the trachea. Unlike the right main bronchus, it then splits into an upper and a lower division.

The upper division divides into two branches: one supplies the anterior segment, and the other supplies the apical-posterior segment of the upper lobe. The anterior segment of the left upper lobe corresponds to that of the right upper lobe, whereas the apical-posterior segment corresponds to both the apical and posterior segments of the right upper lobe.

The lower division supplies the lingula, which, although actually a part of the left upper lobe, corresponds morphologically to the right middle lobe. The bronchus to the lingula divides into two branches, which are situated one above the other and supply the superior and the inferior segments of the lingula.

The lower division of the left main bronchus continues its downward course as the left lower lobe bronchus. It divides into four branches, which supply the superior, or apical, segment, the anterior medial basal segment (which corresponds to both the anterior basal and the medial basal segments of the right lung), the lateral basal segment and the posterior basal segment.

The various bronchopulmonary segments and the roentgenologic appearance of infiltrations in them on the posteroanterior and lateral projections are illustrated in Figure 85.

THE DIAPHRAGM

The two hemidiaphragms are rounded, smooth, sharply defined shadows, the right one being normally situated one interspace higher than the left. The right leaf of the diaphragm merges with the shadow of the liver. The costophrenic angles are moderately deep, and they are approximately equal in size on the two sides.

BONY STRUCTURES

The ribs, the clavicles, the scapulae and portions of the humeri are reasonably clearly outlined on most chest roentgenograms. These structures should be carefully examined, for they are important aids in diagnosis.

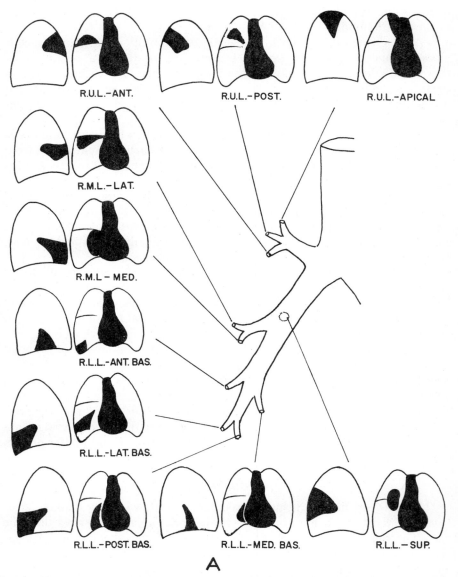

Figure 85. The roentgenographic appearance of infiltrations in the various bronchopulmonary segments on the posteroanterior and lateral chest roentgenograms. **A,** Right lung.

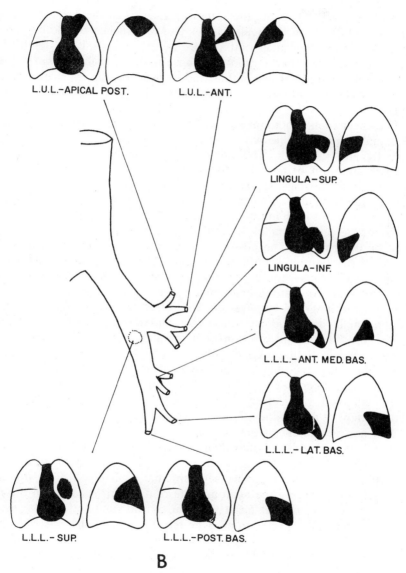

L.U.L.-APICAL POST.

L.U.L.-ANT.

LINGULA-SUP.

LINGULA-INF.

L.L.L.-ANT. MED. BAS.

L.L.L.-LAT. BAS.

L.L.L.-SUP.

L.L.L.-POST. BAS.

B

Figure 85. *Continued.* **B,** Left lung.

EXAMINATION OF THE CHEST ROENTGENOGRAM

It is important that the chest roentgenogram be of high quality and not be either overexposed or underexposed. The patient should be well centered before the exposure is made; the spinous processes of the vertebrae should be in the middle of the tracheal shadow, and the trachea should be midway between the sternoclavicular joints. There should be good bony detail of the ribs, and the vascular markings in the lungs should be visible from the hilum to the periphery. The cardiac outline and, if possible, the transverse fissure, the left subclavian artery and the inferior vena cava, should be sharply defined.

The chest roentgenogram should be examined in a systematic fashion. The actual sequence followed is probably not important as long as it is systematic and thorough. The bony structure should be examined, with particular attention being given to the density of the ribs bilaterally, the vertebrae, both clavicles, the scapulae and humeri; any opacities should be noted. In addition, other abnormalities may be very important. For instance, notching of the ribs is an important manifestation of coarctation of the aorta. The size of the cardiac shadow and the mediastinum as well as their contours should be determined. The position of the trachea and the bronchi and, if possible, their contours should be assessed. The position and shape of the two hemidiaphragms should be noted, as well as the depth, clarity and position of the two costophrenic angles and the appearance of the lateral borders of the lungs. In *emphysema,* the retrosternal space is characteristically abnormally increased and translucent, and the diaphragms are flattened.

The size, shape and position of both hilar shadows should be noted. Enlargement of both hila suggests either pulmonary hypertension or enlarged lymph nodes. Enlarged and butterfly-shaped hila associated with increased pulmonary markings are indicative of pulmonary congestion. If only one hilum is enlarged, particularly in association with a pulmonary lesion in an elderly patient, a malignancy should be considered.

The size and extent of the pulmonary markings and the appearance of the lung fields bilaterally should then be examined with special reference to any abnormal shadows. If a lesion is seen, it is important to localize it to the particular bronchopulmonary segment that is involved. The *silhouette sign* is helpful in placing the anatomic site of a lesion. A lesion of the right middle lobe or the medial basal segment of the right lower lobe usually obliterates the right heart border, whereas a lesion of the posterior basal segment does not. Similarly, a lesion in the lingula or the lateral basal segment of the left lung may obliterate the left heart border.

ADDITIONAL RADIOGRAPHIC TECHNIQUES

In some cases, despite a systematic examination of the chest roentgenogram, further special radiographic techniques may be required in order to conclusively establish the diagnosis. The following techniques are not discussed in order of priority.

Fluoroscopy

Fluoroscopy may be a useful adjunct to the diagnostic roentgenogram, for it may provide information about the function of the respiratory system in addition to the location and nature of a lesion. Although this examination also yields considerable information about the heart, this will not be discussed except as it is related to respiratory disease.

During fluoroscopy, the position of the trachea and the hilar markings should be noted. The extent of aeration and deflation of the lungs should be assessed during quiet breathing, deep breathing, and a cough. Failure of the lungs to become less translucent during expiration suggests either a loss of elasticity or bronchiolar obstruction of the check-valve type. Localization of this phenomenon to one side indicates the presence of trapped air, and obstruction of a bronchus by a malignant process or a foreign body should be considered.

Diminished movement of the diaphragm may be associated with either localized or diffuse pulmonary disease. If one or both of the leaves of the diaphragm is paralyzed, a sniff or even a normal inspiration may result in paradoxical movement of the affected diaphragm; i.e., it rises during inspiration.

Inspiration-Expiration Roentgenograms

Posteroanterior roentgenograms taken at maximum inspiration and maximum expiration, like fluoroscopy, are particularly useful in determining the presence or absence of mediastinal shift or localized air trapping caused by a foreign body or bronchogenic carcinoma. The expiration film may also be useful in demonstrating the presence or absence of a small *pneumothorax,* because there is less radiolucency in the lungs at full expiration and a pneumothorax is then more readily evident. Clearly, this type of study also provides a measure of the extent of movement of the hemidiaphragms.

Oblique Roentgenogram

Oblique views of the chest, which are taken with the corresponding shoulder against the x-ray cassette, are most useful in the assessment of cardiac chamber size; they are occasionally also useful in localizing a pulmonary abnormality involving a lobe or a bronchopulmonary segment. The appearance of the chest roentgenogram in the two oblique portions is shown in Figure 86. In the right anterior oblique roentgenogram, the lingula of the left lung is visualized in front of the heart and the right lower lobe is behind the heart. In the left anterior oblique view, the right middle lobe is visualized in front of the heart and the left lower lobe is behind it.

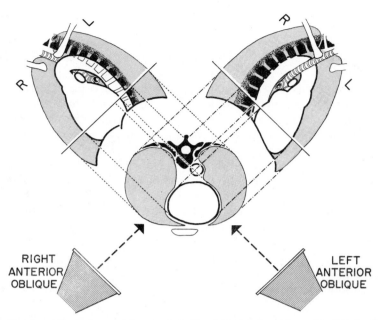

Figure 86. The oblique views of the chest. In the right anterior oblique, the lingula of the¯left lung and right lower lobe are visualized; in the left anterior oblique, the right middle lobe and the left lower lobe are visualized.

Apical Lordotic Roentgenogram

In the apical lordotic view, the clavicles are projected above the lung apices. This view can be particularly helpful when a pulmonary lesion is obscured on the posteroanterior chest film because of overlapping of the ribs.

Tomography

Although not used as extensively nowadays, tomography can be useful in delineating the characteristics of a radiologic shadow, especially a *cavity,* particularly when it is deep seated or underlies the clavicle or a rib. This involves radiographing a single plane, whose thickness can be at various depths in the lung.

Stereoscopic Roentgenogram

Stereoscopic x-ray films are occasionally used to localize pulmonary lesions. In this technique, two chest roentgenograms are taken at the same time. By making them overlap, a three-dimensional impression of the chest is obtained when they are viewed stereoscopically.

Lateral Decubitus Roentgenograms

These views are useful when the presence of fluid in the pleural space is suspected but is not grossly evident in the ordinary film or when one wishes to differentiate fluid above the diaphragm from an *infrapulmonary effusion,* or fluid in an emphysematous bulla from a hydropneumothorax. When an x-ray is taken in the lateral decubitus position (with the patient lying on the suspected side) fluid in the pleural space shifts to the most dependent position and lies along the border of the heart.

Bronchography

An x-ray film of the chest after radiopaque solutions are instilled into the tracheobronchial tree is called a bronchogram. The radiopaque iodized substances reveal in great detail the size and appearance of the tracheobronchial tree. In *bronchiectasis* the bronchi are dilated, have an irregular outline, and may be unable to conduct the material to the periphery of the lungs because of obstruction by secretions, organic narrowing or obliteration of bronchioles. The dilatation may be fusiform, tubular or cystic and may be slight in extent or quite gross. This form of investigation is now rarely carried out unless surgery is contemplated.

Esophagogram

The esophagogram is a useful procedure, particularly when involvement of the mediastinum by a pulmonary malignant process is suspected. Displacement of the esophagus or abnormal impressions on the esophagus may indicate the presence of enlarged mediastinal lymph nodes or metastatic involvement of the esophagus.

Radioactive Isotope Scan

Perfusion of the lungs can be assessed by scanning the lungs in the anterior, posterior and lateral positions after the intravenous injection of I^{131}-tagged macroaggregates of human serum albumin. Diminished perfusion to an area of lung, particularly if there is no lesion except perhaps an increased radiolucency in this area on the chest roentgenogram, suggests *pulmonary thromboembolism.* This technique is simple to perform and can be repeated at frequent intervals, so that it may be used to assess progress of the disturbance. Under all circumstances, the interpretation of radioisotope scans of the thorax must take into account the extent of ventilation of the area of lung being scanned.

The relationship between ventilation and perfusion over various regions of the lung can be estimated by comparing count rates over the lungs obtained following the inhalation of Xe^{133} with that obtained following the intravenous injection of the same isotope. In addition, Ga^{67} scanning has been recommended in patients with *interstitial lung disease* in order to assess the extent of cellularity present and thus determine the stage of the disease process.

Angiography

In patients suspected of having pulmonary **thromboembolism,** roentgenograms are taken during the passage of a radiopaque substance through the right side of the heart, the pulmonary circulation, the left side of the heart and then the aorta. Dilated major pulmonary artery branches and obstruction of a segmental or lobar branch of the pulmonary artery may be demonstrated in acute episodes, or there may be irregular filling defects along the walls of arteries in more long-standing cases. Angiographic examination is also of value in cardiopulmonary disorders, particularly when there is a right-to-left shunt of blood.

Venography

This technique, which entails antecubital venous injection of a radiopaque material, may be used to demonstrate obstruction of a major vein in the thorax, i.e., the superior vena cava, such as may occur with a **bronchogenic carcinoma.**

Ultrasound

Ultrasound may be useful in assessing lesions of the pleura and the mediastinum, but is of no value in assessing lung lesions, because they are so well aerated.

Computerized Tomography

The current availability of computerized tomographic scanning in most centers has provided an excellent tool for evaluating mediastinal and hilar masses and for determining the anatomic location of other masses in the lung, pleura or chest wall. This technique has largely replaced tomography and other roentgenographic procedures that were previously used for this purpose.

SUMMARY

Assessment of the deviation from the normal chest roentgenogram, along with other ancillary radiologic techniques, enables the examiner to recognize an abnormality in the respiratory system. From knowledge of the anatomy of the lungs, one can establish the exact location of a lesion. Radiographic procedures are also of considerable value in following the course of a disease and its response to therapy.

13

LABORATORY ASSESSMENT

As we have seen, the analysis of a patient's complaints, any abnormal findings detected on the physical examination, and any abnormalities present in the chest roentgenogram usually make it possible to arrive at a presumptive diagnosis and to assess the degree of impairment present. From further physiologic evaluation, the underlying mechanism of disturbance and the extent of disability present may be determined. The clinical diagnosis should be confirmed and the responsible agent or underlying pathology identified, when necessary, by microbiologic, histologic, immunologic and biochemical techniques. In this chapter we shall be concerned with the laboratory techniques that are useful in establishing the etiology of respiratory disease. These assessments are based principally on bacteriologic, cytologic and chemical examination of abnormal secretions, histologic examination of diseased tissues, and skin testing and other immunologic investigation.

ABNORMAL SECRETIONS

The secretions that are most commonly examined in patients suffering from respiratory disease are bronchial secretions, pleural fluid and discharge from draining sinuses.

BRONCHIAL SECRETIONS

Abnormal bronchial secretions result from inflammation of the tracheobronchial tree, of the lung parenchyma, or both. These secretions are usually expectorated as sputum; they may be swallowed and found in the gastric contents; or they may be aspirated from the bronchial tree by suctioning through a catheter or a bronchoscope. It is important that sputum be properly collected. The ideal time to collect sputum is shortly after awakening, because abnormal bronchial secretions tend to accumulate during a night's sleep. One should be certain that the secretions originate in the tracheobronchial tree, and care should be taken to reduce contamination by organisms that normally inhabit the oropharynx. Postnasal secretions can generally be "hawked up" and discarded before a specimen is collected.

The sputum should be expectorated into a sterile container, and the specimen sent to the laboratory with a minimum of delay. If a specimen is collected in a nonsterile container and allowed to remain at room temperature, the culture may be contaminated by saprophytic organisms, and the antibiotic sensitivity tests may be invalidated.

Occasionally some patients are too ill, too old or too young to expectorate sputum, and others may have no cough or expectoration despite roentgenographic evidence of pulmonary infiltrates. In the former group, one may induce a cough by applying a sterile cotton applicator or laryngeal mirror to the base of the tongue or inserting a sterile suction catheter into the trachea. Secretions may also be aspirated directly from an affected bronchus through a bronchoscope, and this is particularly valuable for demonstrating malignant cells, tubercle bacilli and fungi.

When a diagnosis of *tuberculosis* is suspected, *aspiration of gastric contents* while in the patient is in the fasting state after awakening may be useful for the detection of tubercle bacilli. The mere presence of acid-fast organisms in a smear of gastric contents is not significant, because saprophytic acid-fast mycobacteria are frequently seen in gastric secretions. Only a positive culture of a gastric specimen is diagnostic of *tuberculosis. Induction of sputum* by the inhalation of an aerosol of a heated, hypertonic saline solution containing propylene glycol is another technique used to obtain bronchial secretions. Bacteriologic examination of the induced sputum may reveal tubercle bacilli or another microbe, and cytologic examination may point to a *pulmonary carcinoma.*

Whether examination of induced sputum is superior to a culture of gastric contents for detecting tubercle bacilli is controversial. Studies have shown that a culture of induced sputum is more likely to be positive if the secretions are induced immediately after a gastric aspiration, and both techniques are more likely to be positive if the sputum is induced first, probably because some of the induced secretions are swallowed. This suggests that the induction of sputum, followed by aspiration of gastric contents, would be most fruitful in detecting tubercle bacilli.

Macroscopic Examination

Volume. The amount of sputum expectorated during a 24-hour period often provides useful information about the nature of a disease as well as its course and prognosis. A daily volume of over 100 ml. is frequently expectorated in *bronchiectasis* and occasionally in *chronic bronchitis.* The daily volume should gradually decrease if improvement is taking place, but a sudden decrease in volume may indicate obstruction of the draining bronchus, and a sudden increase may indicate a rupture of a *lung abscess* or an *empyema* into the bronchial tree.

Color and Consistency. Mucoid sputum is translucent and glary, has a viscid, tenacious consistency and is often gray in city dwellers and cigarette smokers. In acute pulmonary edema the sputum is pinkish, watery and frothy, whereas purulent sputum is generally yellow or green. If a large collection of purulent sputum is allowed to stand in a conical glass, it often tends to separate into three layers. The top layer is usually frothy and discolored, the middle layer tends to be cloudy and watery, and the lower layer generally consists of a thick sediment of pus. This usually suggests that the patient has *bronchiectasis.*

Blood in the sputum is easily recognized and may be in the form of pure blood or streaks or small clots mixed in the sputum. The color of the blood depends on the interval between the actual bleeding and the expectoration of the sputum. Fresh blood is bright red, but it may become dark if it is not immediately expectorated.

Odor. Most specimens of sputum are odorless, but purulent sputum may occasionally have a sweet odor. A rotten, decomposed stench indicates an anaerobic putrefactive process, although infections by certain coliform organisms are also occasionally associated with a foul odor.

Abnormal Substances. Occasionally, foreign material that is directly related to the underlying disease process may be expectorated, either alone or mixed with sputum. Such substances can sometimes be recognized by their macroscopic appearance alone, but it is usually necessary to identify them microscopically or chemically. Carbon particles may be present in the sputum of city dwellers and particles of coal dust in that of coal miners. The sputum may contain particles of calcium known as *broncholiths,* which originate from calcified tuberculous hilar lymph nodes that have eroded into the lumen of a bronchus or from calcium deposits in the lung parenchyma, as in *silicosis* and *histoplasmosis.*

Dittrich's plugs may occasionally be found in the purulent sputum of patients with *bronchiectasis* or a *lung abscess.* These are yellow-white particles, varying in size from that of a pinhead to a pea, and they represent inspissated, disintegrated, purulent material that consists of fatty acids and fat globules.

Microscopic Examination

Microscopic examination of sputum is essential in order to identify any organisms and their source, as well as any cells or abnormal substances that may be present.

Bacteriology. Microscopic examination of a gram-stained smear of secretions will indicate whether there are organisms present and whether they are predominantly gram-positive or gram-negative; this is of prime importance in order to institute proper antibiotic therapy promptly. A Ziehl-Neelsen stain may reveal the presence of acid-fast bacilli, indicating active *tuberculosis,* and occasionally fungi, such as *Blastomyces dermatitidis,* can be demonstrated on smear. Proper identification of the pathogenic organisms is achieved by culture of the specimen; this will be discussed later.

Cytologic Examination. The cellular composition of the secretions helps to determine whether the specimen is derived from the oropharynx or from the lower respiratory tract. Secretions from the upper respiratory passages contain flat, polygonal epithelial cells. Large round or oval macrophages, often filled with carbon particles, are frequently seen in secretions from the bronchial tree. Ciliated, columnar cells that have been shed from the bronchial mucosa are often seen as well.

The sputum of a tuberculous infection contains numerous lymphocytes, whereas that of a nontuberculous bacterial infection contains predominantly polymorphonuclear neutrophils. There are frequently many eosinophils in the sputum of patients suffering from *asthma.* Large numbers of erythrocytes are indicative of either a recent hemorrhage or exudation of blood, as in the rusty sputum of *pneumococcal pneumonia.*

In a *bronchogenic carcinoma,* examination of the sputum by a technician who has been specially trained in cytologic examination may disclose malignant cells that have been exfoliated into the bronchial tree by the neoplastic process.

Abnormal Substances. Purulent material should be examined for elastic fibers, which are indicative of destruction of pulmonary tissue such as may occur in *tuberculosis, bronchiectasis, lung abscess* or *pulmonary malignancy.* When a fleck of purulent sputum is mixed with sodium hydroxide, which dissolves the cellular material, elastic fibers will be visible under the low-power objective. They are slender, wavy, highly refractile threads of uniform diameter but of varying length, with split or curled ends, and are usually seen either singly or grouped together in small bundles.

Oil droplets in bronchial secretions are easily recognized microscopically because they readily absorb a scarlet red dye such as Sudan III. Their presence suggests *lipid pneumonia* or *fat embolism.* The oil droplets may be in the cytoplasm of the macrophages or they may be extracellular. Vegetable and animal oils stain black and liquid petrolatum stains yellow with osmic acid.

Asbestos bodies, which are formed by the deposit of an iron-containing protein on an asbestos fiber, are frequently found in the sputum of patients with *asbestosis.* These slender, elongated structures with bulbous ends range from 10 to 180 microns in size and stain a brilliant blue with potassium ferrocyanide.

PLEURAL FLUID

Fluid in the pleural cavity should be aspirated in order to determine its nature, and in most cases a pleural biopsy sample should be obtained at the same time for histologic examination.

Collection

Aspiration of pleural fluid, or *thoracentesis,* and pleural biopsy should be carried out while the patient is in the sitting position if this is at all feasible. The site of aspiration and biopsy must be chosen with care. Both the upper limit of the fluid and the level of the opposite normal diaphragm should be determined by percussion. Aspiration should then be carried out at a point midway between these two levels on the posterior wall of the affected side. If the fluid is encapsulated, its borders should be carefully outlined by percussion, and the needle inserted into the center of the area of dullness. In all cases, the needle should be inserted through the intercostal space over the superior border of the rib, thus avoiding accidental injury to the intercostal vessels or nerves. As much fluid as possible should be removed slowly; too rapid a withdrawal may result in acute edema of the underlying lung. Although it is preferable to keep the pleural cavity free of air, it may be necessary to allow air to enter through the needle if the patient should complain of chest tightness during the aspiration. A roentgenogram of the chest taken as soon as possible after the aspiration will help to determine whether there is an underlying pulmonary lesion.

Macroscopic Examination

Appearance. A *transudate* is usually watery, pale yellow and either clear or slightly hazy. An *exudate* is generally deep yellow and turbid and feels thicker and stickier because of its higher protein content. The turbidity of the pleural fluid depends on the number of formed particles it contains, and the fluid may vary from cloudiness to thick, creamy pus. When red blood cells are present, the color of the fluid varies from a reddish tinge to dark red. Fresh blood in the pleural fluid is generally due to trauma, a pulmonary infarction or a neoplastic process. Empyema fluid varies from brown to yellow or green. Chylous fluid has a milky turbidity, and the fluid has an anchovy color in *amebiasis.*

Coagulability. The degree of spontaneous coagulation of the pleural fluid after its aspiration depends on the amount of fibrin present. A transudate rarely coagulates, but exudates and neoplastic effusions can coagulate fairly rapidly.

Odor. Transudates and exudates are usually odorless, but there may be a putrid stench if the pleural effusion is due to anaerobic organisms.

Chemical Examination

Specific Gravity. The specific gravity of a transudate is usually between 1.006 and 1.018. An exudate, because of its greater protein content, generally has a specific gravity considerably higher than 1.018.

Protein Content. The protein content of pleural fluid may vary from 0.1 to 8.0 gm. per 100 ml. The protein content of a transudate is usually less than 2.5 per cent, whereas in an exudate there is more than 2.5 per cent and the pleural fluid–to–serum total protein ratio is greater than 0.5.

Glucose Content. In pleural effusions due to malignancy, pneumonia, fungal diseases and other infections, the glucose content of the pleural fluid is the same as that in the blood. In approximately 60 per cent of tuberculous effusions, the glucose content is less than 60 mg./100 ml. In rheumatoid disease, the glucose content is markedly reduced to less than 30 mg./100 ml.

LDH. A pleural fluid LDH that is greater than 200 I.U. or a fluid/ serum ratio of greater than 0.6 suggests an exudate.

pH. The pH is low in *empyema, rheumatoid disease, tuberculosis* and *carcinoma.*

Amylase. An amylase level that is higher in the pleural fluid than in the blood suggests *acute pancreatitis,* but this may also occur with a *pancreatic pseudocyst, esophageal rupture* or *lung carcinoma.*

Lipids. In a lipid pleural effusion, the supernatant of centrifuged pleural fluid is cloudy. In chylous effusions, the percentage of neutral fats and fatty acids is high, and the Sudan III stain is positive. In pleural effusions secondary to *rheumatoid disease* or other *collagen disorders,* rheumatoid factor or lupus erythematosus cells are present in the fluid.

Microscopic Examination

Although often not diagnostic in itself, the cellular content of pleural fluid is of considerable importance, and the predominant cell type may suggest the causative disease.

Cytology

LEUKOCYTES. Numerous polymorphonuclear neutrophils (greater than 1000/µl.) usually indicates inflammation such as a *bacterial pneumonia, pulmonary infarction* or a *subphrenic abscess.*

LYMPHOCYTES. A predominance of lymphocytes suggests a transudative effusion, but lymphocytes may also be found in *tuberculosis* or other chronic pleural effusion.

EOSINOPHILS. Numerous eosinophils may be found in a pleural effusion caused by a *collagen disorder* or in a *parasitic infection,* such as *hydatid disease.*

ERYTHROCYTES. Numerous erythrocytes may be found in pleural fluids resulting from *trauma, tuberculosis, pulmonary infarction* or *malignancy.*

NEOPLASTIC CELLS. Malignant cells may be found in about 50 per cent of effusions due to a neoplastic process involving the pleural surfaces. These cells are generally difficult to recognize, however, unless there is mitosis or the cells are arranged in a particular tissue pattern.

BACTERIOLOGIC EXAMINATION

Bacteriologic examination of bronchial secretions, pleural fluid or material from draining sinuses should be smeared, stained and examined for bacteria. The offending organism can only be established by cultural methods, whereas the sensitivity of an organism to antimicrobial agents is extremely important in determining the etiology and treatment of a bronchopulmonary infection. The following discussion of the bacteriologic examination pertains to all respiratory infections.

In all cases of pneumonia, a sputum smear that has been stained by both the Gram and Ziehl-Neelsen methods should be examined. Differentiation of a gram-positive from a gram-negative organism enables administration of the appropriate antibiotic while awaiting the results of the sputum culture and antibiotic sensitivity. At all times, however, the bacteriologic report should be assessed critically and in the light of the clinical picture. One must remember that the bacterial growth may be only secondary invaders and not actually responsible for the disease and that organisms that grow profusely on culture may be present in only small numbers in the bronchial secretions.

BACTERIAL INFECTION

Gram-positive Cocci

Gram-positive cocci in pairs or chains in a sputum smear indicate the presence of either **Diplococcus pneumoniae** or another species of streptococci. Although the **hemolytic streptococcus** may produce a primary type of pneumonia, it generally acts as a secondary invader following in the course of some other infection, such as influenza or measles.

Staphylococci are gram-positive cocci that occur in "grapelike" clusters. Because **Staphylococcus aureus** is frequently present in the upper respiratory tracts of healthy, noninfected individuals, a large number of these organisms mixed with pus cells in a sputum smear is more important than their growth in a sputum culture. This organism most commonly is a secondary invader during the course of influenza or some debilitating disease, although much less frequently than the hemolytic streptococcus. A pulmonary infection may also develop as a result of invasion of the blood from a primary focus in some other part of the body such as a **perinephric abscess,** the pneumonia then being a part of a widespread infection.

Gram-negative Bacilli

Klebsiella pneumoniae, also known as **Friedländer's bacillus,** is a very rare cause of pneumonia. It is occasionally found in the healthy oropharynx, where it behaves as a saprophyte, but it can become pathogenic if the body resistance is lowered.

Hemophilus influenzae generally involves the upper respiratory tract, although it may also cause bronchiolitis or a primary pneumonia in infants and children. It is frequently demonstrated in the sputum of patients with chronic bronchitis, and it is often considered to be pathogenic, usually in association with organisms.

Pseudomonas aeruginosa pneumonia is frequently a hospital-acquired infection and occurs after the normal upper respiratory tract flora has been altered by broad-spectrum antibiotics or following excessive use of nonsterilized nebulizers. This organism is also the commonest found in patients suffering from cystic fibrosis.

Gram-positive Bacilli

Actinomyces israelii can be recognized in bronchial secretions or in the discharge from sinuses in the form of *"sulfur granules,"* which are a dense tangle of gram-positive mycelia. These whitish-yellow amorphous masses are often visible to the naked eye if the pus is shaken in normal saline and examined against a dark background. The organism can be grown only under anaerobic conditions, a feature that distinguishes it from *Nocardia asteroides,* which grows only under aerobic conditions and is weakly acid-fast.

Legionella pneumophila is a gram-negative pleomorphic bacillus that stains poorly with ordinary stains but is readily demonstrable with the Dieterle silver-impregnation method.

Anaerobic Bacteria

Percutaneous transtracheal or pleural aspiration may be necessary to collect secretions for anaerobic culture, the common organisms being members of the genera *Bacteriodes* and *Fusobacterium.*

Mycobacteria

All sputum must be examined for acid-fast bacilli, since the radiologic opacities present in any nontuberculous disease can be mimicked by pulmonary tuberculosis.

Mycobacterium tuberculosis. Tubercle bacilli are usually readily demonstrated in active disease, but the organisms may be found only after repeated and persistent searching when the disease is chronic and indolent. The detection of acid-fast mycobacteria, morphologically resembling tubercle bacilli, by the direct microscopic examination of a smear of sputum stained by the Ziehl-Neelsen method is generally accepted as positive proof of the diagnosis of *pulmonary tuberculosis.* However, it has been estimated that at least 100,000 bacilli must be present in 1 ml. of sputum before a single organism can be detected by the direct examination. Even when no tubercle bacilli are demonstrated in the sputum smear, it may be possible to demonstrate bacilli in a concentrated specimen that is derived from a large collection of sputum by adding sodium hydroxide and then centrifuging it. The sediment is then stained by the Ziehl-Neelsen method and examined for acid-fast bacilli.

When sputum containing tubercle bacilli is planted on a solid medium containing a mixture of egg and potato flour or starches and then incubated at 37°C for four to six weeks, a dry, wrinkled, grayish-yellow warty growth results. A Ziehl-Neelsen stain of a smear from this culture will demonstrate thousands of acid-fast mycobacteria. Strong niacin production indicates that the organism is *Mycobacterium tuberculosis;* a negative niacin test indicates that the organism belongs to another species of mycobacteria.

Nontuberculous Mycobacteria. The nontuberculous, "atypical" or "anonymous" mycobacteria resemble *Mycobacterium tuberculosis* morphologically but have different cultural characteristics. They are found in soil, contaminated water and occasionally in human gastric contents. In the past, they were considered to be saprophytes and not pathogenic to man. In recent years, however, it has become clear that some can produce pulmonary disease that mimics tuberculosis.

Several classifications of these mycobacteria have been suggested, but the one used most commonly is the Runyon classification, which divides them into four groups based on distinctive cultural characteristics:

Group I mycobacteria *(photochromogens),* which include *M. kansasii* and *M. marinum,* resemble *M. tuberculosis* when cultured, if kept in the dark. However, they develop a vivid yellow color when exposed to light during the period of active growth.

Group II mycobacteria *(scotochromogens),* of which *M. scrofulaceum* is the best known member, are orange both in the dark and when exposed to light.

Group III mycobacteria *(nonphotochromogens),* which include *M. avium* and *M. intracellulare,* have little pigment, are ivory or buff in color, and are not affected by exposure to light.

Group IV mycobacteria *(rapid growers),* of which *M. fortuitum* is best known, also possess very little pigment and are not affected by exposure to light, but they are distinguished from the other groups by their very rapid rate of growth. In contrast to the first three groups, which require two or three weeks at room temperature to grow, group IV mycobacteria become mature in a matter of two or three days.

Occasionally these organisms are present as saprophytes in patients with other chronic respiratory disease. Before it can be decided that a pulmonary disease is caused by one of the nontuberculous mycobacteria, they must be demonstrated in very large numbers in the smear, and the identical strain should be grown repeatedly.

VIRAL INFECTION

Of the known filterable viruses that are capable of causing pneumonia in man, the most important ones are the *myxoviruses* and *influenza viruses A and B.* Others are the *respiratory syncytial virus,* which has a predilection for children; *adenoviruses 4 and 7;* and *parainfluenza 3. Cytomegalovirus* and *herpes simplex virus* cause pulmonary infections in immunosuppressed or compromised individuals.

Despite improvement in the isolation techniques of viruses, they can still be identified only in approximately 50 per cent of the nonbacterial pneumonias. Viruses can be grown by inoculating the patient's throat washings, taken during the early phase of the illness, into an embryonated egg, as well as into ferrets or mice. A viral infection can also be identified by the *virus neutralization test,* which demonstrates antibodies capable of neutralizing the virus in the serum. Specimens are obtained as early as possible after the beginning of the illness, 14 days later, and again about four weeks after the onset of the disease. A serum viral-antibody titer that rises from the acute phase to the convalescent phase is diagnostic of a viral infection. In practice, however, this method provides a specific diagnosis in less than 25 per cent of paired serum specimens that are submitted to the laboratory, and even then the diagnosis is established long after a pneumonia has run its natural course. A viral etiology can also be established by the *hemagglutination inhibition test,* which is based on the ability of the virus to agglutinate erythrocytes, a reaction that can be inhibited by a specific antiserum.

MYCOPLASMAL INFECTION

Mycoplasma pneumoniae is the most frequent cause of nonbacterial pneumonia in the civilian population. This organism shares the characteristics of both a virus and a bacterium; its particle size is similar to that of viruses, but it also possesses enzyme systems similar to those of bacteria. *Mycoplasmal pneumonia* is diagnosed by isolating *Mycoplasma pneumoniae* in the sputum. The demonstration of an increased specific antibody in the serum is also of value, but this procedure takes two to three weeks. In about 40 per cent of proven cases, a substance capable of agglutinating human group O erythrocytes is present in the serum at low temperatures but not at body or room temperature. These *cold hemagglutinins* frequently appear only during convalescence and may reach a titer of 1:32 in the average case. However, the demonstration of cold hemagglutinins is not specific for mycoplasmal pneumonia, because they may be elevated in about 20 per cent of the pneumonias caused by adenoviruses and also occasionally in *pneumococcal pneumonia, tuberculosis* or *bronchogenic carcinoma.* Agglutinins to the streptococcus MG antigen may also be present in patients suffering from *mycoplasmal pneumonia,* but these are even less specific than the cold agglutinins.

FUNGAL INFECTION

Although mycotic infections of the respiratory tract are rare compared with other pulmonary infections, they do occur with sufficient frequency to warrant consideration in the differential diagnosis of an obscure pulmonary lesion, particularly if the patient is known to have resided in a geographic area in which a particular fungal infection is endemic. Diagnosis of a mycotic infection can be established only by isolation and identification of a fungus in bronchial secretions or by histologic examination of diseased tissues.

Most pathogenic fungi can be identified only by cultural methods. They may be isolated by culturing the sputum on either Sabouraud's agar at room temperature or on blood agar at 37°C. However, the presence of fungi in the sputum does not necessarily imply that they are the primary or sole cause of the disease. They may be saprophytic, they may have secondarily invaded some other pre-existing disease, or they may have accidentally contaminated a specimen. This applies particularly to yeasts, which are frequently found in the sputum of patients with such chronic diseases as *tuberculosis, bronchiectasis* or *bronchogenic carcinoma.*

Candida albicans and other members of the Candida genus are inhabitants of the mouth normally. For this reason, the diagnosis of pulmonary candidiasis is often difficult, especially since the advent of the widespread use of antibiotics and corticosteroids, which has increased their incidence in sputum cultures. On the other hand, certain other fungi, when isolated from the bronchial secretions, can definitely be considered to be responsible for pulmonary disease, particularly *Histoplasma capsulatum, Coccidioides immitis, Blastomyces dermatitidis, Cryptococcus neoformans* and *Aspergillus fumigatus.*

Histoplasma capsulatum, which causes *histoplasmosis,* differs from other pathogenic fungi in that it is an intracellular organism and is confined to the cells of the reticuloendothelial system so that it is rarely found in the sputum. *Coccidioides immitis,* the cause of *coccidioidomycosis,* exists in nature in a mycelial form, but it becomes a large spherule once it invades the tissues. *Blastomyces dermatitidis,* the fungus responsible for *North American blastomycosis,* is a large, yeastlike cell. *Cryptococcus neoformans* is responsible for *cryptococcosis,* which initially affects the lungs. These organisms are difficult to differentiate from *Histoplasma capsulatum* with hematoxylin and eosin stains, but mucicarmine stains are diagnostic. *Aspergillus fumigatus* is responsible for the *aspergillus mycetoma,* which is occasionally found in a pre-existing cavity or in a bulla. This aspergillus grows in the mycelial form, and branching septate hyphae are usually seen in the tissue.

PROTOZOAL INFECTION

Pneumocystis carinii is now a common cause of infectious pneumonitis in immunodeficient patients, and recently pneumonia due to this organism has been described in epidemic proportions in homosexual men. Groups of encysted organisms may be seen in lung tissue and rarely in sputum when stained with methenamine silver. *Toxoplasmosis,* which is caused by *Toxoplasma gondii,* may also cause an interstitial pneumonitis in the immunocompromised host. *Entamoeba histolytica* causes *amebiasis,* which is always secondary to intestinal and hepatic infection. Trophozoites with clear pseudopods may be seen in fresh sputum. The indirect hemagglutination, indirect fluorescent antibody, and gel diffusion precipitation are valuable tests in the diagnosis of invasive amebiasis.

RICKETTSIAL INFECTION

Coxiella burnetii, which is responsible for the pneumonia in *Q fever,* çan occasionally be isolated by the injection of a specimen of a patient's blood or urine into a guinea pig or the yolk sac of a chick embryo. The diagnosis is usually made serologically by the complement-fixation and agglutination tests using *C. burnetii* yolk sac antigen. Complement-fixing antibodies usually appear during the first week of the illness, and agglutination antibodies usually appear during the second or third week.

The *Weil-Felix reaction,* an agglutination test using *Proteus X-19, X-2 and X-K,* is frequently positive in most of the rickettsial diseases except for *Q fever.*

HISTOLOGIC EXAMINATION

In certain conditions, an accurate diagnosis of the respiratory disease present can be established only by histologic examination of the tissue. As pointed out above, some pulmonary infections may be diagnosed only by special stains of tissue. In addition, histologic examination of tissue is essential to establish the diagnosis of many bronchial, parenchymal and pleural conditions. The tissue can be obtained by bronchial biopsy, transbronchial tissue biopsy through a bronchoscope, percutaneous needle aspiration of a solitary pulmonary lesion, biopsy of diseased pulmonary tissue through an open thoracotomy or biopsy of enlarged mediastinal lymph nodes by mediastinoscopy.

BRONCHIAL BIOPSY

Endobronchial biopsies of the trachea and the major bronchi as well as the orifices of their larger subdivisions are performed through a bronchoscope. The smaller bronchi and their peripheral radicles cannot be visualized, but one may obtain valuable information by brushing or aspirating secretions from these areas for bacteriologic and cytologic studies.

Bronchoscopy is indicated whenever there are any symptoms or signs of a localized bronchial obstruction. This should be carried out if there is the least suspicion of a *bronchogenic carcinoma,* because more than 50 per cent of these tumors can be visualized with the bronchoscope and many more are diagnosed from examination of aspirated bronchial secretions.

LUNG BIOPSY

A lung biopsy is often necessary to establish the diagnosis when there is roentgenologic evidence of diffuse pulmonary infiltrations or certain types of solitary lung lesions. The most satisfactory means of obtaining adequate tissue for histologic examination is by open thoracotomy, although there is a degree of morbidity associated with this procedure.

Lung tissue can also be obtained through a bronchoscope *(transbron-*

chial biopsy) by means of a long flexible forceps that is inserted into the diseased area under fluoroscopic control. Although the amount of tissue obtained is very small, many specimens may be obtained from different lobes.

Percutaneous needle biopsy or drill biopsy of the lung have also been used in *interstitial lung disease,* but they have limitations, because diseased lung tissue may be missed and occasionally *pneumothorax, hemothorax* or pleural infection may occur. A percutaneous aspiration biopsy of a solitary lesion, under fluoroscopic control, may also yield a cytologic or a bacteriologic diagnosis.

LYMPH NODE BIOPSY

Enlarged lymph nodes should be examined histologically to establish whether they are due to granulomatous disease such as *sarcoidosis* or *tuberculosis,* a *lymphoma* such as *Hodgkin's disease,* or *carcinoma.* Even when the diagnosis of *bronchogenic carcinoma* has been established, the lymph nodes should be examined to decide whether the lesion is surgically resectable. Biopsy of the scalene nodes, which are situated in a pad of fat lying anterior to the scalenus anticus muscle in the neck, has been used, but mediastinoscopy and biopsy of mediastinal lymph nodes is generally accepted as yielding the highest number of positive results.

PLEURAL BIOPSY

In many cases, the etiology of a pleural effusion can be determined by clinical assessment of the patient's illness or by laboratory examination of the fluid, but these methods may not be adequate in a significant number of patients. Examination of a pleural biopsy will establish the diagnosis of *tuberculosis* in a high percentage of patients who suffer from an acute serous pleurisy, and occasionally a *mesothelioma* may be diagnosed. A specially designed needle is used to aspirate the pleural effusion and to obtain a biopsy from the parietal pleura. Since it is possible to take a biopsy from a relatively normal area and miss a pathologic lesion, several pleural biopsies should be taken at different sites. In certain selective cases, particularly if a malignancy is suspected, it may be necessary to carry out an exploratory thoracotomy. This enables the surgeon to visualize the pleura and thus to detect a lesion that may have been overlooked by the needle biopsies.

TESTS OF IMMUNE FUNCTION

IgE ANTIBODIES

A semiquantitative assessment of the levels of allergen-specific *IgE antibodies* in the serum can be obtained by a radioimmunoassay called the radioallergosorbent *(RAST)* test. This test is particularly useful when skin testing is difficult to perform or interpret and in the evaluation of allergic chíldren. The clinical implication of a positive RAST test is no different from that of positive skin tests. Both indicate the presence and the relative amount of allergen-specific IgE antibodies in a given patient.

The amount of IgE in the serum is usually measured by the radioimmunosorbent test *(RIST)* and the *double-antibody radioimmunoprecipitation assay.* The *single radioimmunodiffusion method* is another simple test that can be used to detect high levels of serum IgE (greater than 400–500 I.U.). The RIST is based on the competition between radioactively labeled IgE and IgE protein in the serum for binding with anti-IgE, which is attached to insoluble particles or paper discs *(PRIST,* paper radioimmunosorbent test). A high serum IgE level is seen in *hypergammaglobulinemia E syndrome* (elevated IgE level, increased susceptibility to infection and dermatitis) and during the active stages of *allergic bronchopulmonary aspergillosis.*

LEUKOCYTE HISTAMINE RELEASE

This test measures the amount of histamine released after the *in vitro* incubation of peripheral blood leukocytes with a specific antigen. The assay detects the presence of basophil-fixed IgE antibodies and also measures the capacity of the basophils to release histamine when challenged with the appropriate antigen.

IgG BLOCKING ANTIBODIES

There is a significant rise in the serum level of allergen-specific IgG antibodies following allergy hyposensitization treatment *(immunotherapy),* such as with pollen extracts, for *allergic rhinitis.* However, no clear correlation between serum IgG levels and the degree of symptomatic improvement following immunotherapy has been established.

ANTI–BASEMENT MEMBRANE (BM) ANTIBODIES

The presence of *anti–BM antibodies* in the circulation and along the glomerular and pulmonary alveolar basement membranes is the hallmark of *Goodpasture's syndrome.* Fixation of these antibodies on the BM of these two organs can be demonstrated by direct immunofluorescent staining of renal or lung biopsy tissue with a fluorochrome-conjugated anti-immunoglobulin or anti-IgG reagent. Anti-BM in the serum can be detected by an indirect immunofluorescent test or by a more sensitive double-antibody radioimmunoassay.

CIRCULATING IMMUNE COMPLEXES

A number of procedures may be used to demonstrate the presence of circulating immune complexes indirectly. There are increased circulating immune complexes in *lupus erythematosus,* and it has been suggested that there are elevated circulating immune complexes in patients with active *interstitial lung disease.*

PRECIPITINS

Precipitating antibodies to specific antigens are present in *hypersensitivity lung disease,* such as *farmer's lung* and *bird fancier's disease.* Using gel-diffusion techniques, a line of precipitate will form between specific antigens and the patient's serum if it contains antibody to the antigen.

SERUM COMPLEMENT

The presence of circulating immune complexes may be associated with depressed total serum complement or some of the early complement components (e.g., C4 and C3).

COMPLEMENT FIXATION

Complement fixation and precipitin tests may be helpful in establishing a diagnosis of a mycotic infection. These tests become positive only after the development of a hypersensitivity reaction in the tissues. The complement-fixing antibodies appear later than the precipitins and persist for a longer time, so that the precipitin test is of more value in the early phase of the disease. A negative reaction to either test, however, does not imply absence of a mycotic infection. The complement fixation test is positive in about 75 per cent of cases of *hydatid disease,* but it may be negative if the cyst is walled off or if the cysts are inactive.

SERUM CRYOGLOBULIN

Immune complexes in the serum may become insoluble at low temperature and may be detected as cryoglobulins. Cryoglobulins are present in about half of the patients with immune complex vasculitis (e.g., *periarteritis nodosa).*

LE CELLS

The *lupus erythematosus cell* (LE cell), a polymorphonuclear leukocyte that contains a phagocytosed, homogeneous, structureless inclusion body, can be demonstrated in special preparations of the blood and bone marrow. The inclusion body is apparently nuclear protein that has been altered by the LE factor in the serum, an immunoglobulin apparently with specificity against nucleoprotein. Demonstration of LE cells on two or more occasions is thought to establish the diagnosis of *systemic lupus erythematosus.*

RHEUMATOID FACTOR

This is an autoantibody against immunoglobulin G (IgG). The *rheumatoid factor* itself is usually IgM, but it may also be IgG, IgA or even IgD. A titer greater than 1:80 with the latex agglutination test or 1:32 with the sheep cell agglutination test (SCAT) is generally considered significant. The rheumatoid factor test is positive in *rheumatoid disease,* but may also be positive in patients with other forms of connective tissue diseases, such as *Sjögren's syndrome, systemic sclerosis, systemic lupus erythematosus,* and in patients with *pneumoconiosis* or *idiopathic pulmonary fibrosis.* Rheumatoid factor may also be present in a variety of diseases characterized by prolonged antigenic stimulation, such as chronic parasitic and bacterial infections, or in patients who have undergone organ transplants.

ANTINUCLEAR ANTIBODIES (ANA)

In *systemic lupus erythematosus* there is a tendency to form autoimmune antibodies against a variety of self tissue constituents, particularly components of nuclear antigens. Four patterns of immunofluorescence may be seen: localization of the fluorescence in the periphery of the nuclei *(ring pattern),* which indicates antibodies against the deoxyribonucleic acid component of the nuclear antigens (anti-DNA); a *nucleolar pattern,* which indicates antibodies against ribonucleic acid (RNA) or ribonucleoprotein; a *homogeneous pattern,* which is distributed evenly in the nuclei and indicates antibodies against deoxyribonuclear protein; and a *speckled pattern,* which indicates antibodies against extractable, soluble nuclear antigens (ENA).

Hepatitis B surface antigen (HB_sAg) has been detected in 20 to 30 per cent of patients with *periarteritis nodosa.* Serum autoimmune antibodies such as rheumatoid factor and antinuclear antibodies may be present in *rheumatoid arthritis* or *systemic lupus erythematosus* (SLE) with pulmonary involvement.

DIAGNOSTIC SKIN TESTS

Skin tests may be used to demonstrate the presence of allergen-specific IgE antibodies and thus to help determine whether an individual is allergic, or they may demonstrate exposure to various infectious agents and cellular immunity.

When the history is suggestive, skin tests may be performed with extracts of inhalant allergens, such as animal dander, feathers, house dust, house dust mites, saprophytic mold spores, tree pollens, grass pollens and weed pollens. The reponse to allergenic extracts that are prepared from antigenic materials suspected of causing an allergic reaction is compared with the response to diluent (such as phosphate-buffered saline) to distinguish false-positive skin reactions.

The *prick skin test* is simple to perform and correlates well with the *in vitro* detection of IgE antibodies (the *RAST* test) and with bronchoprovocation. It is carried out by placing a drop of undiluted allergenic extract prepared in 50 per cent glycerine on the skin surface, and then puncturing the skin directly under the drop with a sterilized sharp needle. The drop of extract is removed 10 to 15 minutes later, and the reaction is recorded.

The *intradermal skin test* consists of injection of a very small volume (about 0.02–0.03 ml.) of an allergenic extract (1:100 dilution of the original concentration) so as to raise a tiny visible bleb on the skin surface; the reaction is read in 10 to 15 minutes. Since more antigenic material is injected in this case, an immediate reaction as well as a delayed or late reaction may occur.

THE SKIN REACTION

The Immediate Reaction

The **immediate-type hypersensitivity skin reaction** is associated with antibody formation and is characterized by the development of a wheal and flare at the test site within 10 to 15 minutes. There are no uniform criteria for the grading of the reaction, but one generally grades it according to the size of the wheal: one-plus for wheals smaller than 5 mm., two-plus for 5- to 8-mm. wheals, three-plus for 9- to 12-mm. wheals, and four-plus for larger wheals or those with pseudopod formation.

A positive immediate wheal-and-flare reaction indicates the presence of specific IgE antibodies to the allergen being tested in the subject. On the other hand, it is important to note that this does not necessarily mean clinical disease, and the skin test results must be considered in conjunction with the history, physical findings, and other laboratory tests.

The Late Reaction

An immediate reaction may be followed by a **late reaction** 4 to 8 hours later. This reaction is manifested by more diffuse erythema and swelling, and the skin site is warm and often itchy. The late reaction is seen in allergic subjects after testing with a variety of allergens such as fungi, pollens, or **Bacillus subtilis enzyme.** Since it is more common when larger amounts of allergens are injected, it is seen more frequently with intradermal tests than with prick tests.

The Delayed Reaction

A **delayed skin reaction** is due to hypersensitivity that is not associated with the formation of antibodies but is mediated by specifically sensitized lymphocytes. This kind of reaction is usually manifested within 48 to 72 hours after infection. It occurs in association with mycobacterial infection and some fungal infections and is indicative of a previous exposure or infection with the offending organism.

Mycobacterium tuberculosis

Because of potential cross-reactivity with the nontuberculous mycobacteria, only erythema greater than 10 mm. in diameter along with induration 48 to 72 hours after injection of Old Tuberculin (1:2000 dilution containing 5 tuberculin units) or its active principle, purified protein derivative (PPD) (0.0001 mg.) is considered significant. The tuberculin skin reaction is almost always positive after a primary infection, but it may be negative early in the course of the illness or when the condition is disseminated. The incidence of positive reactivity falls with advancing age. In addition, certain conditions, such as viral infections (e.g., *measles*) or the administration of some vaccines (e.g., *poliomyelitis* or *yellow fever*), may reduce the skin reactivity. The skin sensitivity may also be lost temporarily in *sarcoidosis* and in immunosuppressed individuals, such as those suffering from *renal* or *hepatic failure* or *Hodgkin's disease* or those receiving immunosuppressant drugs such as steroids or cytotoxic drugs.

Nontuberculous Mycobacteria

Antigens of the *nonphotochromogen* (PPD-B), the *photochromogen* (PPD-Y) and the *scrotochromogen* (PPD-G) strains of mycobacteria can be injected intradermally in a manner similar to that used for PPD; again reactions are noted after 48 hours. A reaction to one of the nontuberculous mycobacteria is considered positive only if it results in an area of induration that is at least 5 mm. greater than that produced by standard tuberculin.

Fungal Disease

A delayed skin reaction following the intradermal injection of the appropriate antigen may also be seen in persons suffering from a fungal disease. Skin tests for *coccidioidomycosis, histoplasmosis* and *blastomycosis* use antigens derived from the mycelial phase of the fungus, i.e., *coccidioidin, histoplasmin* and *blastomycin.*

Fungal skin tests, particularly the histoplasmin skin test, should be performed after measurement of the complement fixation and precipitin tests, because the injection of the antigen may have a "boosting effect" on the circulating antibodies.

As with tuberculosis, a positive skin reaction (10 mm. or more of induration) to a 1:10 to 1:100 dilution of coccidioidin or histoplasmin indicates exposure to the fungus or active disease. However, it does not indicate whether this was recent or in the remote past. In addition, it does not necessarily mean that the pulmonary disease under study is caused by that fungus. Like the tuberculin test, it may be negative in disseminated disease. The blastomycin skin test may not be positive in 50 per cent of patients with active disease, and conversely it may be positive in patients who are infected with *Histoplasma capsulatum.* Histoplasmin may also cross-react with coccidioidin. Usually, the antigen of the fungus responsible for the disease generally produces the strongest reaction.

Hydatid Disease

A positive response to an antigen consisting of fluid from an uncomplicated *hydatid cyst* that has been passed through a Berkefeld or Seitz filter (i.e., the *Casoni skin test*) is present in 90 per cent of infected patients. This persists for a lifetime, so that a negative reaction generally means that the patient has not been infected by the *Echinococcus granulosus.* There are two phases to a positive reaction: an immediate wheal that enlarges in size, develops pseudopodia and is surrounded by a zone of erythema, reaching its maximum within one-half hour; and a late response occurring about 24 hours later and consisting of an indurated area surrounded by a zone of erythema.

Sarcoidosis

The diagnosis of *sarcoidosis,* a systemic granulomatous disease of unknown etiology that primarily affects the reticuloendothelial system, is established by the demonstration of a noncaseating epithelioid cell granuloma in lymph nodes, skin, liver, lung or conjunctiva. The *Kveim skin test,* in which a small amount of a suspension of a sarcoid spleen is injected intracutaneously, may be valuable when histologic confirmation is not available. The intracutaneous injection results in a specific granulomatous skin reaction in patients who are suffering from an active form of the disease. Unfortunately, it requires 6 to 8 weeks or even longer before a positive reaction (a reddish papule) appears. The injection site is excised after 8 weeks and examined microscopically, whether or not a papule develops.

ANERGY

It is important to point out that patients with *sarcoidosis* and immuno-suppressed patients may have a negative tuberculin skin test because of a state of anergy associated with active *sarcoidosis.* In the presence of complete anergy, *tuberculosis* cannot be excluded by a negative skin test, and a careful search for mycobacteria as well as the cause of the anergy must be carried out. If a state of anergy is suspected, the intracutaneous injection of other reagents capable of inducing delayed skin reactions, such as *candida, mumps, streptokinase,* or *trichophyton,* will help to determine whether *cellular immune function* is intact.

BRONCHOPROVOCATION STUDIES

Inhalation challenge is particularly useful in individuals who demonstrate a positive skin reaction to specific allergens or who have symptoms that appear to be related to a particular occupational exposure. By assessing bronchial reactivity, one can determine the clinical significance of these specific allergens or irritants. Inhalation challenge with a suspected agent or antigen is particularly important when, despite a very suggestive history, no method of demonstrating specific antibodies against the putative agent is available.

To date, a large number of chemical agents, such as toluene diisocyanate; wood dusts, such as western red cedar; and flour, such as soybean, have been implicated in occupational asthma. Commercially available or specially prepared allergenic extracts, which are usually prepared in phosphate-

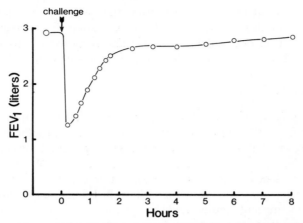

Figure 87. The immediate bronchial reaction to inhaled antigen. The FEV₁ falls within minutes after the bronchoprovocation.

buffered saline with a pH of 7.0 and containing 0.4% phenol, may be used for the inhalation challenge. In addition, bronchoconstricting mediators such as *histamine* or a neurotransmitter such as *acetylcholine* (or its analog, acetyl-beta-methylcholine chloride, *methacholine*) are generally used to assess nonspecific airway reactivity. As indicated earlier, one can also use exercise as a nonspecific bronchoprovocation test.

The bronchoprovocation is carried out while the subject is asymptomatic and has relatively good lung function (e.g., the FEV_1 is more than 80 per cent of the best value previously recorded from the subject). Since bronchodilators, antihistamines, anticholinergics and disodium cromoglycate may affect the bronchial response to provocation, these drugs are withheld before

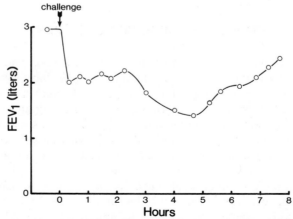

Figure 88. The dual (immediate and late) bronchial reaction to inhaled antigen. There is an immediate fall in FEV₁, followed hours later by another fall.

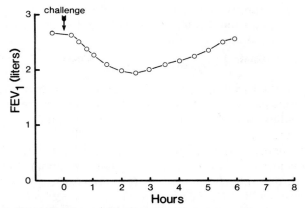

Figure 89. The late bronchial reaction to inhaled antigen. The response to bronchoprovocation is delayed and occurs hours after the inhalation.

the procedure. A drop in FEV_1 of 20 per cent or in R_{aw} of 35 per cent is generally considered to be a positive response to bronchoprovocation.

The bronchoconstriction may develop immediately (Fig. 87), and, as shown in Figure 88, this may be followed by a late reaction 4 to 8 hours later (i.e., a dual reaction). In other cases, only the late reaction may develop (Fig. 89). Such a late reaction is seen in patients with allergic bronchopulmonary aspergillosis following inhalation of aspergillus extract. Clearly then, a subject should be observed closely following bronchoprovocation with an antigen or irritant, and lung function assessed not only at frequent intervals over the first hour, but also at hourly intervals for 8 to 10 hours, as well as 24 hours later in order to detect a late asthmatic response. Repeat antigenic challenge, if necessary, should not be done for at least 24 hours after the last challenge.

BIOCHEMICAL STUDIES

There are a number of biochemical estimations that contribute to the assessment of respiratory disorders and may help in the diagnosis. The tests will not be described in great detail here and will be commented on only briefly.

SWEAT CHLORIDES

In most patients suffering from *cystic fibrosis,* the levels of sodium and chloride in the sweat are markedly elevated because the sweat glands are unable to conserve salt. This electrolyte abnormality has also been found in untreated *adrenal insufficiency.* It is being found with increasing frequency in adult patients who have *bronchiectasis,* presumably because they have a form of *cystic fibrosis.* Many patients with *cystic fibrosis* also have pancreatic insufficiency, and this is manifested by an absence of trypsin, lipase and amylase in the duodenal contents, as well as by an excess of fat and nitrogenous matter in the feces.

SERUM PROTEINS

There is normally between 6.0 and 8.5 grams of protein per 100 ml. of serum. The principal components of the serum proteins are albumin; alpha and beta globulins, which are produced in the liver; and gamma globulin, which is formed by the lymphocyte–plasma cell system. By means of immunoelectrophoresis the various globulins can be separated into groups that are antigenically distinct from each other. Gamma globulin may be elevated in chronic infection, such as **bronchiectasis,** and in **sarcoidosis,** whereas hyperglobulinemia may be present in connective tissue disorders, such as **lupus erythematosus** and **rheumatoid disease.** Low levels of gamma globulin, either congenital or acquired, and high levels of an abnormal nonfunctional globulin, as in **myelomatosis,** predispose the patient to frequent bacterial infections or recurrent pneumonias.

Alpha-1-Antitrypsin

Alpha-1-antitrypsin is the major circulating proteolytic enzyme inhibitor **(antiprotease)** in the body, and it forms the major component of the alpha-1-globulin fraction of the serum. A genetically determined deficiency of alpha-1-antitrypsin in the serum with an antitrypsin activity of less than 10 per cent **(homozygotes)** is associated with the development of **panlobular emphysema.** Those with a ZZ phenotype (i.e., homozygotes) are particularly prone to the development of **emphysema,** whereas those with MZ phenotype (i.e., heterozygotes) have an only slightly increased incidence of the disease. Recently, it has been shown that the ability of the alpha-1-antitrypsin to function effectively may be reduced in cigarette smokers.

SERUM ENZYMES

Certain tissues contain characteristic enzymes that enter the blood when the tissues are damaged or destroyed. The level of lactic dehydrogenase in the serum can be elevated by damage to nearly any tissue. It was previously thought that an elevated serum lactic dehydrogenase without a concomitant increase in glutamic oxaloacetic and glutamic pyruvic transaminases was indicative of pulmonary embolism and infarction, but this may not be specific. As indicated earlier, an elevated serum amylase ordinarily indicates pancreatic disease, and the finding of a higher level in the pleural fluid indicates an **acute pancreatitis.**

OTHER BIOCHEMICAL STUDIES

Some blood and serum determinations are helpful in the differential diagnosis of pulmonary infiltrates. The **blood urea nitrogen** may be elevated because of functional impairment of the kidneys in **chronic nephritis.** **Hyperglycemia** is indicative of **diabetes mellitus,** and **hypercalcemia** may be a feature of active *sarcoidosis.* Significant elevation of the *serum acid phosphatase* suggests a *prostatic carcinoma* that has metastasized. *Amyloidosis,* a complication of long-standing suppuration, can be demonstrated by the intravenous injection of Congo red, a dye that has an affinity for amyloid tissue.

HEMATOLOGIC STUDIES

Anemia may result because of depression of the bone marrow in chronic infections such as *tuberculosis.* A neoplasm that has metastasized to the bone marrow may cause anemia by mechanical interference with blood formation, and it may result from hemolysis in certain bacterial infections, particularly those caused by the *hemolytic streptococcus. Secondary polycythemia* may occur in diseases with associated chronic hypoxemia.

A *neutrophilic leukocytosis* is generally present in acute infections produced by pyogenic organisms, such as *Staphylococcus aureus, hemolytic streptococcus* organisms and *Diplococcus pneumoniae.* The degree of leukocytosis is governed by the resistance of the patient as well as the virulence and the number of the invading organisms. A severe leukocytosis, called a *leukemoid reaction,* may occasionally be seen in malignant pulmonary conditions, particularly those with associated infection and necrosis. An *eosinophilia* in the blood most commonly occurs in allergic disease. Beta-adrenergic blockade enhances the release of mature eosinophils from the marrow, and this has been proposed as the mechanism of the eosinophilia in patients with *asthma. Eosinophilia* is particularly severe in the migratory pulmonary infiltrations of *Loeffler's syndrome.* It is also a feature of parasitic infestations such as ascariasis, *amebiasis* and *hydatid disease,* as well as *periarteritis nodosa* and *Hodgkin's disease.*

A relative *lymphocytosis* may occasionally be seen in diseases with generalized lymphadenopathy, such as *Hodgkin's disease* and *lymphosarcoma.* A high degree of relative lymphocytosis may be found in *pertussis.*

In contrast to the bacterial pneumonias, the leukocyte count is rarely greater than 15,000 per mm.^{3} in *viral and mycoplasmal pneumonias.* Various degrees of *neutropenia* may be found in such viral diseases as *measles* and *influenza* and in some overwhelming bacterial infections, probably because of bone marrow depression by the organisms or their toxins.

The erythrocyte sedimentation rate frequently provides an indication of the activity of the disease process. In acute infective processes, the sedimentation rate is accelerated in the early part of the disease and gradually falls to normal levels as recovery takes place.

URINE ANALYSIS

Examination of the urine is an essential component of the assessment of all patients. A small percentage of patients suffering from *pulmonary tuberculosis* develop *genitourinary tuberculosis,* particulary when the disease has apparently become inactive. Chronic suppurative diseases may become complicated by the development of *renal amyloidosis. Carcinoma of the kidney* may metastasize to the lung or produce a *secondary polycythemia.* Patients suffering from *diabetes mellitus* are more liable to develop *pulmonary tuberculosis.*

ELECTROCARDIOGRAPHY

The typical electrocardiographic changes of *right ventricular hypertrophy and strain* and *"P pulmonale"* are found in patients suffering from chronic pulmonary diseases who have developed an increased pulmonary vascular resistance. In addition, respiratory insufficiency is frequently associated with *supraventricular,* and sometimes *ventricular, arrhythmias.*

THE PATTERNS OF RESPIRATORY DISEASE

- AIRWAY DISEASE
- LUNG PARENCHYMAL DISEASE
- PULMONARY VASCULAR DISEASE
- PLEURAL DISEASE
- CHEST WALL AND DIAPHRAGMATIC DISEASE

14

AIRWAY DISEASE

The airways are involved in most pulmonary diseases. In some the bronchi are diffusely involved, whereas in others only a single bronchus or one of its subdivisions may be affected. Even when the lung parenchyma is primarily involved, there may be inflammation of the bronchiolar walls, and the lumen of the bronchus draining the diseased area may be narrowed by mucosal swelling or inflammatory exudate, so that air movement into and out of the alveoli and drainage of secretions may become impaired.

The term "airway obstruction" is relative, for the amount of obstruction of an affected bronchus will vary inversely with the diameter of its lumen. Clearly, mucosal swelling of large bronchi will not produce the same degree of obstruction as will swelling in one of the finer bronchi. In the infant, where the bronchial diameters are small, inflammatory swelling of even the large bronchi may produce serious obstruction. Even in persons with normal lungs, there may be a degree of airway narrowing, particularly in the dependent lung regions, under certain circumstances, such as when obesity is present.

GENERAL FEATURES OF AIRWAY OBSTRUCTION

Figure 90 depicts three mechanisms by which an airway lumen may be narrowed. In an ***extramural obstruction,*** the airway narrowing is due to

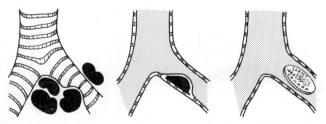

Figure 90. The causes of bronchial obstruction. *Left,* Extramural; *middle,* intramural; *right,* intraluminal.

external pressure, such as by enlarged lymph nodes resulting from *carcinoma,* a *lymphoma* or *tuberculosis.* An obstruction may be due to an *intramural* lesion within the confines of the bronchial wall, such as a neoplasm projecting into the lumen of the bronchus. *Intraluminal obstruction* may result from an inhaled foreign body, thick bronchial secretions or mucoid impaction.

Whatever the mechanism of the obstruction, it may be either partial or complete. In a partial obstruction, airflow and drainage of secretions are impaired whereas in a complete obstruction, both airflow and drainage of secretions can no longer occur.

PARTIAL OBSTRUCTION

A partial airway obstruction always acts as either a *bypass valve* or a *check valve,* depending on the degree of narrowing of the airway lumen and the nature of the pathologic process producing it.

Bypass Bronchial Obstruction

In a bypass type of obstruction (Fig. 91), air is able to move in and out of a narrowed airway and the airflow resistance is increased. A bypass bronchial obstruction often results in overdistention of the alveoli distal to the obstruction, because the airways narrow further during expiration so that the flow resistance is greater than it is during inspiration. If the bronchi are diffusely involved, generalized overdistension of the lungs will result.

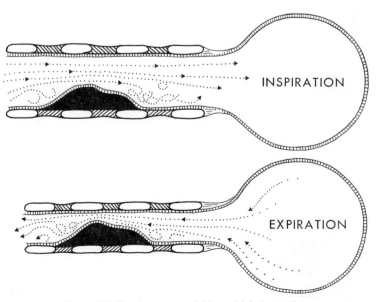

Figure 91. The bypass partial bronchial obstruction.

The increased lung elastic retractive force associated with an increase in lung volume helps to overcome the increased flow resistance during expiration.

Check-Valve Bronchial Obstruction

This type of bronchial obstruction differs from a bypass obstruction in that the bronchial lumen becomes completely occluded during expiration so that the egress of air is prevented. As is seen in Figure 92, widening of the bronchial lumen during inspiration allows air to pass into the alveoli, but occlusion of the lumen during expiration leads to air trapping in the affected area, and overdistension of the alveoli. An endobronchial tumor attached to the bronchial wall by a pedicle can produce this type of obstruction.

COMPLETE AIRWAY OBSTRUCTION

In the complete, or *stop-valve,* type of obstruction, illustrated in Figure 93, the airway is completely occluded so that air cannot move in or out. The consequence of this type of obstruction is *atelectasis* of the affected portion of the lung.

Atelectasis

The term "atelectasis," which is derived from the Greek words "ateles," meaning imperfect, and "ektasis," meaning expansion, implies that the alveoli in the affected area of the lung have collapsed and become airless.

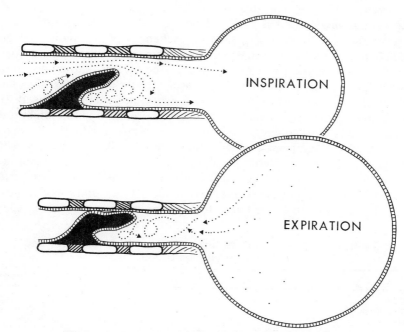

INSPIRATION

EXPIRATION

Figure 92. The check-valve partial bronchial obstruction.

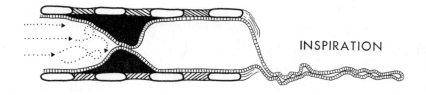

INSPIRATION

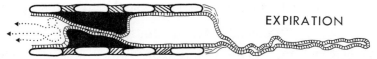

EXPIRATION

Figure 93. The complete bronchial obstruction.

Although it is usually the consequence of a completedly obstructed bronchus, it will occur only if there is blood flow to the affected alveoli; it will not occur if the pulmonary artery supplying the affected lobe is ligated before its bronchus is blocked.

When a bronchus supplying perfused alveoli is completely obstructed, the alveolar gases are absorbed into the pulmonary capillary blood, because the total pressure of the gases in the alveolar air is higher than that in the mixed venous blood (Table 14). Although the gases move in and out of the alveoli simultaneously, it is easier to describe the process of absorption of air from the alveoli as a sequence of exchanges of the individual gases. Initially, because of the partial pressure differences, slightly more oxygen moves into the pulmonary capillaries from the alveoli than carbon dioxide moves in the opposite direction. As a result, the volume of the alveolar gas is reduced. The lung, by virtue of its elasticity, accommodates itself to the new volume, so that the alveolar gases are compressed and the total pressure is maintained. Consequently, the partial pressure gradient between the alveoli and the blood is maintained, and eventually all of the gas is absorbed and the alveoli are completely collapsed. This process takes several hours, because initially there is little difference in partial pressure of nitrogen between the alveoli and the pulmonary capillary blood and it is the nitrogen that is the major contributor to the total gas pressure in the alveoli. Clearly,

**TABLE 14. The Partial Pressures of Gases in Alveolar Air and
Mixed Venous Blood**

	Alveolar Air	Mixed Venous Blood
Oxygen	110	40
Carbon dioxide	40	46
Nitrogen	563	563
H_2O	47	47

if the alveoli contained pure oxygen rather than nitrogen, complete atelectasis could occur within a few minutes, because there would be a marked partial pressure difference of oxygen between the alveoli and the blood.

Atelectasis may not develop following complete obstruction of a bronchiole, because there may be collateral ventilation through minute apertures in the interalveolar septa between neighboring lobules. Thus, even though a terminal bronchiole becomes obstructed, the primary or secondary lobule may continue to contain air because it is supplied from the alveoli or neighboring lobules.

Atelectasis or collapse of alveoli may also occur as a result of compression of alveoli by air or fluid in the pleural cavity or by marked elevation of the diaphragm. In these situations, lung volume may be reduced to the point at which airway closure occurs, and if this is maintained it will be followed by the sequence of absorption of gas, reduction of alveolar size, and finally complete emptying of alveoli. Similarly, an increase in the surface tension at the air-liquid interface of small bronchioles and alveoli can result in atelectasis. As was discussed in Chapter 1, according to LaPlace's equation, a very high transmural pressure is necessary to maintain patent alveoli when the surface tension is increased. The converse is also true, in that expansion of an atelectatic lung requires a very high transpulmonary pressure to overcome the resistance to expansion that results from the forces of surface tension, a situation that is analogous to the inflation of the degassed lung that was described in Chapter 1.

OBSTRUCTION OF THE TRACHEA AND LARGE AIRWAYS

Obstruction of the trachea and large bronchi may occur suddenly or develop gradually. It is encountered most commonly in patients who have previously been intubated, and it can also occur with infection, tumors, and inhaled foreign material. The chief symptom is dyspnea, although hoarseness may also be present. In acute situations, the onset of the dyspnea is immediate; in chronic disorders, it may develop gradually.

Complete obstruction of the trachea results in asphyxia and death. When there is a partial obstruction of the trachea, inspiration becomes forceful and prolonged and a musical or crowing sound *(stridor)* can be heard during both inspiration and expiration. There is visible in-drawing over the sternal notch, the supraclavicular spaces, the intercostal spaces and the epigastrium. If the obstruction is fixed, inspiration and expiration are affected equally. If the obstruction is variable and extrathoracic, expiration is less affected than inspiration, because the pressure in the airway is greater than that surrounding it during expiration, and the reverse is true during inspiration. If the obstruction is variable and intrathoracic, the obstruction is worse during expiration because the pressure in the airway is less than that surrounding it. Assessment of the respiratory phase most affected clinically and, as discussed in Chapter 7, measurement of the maximal rate of airflow during forced inspiratory and expiratory vital capacity maneuvers, help to differentiate the site of upper airway obstruction.

POSTINTUBATION OBSTRUCTION

Upper airway obstruction is most frequently encountered in patients who were intubated with an endotracheal tube or in whom a tracheostomy tube was instilled for a prolonged period of time, particularly if extreme care was not taken during inflation of the cuff or during the suctioning process. Removal of the tube may be followed by severe respiratory distress because of edema of the vocal cords or tracheal wall damage.

FOREIGN BODY OBSTRUCTION

Obstruction of the large airways by a foreign body is commonest in children, but adults may also experience tracheal obstruction, as a result of compression by impacted food in the upper esophagus (the *"cafe coronary"*). With aspiration, the first symptoms are usually choking, gagging, temporary aphonia, cough, respiratory distress and wheezing. Laryngospasm lasting a few seconds is common. If the object lodges in the larynx, hoarseness or aphonia and a brassy cough are usually present. If the foreign body lodges in the trachea, signs and symptoms similar to those of laryngeal lodgement may be produced, or there may be a relatively symptomless period after the aspiration.

LARYNGOTRACHEOBRONCHITIS

Inflammation of the upper airway occurs in both children and adults, but it is particularly important in children, where it produces a clinical syndrome often called *croup*. This consists of inspiratory stridor, a brassy and barking cough and hoarseness as a result of varying degrees of laryngeal obstruction. Upper respiratory infection is followed in 3 to 4 days by inflammation, edema and spasm of the true cords and subglottic structures. In severe obstruction, marked supraclavicular, suprasternal and subcostal retractions may be seen. Most cases occur during cold weather, when there is an increased incidence of respiratory infection. A viral etiology has been implicated in 85 per cent of patients, the parainfluenza viruses 1, 2 and 3 being the commonest agents isolated, though influenza, respiratory syncytial virus and adenoviruses are also found. The majority of patients with viral croup are between 3 months and 3 years of age.

EPIGLOTTITIS

This acute infection of the epiglottis, aryepiglottic folds and surrounding tissue is usually due to infection with *Hemophilus influenzae* type B. This serious illness has a fulminant course over a few hours, and the inflammation may spread to involve the remainder of the supraglottic as well as the subglottic areas. The presenting symptoms are usually a high fever, sore throat, dyspnea, drooling, dysphagia, cough, and occasionally a low-pitched stridor. Examination of the pharynx reveals a fiery red swollen, edematous epiglottis. A lateral roentgenogram of the neck often reveals a swollen epiglottic shadow, and the hypopharynx is often filled by the swollen epiglottis and aryepiglottic folds.

LOWER AIRWAY OBSTRUCTION

FOREIGN BODY OBSTRUCTION

About 2 per cent of foreign bodies inhaled into the tracheobronchial tree are spontaneously expelled by coughing, but the rest usually result in complications. Because the orifice of the right main stem bronchus is slightly wider than the left and lies in a more direct line with the trachea, the majority of aspirated foreign bodies enter the right main bronchus.

If a large airway becomes obstructed abruptly, intense dyspnea is usually experienced; if it develops gradually, there may be no symptoms, aside from a cough. Either local or diffuse airway obstruction may be produced. Aspiration of peanuts or seeds may cause a localized airway obstruction in children under 4 years of age. Because of its hydrophilic nature, an aspirated peanut is particularly dangerous, because it swells in addition to causing a marked local inflammatory reaction and mucosal edema. A foreign body that lodges in a major bronchus usually produces unilateral signs. Inspiratory and expiratory rhonchi may be heard if it is a bypass obstruction; a check-valve obstruction may produce hyperinflation of the affected lung; and complete obstruction an *atelectasis.* Not uncommonly, a partial obstruction will progress to complete obstruction because of mucosal swelling and edema. Cough, chest tightness and intense dyspnea may be experienced if there is acute obstruction of the finer bronchi and bronchioles, as in *asthma,* whereas obstruction of the small airways, if localized, may produce no symptoms. Indeed, the commonest symptom associated with all types of bronchial obstruction is cough, and it increases as the degree of obstruction becomes greater. Interference with bronchial drainage is a frequent consequence of bronchial obstruction, and because bacteria grow readily in retained secretions, severe and prolonged infection may develop in the affected area of the lung. This can create a vicious circle, with the production of more secretions and more cough, or a *lung abscess* or *bronchiectasis* may develop.

The roentgenologic abnormalities associated with a localized bronchial obstruction depend on the type and degree as well as the site of obstruction. Since most foreign bodies aspirated by children are of vegetable or plastic origin, they are unfortunately frequently not visualized in the chest roentgenogram. If there is a localized check-valve obstruction, the affected portion of lung will be hyperinflated and the medastinum will be shifted toward the

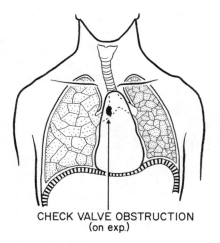

Figure 94. Overinflation due to a check-valve obstruction.

CHECK VALVE OBSTRUCTION
(on exp.)

unaffected side (Fig. 94). This will be particularly evident during expiration, so that it is best demonstrated during fluoroscopy or on inspiration-expiration chest roentgenograms. With diffuse partial obstruction of the smaller bronchi, the hyperinflation of the lungs is usually generalized.

Atelectasis following a complete bronchial obstruction produces characteristic radiologic signs. The airless lobe tends to become wedge shaped with concave borders, the apex being at the mediastinum and the base in apposition to the chest wall. As is seen in Figure 95, when there is a reduction in lung volume, the mediastinum will be shifted to the affected side.

ACUTE BRONCHITIS

In *acute bronchitis* there is diffuse inflammation of the bronchial tree and an excessive production of mucus. This condition is moderately common

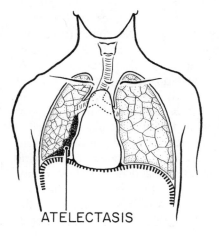

Figure 95. Atelectasis of the right lower lobe.

ATELECTASIS

and usually leads to little permanent disability. Most commonly, it develops as a consequence of a viral infection, such as influenza, but it may occur as a primary manifestation during the course of such infectious diseases as *measles* and *typhoid fever* or as a concomitant of an acute bacterial pneumonia.

The onset of acute bronchitis is heralded by a substernal burning discomfort, which is due to an associated tracheitis, and a harassing, rasping, painful cough. Paroxysmal attacks of cough and wheezing may be precipitated by the inhalation of irritants such as cigarette smoke or by exposure to cold air. Initially, there is a scanty expectoration of mucus, but later this may become more abundant and mucopurulent.

BRONCHIOLITIS

Inflammation of the bronchioles occurs in both adults and children and is caused by a variety of agents, most commonly *respiratory syncytial virus* (RSV), *parainfluenza virus* (PV) and *adenovirus* (AV). Obliterative bronchiolitis may develop in adults after exposure to nitrogen dioxide fumes. Since airflow resistance is inversely related to the fourth power of the radius of the airways involved, bronchiolitis is particularly serious in infants and children, whose airways are relatively small. Damage to the bronchioles consists of necrosis of the epithelium and destruction of the cilia, along with peribronchiolar infiltration by inflammatory cells. Bronchiolar obstruction results because of edema and lymphocytic infiltration of the bronchiolar walls as well as obstruction of the lumen with mucus and cellular debris. In its most severe form there may be widespread necrotizing lesions of the mucosa of the entire respiratory tract and destruction of the walls of bronchi and bronchioles.

In children under 2 years of age, the first sign of acute bronchiolitis is a coryza, which may last for several days or may rapidly progress to a paroxysmal cough, an audible expiratory wheeze and occasionally an expiratory grunt. In the more severe cases the respiratory rate may be as high as 80 per minute, and cyanosis may be evident. The anteroposterior diameter of the chest is increased, and there are subcostal, intercostal and suprasternal retractions. The chest is hyperresonant to percussion, and on auscultation, breath sounds are diminished bilaterally, with a prolonged expiration. Wheezing is always present, and fine inspiratory and expiratory crackles may be heard. The $P_{A-a}O_2$ is increased in the majority of patients, and the P_aO_2 is low because of gross mismatching of ventilation and perfusion. In severe cases carbon dioxide retention may be associated with the hypoxemia.

Roentgenograms demonstrate hyperinflation with depressed and flat diaphragms, an increased anteroposterior diameter of the thorax, abnormally translucent lung fields and an increase in the size of the retrosternal air shadow. Thickened bronchioles are often visible, and frank infiltrates or areas of linear atelectasis may also be present. The disease is usually self-limited and is over in one to two weeks. However, bronchiolitis is thought to be a potential forerunner of hyperreactive airway disease in later life.

CHRONIC AIRFLOW LIMITATION

It has been estimated that more than 16 million persons in North America suffer from some degree of chronic airflow limitation. This term is used because airflow in the tracheobronchial tree may be limited, particularly during a forced expiration, by airway obstruction or a reduction in the driving pressure (i.e., lung elastic recoil). Chronic airflow limitation is a predominant feature in **asthma, chronic bronchitis, emphysema, bronchiectasis,** and **cystic fibrosis.**

ASTHMA

Asthma, which literally means "different breathing" affects almost 7 million people in the United States. The *sine qua non* of this condition is airway hyperreactivity, which is manifested by widespread but reversible narrowing of the airways in response to a wide variety of factors. Many physicians consider wheezing to be synonymous with asthma, but it is obvious from the earlier discussion of bronchial obstruction that, although patients suffering from asthma are subject to wheezing, not all patients who wheeze necessarily have asthma.

Bronchospasm may be induced by nonspecific irritants such as infection or exercise, specific irritants such as fumes, dust, smoke or drainage from an upper respiratory tract infection, and physical agents such as extremes of temperature, particularly cold air, or exercise. Many allergens may also lead to bronchoconstriction, the most important ones being inhaled pollens, mold spores, animal danders, feathers and common house dust. Recent evidence suggests that allergy to house dust may be due to the common household mite of the **Dermatophagoides genus,** which has been detected in most house dust samples, particularly mattress dust. Attacks of bronchoconstriction during the spring and summer months suggest that a pollen or a mold spore may be the offending allergen. Attacks in the spring are usually due to tree pollens, in the early part of the summer to grass pollens, and in the late summer to weed pollens.

Practically any food may induce bronchospasm, particularly in children, and even drugs, such as morphine or aspirin, may precipitate attacks. Airway hyperreactivity has also been shown to develop in an ever-increasing list of occupations that involve exposure to particular allergens (or irritants) such as fumes, wood dusts and metal dusts, and very unusual agents, such as odors of cosmetic agents or hair spray. Recently metabisulfites, which are used as a preservative for vegetables or fruit and in beer and wine bottles, has been shown to cause respiratory difficulty. Even emotional upsets are capable of "triggering" an attack of bronchospasm in an already hyperirritable bronchial tree. It has been suggested that this is due to hyperventilation, which in itself may precipitate an attack of bronchospasm.

Pathogenesis

The mechanisms underlying airway hyperreactivity are not clearly understood, but two theories have been proposed: an intrinsic abnormality of beta-adrenergic receptors and an alteration of parasympathetic control of the airways.

Altered Beta-Adrenergic Receptors. Beta-adrenergic stimulation (for instance by isoproterenol) results in bronchodilation. Conversely, beta-adrenergic blockade by a drug such as propranolol may precipitate acute bronchospasm in individuals with *hay fever* or *asthma* or enhance the bronchial response to bronchoconstricting agents such as acetylcholine. It is believed that modulation of bronchial smooth-muscle contraction depends on the balance between cyclic 3′,5′-adenosine monophosphate (cyclic AMP) and cyclic 3′,5′-guanosine monophosphate (cyclic GMP). As seen in Figure 96, increases in intracellular cyclic AMP lead to bronchodilation, and decreases cause bronchoconstriction; changes in cyclic GMP appear to have the opposite effects. The state of beta-adrenergic blockade appears to extend beyond the respiratory organs, particularly in severe clinical asthma, where it has been shown that the cyclic AMP response of lymphocytes and leukocytes to beta-adrenergic stimulation is impaired. This appears to correlate with the degree of bronchial reactivity to inhaled histamine.

Altered Parasympathetic Control. It has also been suggested that hyperreactive airways are due to a functional abnormality of the rapidly adapting or irritant receptors in the airways. Stimulation of the distal end of a cut vagus leads to bronchoconstriction and mucus production. In addition, the inhalation of histamine, mechanical irritation of the irritant receptors, or exposure to irritant gases or cigarette smoke induces hyperpnea and bronchoconstriction through vagal reflexes. Bronchial reactivity increases in healthy individuals during a viral respiratory infection and, in both animals

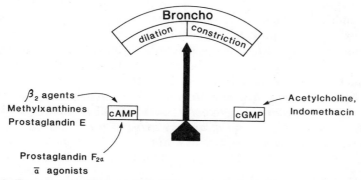

Figure 96. The balance between cyclic AMP and cyclic GMP appears to control bronchial caliber. A decrease in cAMP or an increase in cGMP results in bronchoconstriction. Note the effect of various mediators and therapeutic agents.

and humans, after exposure to ozone. It is also increased following antigenic bronchoprovocation in the laboratory or during the pollen season in asthmatics with a pollen allergy. This has led to the suggestion that functional disturbance of the irritant receptors leads to bronchial hyperreactivity. It is thought that the irritant receptors are stimulated as a result of damage to the bronchial epithelium by viral infection, allergic reaction or other factors.

Immediate Hypersensitivity Reaction. Asthma may also have a hereditary basis. The term *atopy* (meaning "strange" or "unusual" in Greek) or *atopic diseases* has been used to refer to several diseases, including *allergic rhinitis, asthma, eczema* and *urticaria,* that commonly occur together in certain individuals and families. The property that is inherited is probably not the specific allergy, but rather a tendency to develop a sensitivity to any of the antigens to which one may be exposed and to which a normal person's immune system is tolerant. A specific antigen does not produce a unique clinical picture; the same antigen may produce bronchoconstriction in one person, rhinitis in another, urticaria in a third, purpura in a fourth, and even different symptom complexes in the same person at different times. Nevertheless, certain "shock organs" show a greater degree of reactivity to contact with the antigen, presumably because of greater concentration of cells coated with reaginic antibodies in these areas.

In allergic patients, as we have seen in Figure 87, bronchoconstriction may come on immediately (within a few minutes or even seconds) following exposure to an antigen (a foreign substance). This is thought to be precipitated by pharmacologically active substances that are released when the antigen combines with an antibody capable of combining specifically with it. The antibodies that are responsible for allergic asthma and the other atopic sensitivities belong to the class of immunoglobulins known as IgE, which is fixed to the mast cells in the tissues or the basophils in the peripheral blood. Subsequent exposure to the same antigen is thought to evoke a reaction that leads to degranulation of the mast cell with release of lysosomal granules and a number of chemical mediators that induce airway smooth-muscle constriction, accumulation of inflammatory cells with a predominance of eosinophils, mucosal edema, hypersecretion of thick, tenacious mucus, and increased vascular permeability. The chemical mediators that are released as a direct result of the IgE-mediated immunologic reaction are called *primary mediators* and include *histamine, slow-reacting substance of anaphylaxis* (SRS-A), *platelet aggregating factor* (PAF), and *eosinophil and neutrophil chemotactic factors of anaphylaxis* (ECF-A and NCF-A). There are also *secondary mediators,* such as *kinins* and *prostaglandins,* which may be generated as a result of the tissue-inflammatory reactions induced by the primary mediators.

For the bronchoconstriction to occur as rapidly as it does in the immediate hypersensitivity reaction, the inhaled allergens must come in contact with IgE antibodies on the surface of mast cells in the very superficial layers of the respiratory mucosa. It is thought that the chemical mediators that are released from the mast cells also alter the tissue permeability, and as a result, the diffusion of inhaled allergens to the deeper layers of the respiratory mucosa is favored. Once in the deeper layers of the bronchial wall, they can react with more mast cells.

Late Hypersensitivity Reaction. Some allergic individuals also develop a *late reaction* with or without *an immediate reaction* (see Figs. 88 and 89). This reaction, 4 to 10 hours after exposure, has been attributed to the combination of the antigen with a precipitating antibody (usually an IgG, although IgE and IgM may also contribute), which in turn activates the complement cascade and leads to the influx of inflammatory cells and then mediator release. The commonest cause of this type of reaction is *Aspergillus fumigatus,* and it is also seen following exposure to a number of occupational allergens or irritants.

Clinical Manifestations

Asthma is characterized by recurrent, paroxysmal attacks of cough, chest tightness and difficult breathing, often accompanied by wheezing. The attacks may be precipitated by direct exposure to a specific agent or by any of the nonspecific factors indicated earlier. They may last only a few minutes or for hours, and some patients may remain in a state of continuous severe respiratory distress for days. Thick gelatinous mucus, which is exceedingly difficult to expectorate, is frequently present.

In the lungs of patients dying from severe asthma there is massive air trapping with occlusion of bronchi and bronchioles by thick, tenacious mucous plugs that contain shed mucosal epithelium. Bronchiolar muscle is prominent, the epithelial basement membrane is greatly thickened, and there is a heavy infiltrate of eosinophilic granulocytes in bronchial and bronchiolar walls up to the preterminal or terminal bronchioles.

A patient with uncomplicated asthma often has no symptoms between the paroxysms of difficulty. In about one-quarter of the cases beginning in childhood, the attacks may cease spontaneously after adolescence. A considerable number of patients, however, remain in a chronic state of mild asthma, with symptoms particularly noticeable during periods of exertion or emotional excitement. *Chronic bronchitis* may be associated with asthma, because recurrent bronchial infection is a common manifestation. However, it is extremely unlikely that asthma ever leads to the development of *emphysema.*

The physical signs are characteristically those of diffuse partial airway obstruction. The lungs are usually hyperinflated, so that a hyperresonant note is obtained on percussion, and the breath sounds are distant. Expiration is prolonged, and high-pitched wheezes may be present throughout both lungs.

Radiologic Manifestations

The are no characteristic roentgenologic changes in asthma. The bronchial markings may be prominent and the lungs hyperinflated, just as in other cases of chronic airflow limitation. The degree of overinflation is variable, depending on the severity of the airway obstruction. The normal caliber and tapering of the pulmonary vasculature is preserved, and the pulmonary vessels extend to the periphery of the lung.

If *bronchopulmonary aspergillosis* complicates the *asthma,* there may be infiltrations that are fleeting in nature. Although not usually performed, bronchography in this condition reveals cylindrical *bronchiectasis* involving the proximal airways and sparing the distal branches.

Functional Manifestations

Although a patient may appear clinically to be free of difficulty between attacks, airflow resistance is usually increased and maximal expiratory flow rates are lower than expected. Even in remission, the distribution of inspired gas is usually impaired and the dynamic lung compliance falls with increasing respiratory frequency. This suggests that there are abnormalities in the small airways in asthma even when the patient is relatively free of symptoms.

During an acute attack of bronchospasm, airflow resistance rises and the FEV_1, FEF_{25-75} and $\dot{V}_{max}$ at all lung volumes are markedly reduced. The pressure-volume characteristics of the lung are altered; the P-V curve is shifted upward and to the left (i.e., lung volume is increased and lung elastic recoil pressure at any particular volume is reduced), but the shape of the curve is the same as that seen in healthy individuals (see Fig. 15). Total lung capacity is usually increased, and the vital capacity is often considerably reduced, because of the hyperinflation (i.e., an increased residual volume). Hypoxemia is present, the severity being related to the degree of flow limitation present. In moderate obstruction, hypocapnia is usually associated with the hypoxemia because there is compensatory hyperventilation of well-ventilated alveoli. When the airflow limitation becomes severe, the hypoxemia increases and hypercapnia may devleop. In patients with acute bronchospasm, even a rising P_aCO_2 into the normal range is indicative of a serious and grave situation, for it usually means the patient is getting worn out.

CHRONIC BRONCHITIS

Chronic bronchitis is characterized by a chronic cough with excessive mucus in the bronchial tree that is not due to known specific causes, such as bronchiectasis or tuberculosis, and that is present on most days for at least three months of the year for two or more successive years. It is commoner in males and outranks all other respiratory diseases as a crippler and a killer (about 7.5 million individuals are affected in the United States). In a well-established case there is an increase in the number and size of the mucus-secreting glands and goblet cells in the bronchi, and the cilia may become inefficient so that drainage is impaired. The finding of a high bronchial gland/bronchial wall ratio *(Reid index)* is very suggestive of chronic bronchitis, but there is only a fair correlation between clinical bronchitis and the amount of mucous gland hyperplasia present, and there is considerable overlap between bronchitics and nonbronchitics.

Pathogenesis

The factors involved in the etiology of chronic bronchitis are continually undergoing considerable scrutiny, but the picture is still not completely understood. Irritation of the tracheobronchial tree is common to all cases of bronchitis, and it appears that cigarette smoking is the single most important determinant. However, not all cigarette smokers develop bronchitis, and it is possible that immunologic or familial susceptibility may play an important part in some persons. Epidemiologic studies have uniformly shown that there is a higher prevalence of cough and phlegm in smokers than in nonsmokers, that heavy smokers are more seriously affected than light smokers, and that the symptoms are worse if there is a long history of cigarette smoking.

Cigarette smoking has a profound effect on mucociliary clearance. The majority of particulate matter in cigarette smoke is deposited on the bronchial mucus blanket, and the ciliary activity is inhibited. Therefore, movement of the bronchial mucus blanket is diminished considerably, and the irritating effect on the underlying bronchial epithelium is enhanced. The mucous glands and goblet cells are stimulated to produce more mucus, and this, together with the altered ciliary activity, leads to the development of chronic cough and expectoration. The bronchial mucus that is secreted in chronic bronchitis is apparently no different from normal bronchial mucus biochemically. However, the hypersecretion of mucus increases the liability to infection and delays the tendency to recovery; as a result a vicious circle of hypersecretion, infection and more hypersecretion results.

Another major important effect of inhaled cigarette smoke is bronchoconstriction, which is apparently due to irritation of nerve endings in the bronchial tree. Airflow resistance may double following a single cigarette, and this may persist for as long as 30 minutes. The inhalation of an aerosol of carbon particles produces a similar effect, but an aerosol of nicotine does not. Recently it has been suggested that chronic smoking is associated with constriction of the peripheral airways and the alveolar ducts, and that this is reversed by inhaled bronchodilator or smoking cessation.

The role of infections in chronic bronchitis is not clear. The lower respiratory tract is essentially sterile even though many bacteria that normally inhabit the mouth and nasopharynx are probably inhaled during respiration, because they adhere to the tracheobronchial mucus blanket and are removed by ciliary activity or coughing. In patients with chronic bronchitis, however, many of these organisms can be isolated from the sputum, although the relationship of these organisms to acute exacerbations of the disease is controversial. Many of the acute episodes of bronchitis that develop in patients with chronic airflow limitation are probably caused by a virus infection, but the resulting damage to the bronchial mucosa may encourage the growth of bacteria. ***Hemophilus influenzae*** and ***Diplococcus pneumoniae*** seem to be the important organisms, although occasionally ***Staphylococcus aureus*** and ***Friedländer's bacillus*** may have pathogenic significance.

The role of occupation in the etiology of chronic bronchitis is difficult to assess. The prevalence of the condition is highest in industrial areas, particularly among men who work in dusty occupations, such as miners, but no close relationship with the duration of exposure to dust has been demonstrated. Recently, it has been demonstrated that there is an additive effect between cigarette smoking and exposure to occupational dusts in the mining community. It is interesting that the incidence of bronchitis among the wives of these workers is also high, suggesting that an environmental cause, i.e., atmospheric pollution, may be implicated.

Similarly there is no doubt that air pollution aggravates and may influence the progression of bronchopulmonary disease, but whether it can actually cause chronic bronchitis has not been established. Large particles of pollution, such as droplets in wet fog, are usually trapped in the nose and pharynx, and medium-sized particles are generally trapped in the large bronchi, but the small particles penetrate deep into the bronchial tree. The inhalation of inert dust particles or a very low concentration of sulfur dioxide causes a twofold increase in the airway resistance, even in healthy human subjects, and in major cities there is a significant correlation between the day-to-day condition of patients suffering from bronchitis and the average concentration of sulfur dioxide in the atmosphere.

Another important source of bronchial irritation is drainage from the upper respiratory tract. Although it may be difficult to sort out which comes first, infection in the upper respiratory tract and postnasal discharge are common concomitants of chronic bronchitis. Drainage from the upper respiratory tract (*postnasal discharge*) is usually expectorated during the awake hours, but the secretions may be aspirated into the tracheobronchial tree during sleep, because the larynx and the cough reflex are depressed.

Clinical Manifestations

The onset of chronic bronchitis is generally insidious, a chronic cough often being attributed to cigarette smoking. However, it is important to understand that the so-called cigarette cough is not a normal event but is an early manifestation of bronchitis. It may disappear if cigarette smoking is given up early enough. Often there is an associated chronic rhinitis or sinusitis, which also improves if one stops smoking. Respiratory difficulty may become apparent to the patient only after about 30 years of smoking. Many patients trace the onset of symptoms to some acute infective episode, such as pneumonia. The clinical condition may vary from day to day, the symptoms being aggravated by irritants and cold, damp or foggy weather and punctuated by recrudescence of infection. In many persons the condition progresses to become a year-round affliction, with intercurrent acute exacerbations. Death resulting from bronchopneumonia, respiratory insufficiency, and right-sided heart failure may occur 20 to 35 years after the onset of symptoms.

The sputum is usually clear and mucoid and is commonly expectorated in the morning. However, it becomes more copious and purulent during acute infections. Exertional dyspnea often begins 5 to 10 years after the onset of the chronic cough, and it may remain fairly stationary, but usually the breathlessness is aggravated during episodes of acute bronchitis and progressively increases in severity. Wheezing may be present, particularly during acute exacerbations or on exertion, and later may become persistent. Cough, wheezing and breathlessness may awaken the patient, thus mimicking an attack of paroxysmal nocturnal dyspnea or asthma, but in this case the symptoms are generally relieved by the expectoration of sputum.

The serious complications of chronic bronchitis are intercurrent bronchopulmonary infection, emphysema, and right ventricular heart failure. The link between chronic bronchitis and emphysema is probably the associated bronchiolitis, which may lead to obliteration of bronchioles or weakening and dilatation of their walls, with the resultant development of centrilobular emphysema, which is described later. When hypoxemia and acidemia are present pulmonary hypertension develops because of vasoconstriction of the precapillary arterioles. As a result of the increased pulmonary vascular resistance, the work of the right ventricle increases and the wall of the right ventricle hypertrophies. Later, the right ventricle may fail, and there is the full-blown picture of right ventricular failure.

The physical signs in the lungs will depend on the degree of airflow limitation. Respiratory distress may be evident with minor exertion or even while talking. In the advanced stages, the patient may have a florid appearance and cyanosis of the mucous membranes. The chest cage is often in an inspiratory position, and this, together, with kyphosis of the dorsal spine, increases the anteroposterior diameter of the chest, producing a barrel-like shape. The accessory muscles are used excessively during breathing, and the chest cage moves "en bloc" (the so-called thoracic heave) with inspiratory in-drawing of the lower intercostal spaces. The percussion note is usually hyperresonant and the breath sounds faint. Medium- and high-pitched sibilant wheezes are usually present. Quite often the high-pitched wheezes may be elicited only by having the patient expire forcibly for as long as possible.

A systolic heave in the left parasternal area of the precordium, together with an accentuated second pulmonic sound, suggests the presence of pulmonary hypertension and right ventricular hypertrophy. If this has progressed to congestive heart failure, the external jugular veins will be distended, the liver will be enlarged and tender, and dependent edema will be evident.

Radiologic Manifestations

There may be no roentgenologic abnormality, but usually the lungs are hyperinflated and the diaphragm depressed. Other features are parallel shadows, or "tram lines," especially in the lower lung fields, which are thought to be indicative of thickened bronchial walls, although there is no evidence to substantiate this. Bronchography has demonstrated small spikelike protrusions or diverticula that project outward from the major or segmental bronchi and are probably collections of radiopaque media in the ducts of the enlarged mucous glands. The caliber of the bronchi is often slightly narrowed, and irregularities of the bronchial lumen result from a mixture of stenosis and dilatation. Occasionally, a circular pool is seen at the abrupt ending of a long, narrow branch, giving it a beaded appearance; this probably represents a dilated bronchiole, or it may indicate an area of centrilobular emphysema.

Functional Manifestations

The pattern of altered pulmonary function in chronic bronchitis is quite variable, and there is no correlation between the amount of secretions and the severity of dysfunction. Mild-to-moderate bronchitis and bronchiolitis may not materially affect standard tests of ventilatory function or flow resistance, but physiologic evidence of altered function in the periphery of the lungs can be found in asymptomatic smokers using tests thought to reflect small airway dysfunction. Mucous plugging or inflammation of the small airways leads to an uneven distribution of inspired gas, frequency dependence of dynamic lung compliance, and mismatching of ventilation and perfusion, so that the $P_{(A-a)}O_2$ is increased.

In established but uncomplicated chronic bronchitis, there is airflow limitation, the FEV_1, the FEF_{25-75} and $\dot{V}_{max}$ at all lung volumes being considerably reduced. The pressure-volume curve is shifted upward and to the left (as in asthma), but the shape of the curve is normal (see Fig. 15). The total lung capacity, residual volume and functional residual capacity are all increased. The vital capacity is either normal or low, depending on the relative size of the residual volume and the total lung capacity. Because there is considerable mismatching of ventilation and perfusion, hypoxemia is common, and hypocapnia is usually present because of the hyperventilation induced by the hypoxemia. Each acute exacerbation leaves behind it a legacy of further deterioration in gas exchange; the mismatching of ventilation and perfusion worsens, and hypoxemia increases. Carbon dioxide retention does not develop as long as the perfused areas of lung are capable of being hyperventilated. However, when the alveolar ventilation is no longer adequate to cope with the carbon dioxide being produced in the body because of the elevated work of breathing, carbon dioxide retention develops along with the hypoxemia.

EMPHYSEMA

Emphysema, the Greek word meaning "overinflation," is a pathologic process consisting of permanent overdistension of the air spaces distal to the terminal nonrespiratory bronchioles accompanied by attenuation and destruction of the alveolar walls. Several pathologic types of emphysema have been described; these are based on the anatomic distribution of the air space enlargement and alveolar destruction within the secondary lobule (distal to the terminal bronchiole).

Centrilobular emphysema (CLE) predominantly involves the center of the secondary lobule; i.e., the respiratory bronchioles are enlarged, destroyed or become confluent, the distal portion of the lobule being relatively unaffected. The punched-out areas separated by normal lung parenchyma, which are characteristic of centrilobular emphysema, occur most commonly in the upper zones of the lungs. This condition is much commoner in males and is often associated with *chronic bronchitis;* indeed, CLE rarely occurs in nonsmokers.

Panlobular emphysema (PLE) involves the entire secondary lobule almost uniformly, with enlarged alveoli that are not easily distinguished from the ducts and show abnormal fenestrations in their walls. With progression, there is loss of parenchyma until all that remains are thin strands of tissue around blood vessels. PLE occurs somewhat randomly throughout the lungs but tends to involve the lower zones particularly. PLE is as common in women as in men and is not usually associated with bronchitis. It is the type of emphysema seen in patients suffering from alpha-1-antitrypsin deficiency. It may occur together with CLE, in which case it is usually associated with *chronic bronchitis* and a history of cigarette smoking.

Paraseptal emphysema is a variant of panlobular emphysema. Here the alveolar sacs and associated alveoli are destroyed, though the proximal portion of the secondary lobules may be normal. Since this occurs at the periphery of the lobule and is adjacent to the interlobular septa, bullae may develop in the subpleural area and rupture into the pleural space.

Scar emphysema, or *paracicatricial emphysema,* is usually found in the vicinity of scars. This is the most common form of emphysema found at postmortem, particularly in association with granulomatous disease, but is the least significant clinically.

Bullae are air spaces within the lung parenchyma. They are usually encountered in lungs severely affected by panlobular or centrilobular emphysema. They generally develop because of a check-valve bronchiolar obstruction, which leads to alveolar overdistension. Coalescence of several alveoli occurs because of fragmentation of the interalveolar elastic tissue, and subsequent rupture of the attenuated interalveolar septa.

Blebs are collections of air that lie in the interlobular connective tissue just beneath the pleura. They are formed by ruptured alveoli, the escaped air tracking along the tissue planes of the lungs and finally becoming localized in the subpleural areas. A bleb may persist, or it may rupture through the visceral pleura, producing a spontaneous pneumothorax. On rare occasions, the air may track medially and rupture into the mediastinum. The actual cause of the alveolar rupture is unknown, although it has been suggested that it is caused by a localized check-valve bronchiolar obstruction, which produces alveolar overdistension.

It is thought that there are more than 2 million individuals suffering from emphysema in the United States. However, at postmortem, there is well-defined centrilobular or panlobular emphysema in about two-thirds of lungs of adult males and about one-quarter of females. The incidence rises sharply in the fifth decade and then tends to level off.

Pathogenesis

There have been major advances in understanding of emphysema, but the etiology and mechanism of development of emphysema is still controversial. Laennec, a pioneer in the study of emphysema, thought that the disease could be entirely explained by mechanical factors and claimed that it began as a catarrh of the bronchi, which leads to partial bronchial obstruction during both inspiration and expiration. The failure of the emphysematous lung to collapse when the chest is opened during the postmortem examination, the appearance of atrophied stroma and the fact that the pleural pressure fluctuates in the neighborhood of atmospheric pressure indicate that the elastic retractive force is diminished in this condition. However, the relationship between alveolar distention and loss of elasticity is not necessarily one of cause and effect. Although it is true that a primary loss of elasticity may lead to alveolar distention, it is possible that alveolar distention over a long period of time hastens the loss of elasticity. In other words, each may be the cause or the effect of the other, and the loss of elasticity in emphysema may be the basic defect or a secondary development.

The description of emphysema in individuals suffering from severe *alpha-1-antitrypsin deficiency* (zz phenotype) and the fact that instillation of papain in animals produces the pathologic and physiologic picture of emphysema has led to the hypothesis that emphysema may result from an altered relationship between proteases such as elastase, which may destroy alveolar elastic tissue, and antiproteases such as alpha-1-antitrypsin (Fig. 97). Current thinking suggests that emphysema probably develops as a result of repeated inflammation of the airways (caused by cigarette smoking) and

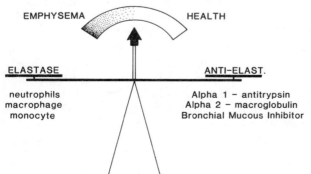

Figure 97. The balance between proteases (elastase) and antiproteases (anti-elastase) appears to control the status of the elastic tissue of lung alveoli. An increase in elastase activity or a decrease of anti-elastase results in the development of emphysema.

the development of partial or complete bronchiolar obstruction, which leads to air trapping. There is a concomitant release of proteases (i.e., elastase) by inflammatory neutrophils, and this results in more and more lung tissue disruption, until finally the clinical picture of emphysema becomes fully developed. It has been further suggested that cigarette smoke may alter the function of antiproteases so that elastase inhibition is reduced.

A relationship between pulmonary emphysema and *asthma* is unlikely. As we have seen, the slope of the pressure-volume curve of the lungs (i.e., lung elastic recoil) is normal in *asthma,* and evidence of emphysema is rarely found in the postmortem examination of the lungs of patients suffering from asthma. Episodes of dyspnea and wheezing may precede the clinical picture of emphysema, but it is not necessary to implicate asthma, for it is more likely that these episodes of dyspnea are due to acute bronchial obstruction by secretions. On the other hand, there seems to be little doubt about the relationship between *chronic bronchitis* and emphysema. Emphysema is more common in bronchitics than in nonbronchitics, and clinical chronic bronchitis and an elevated Reid index are usual in patients with severe emphysema. Many clinicians believe that emphysema always develops as a sequel of chronic bronchitis, but there is a definite group of patients in whom emphysema is heralded by the onset of dyspnea with no preceding chronic cough. Even in these patients, however, pathologic evidence of bronchiolitis is frequently found in the postmortem examination. There also appears to be a relationship between bronchiectasis or other chronic inflammatory diseases of the lung and emphysema, particularly when both lungs are diffusely involved.

Clinical Manifestations

Although emphysema, once severe, has characteristic clinical features, the diagnosis of emphysema on purely clinical grounds can be fraught with error. The chief symptom is dyspnea, which usually begins slowly and is characteristically brought on by exertion. It is aggravated by exposure to cold air and therefore is usually much more severe during the winter months. The dyspnea often progressively increases in severity so that ordinary daily activities such as walking even short distances may induce severe breathlessness. Severe episodes of dyspnea associated with wheezing are usually precipitated by respiratory infections and are accompanied by an increased production of sputum. Conversely, failure to expectorate sputum may, of itself, increase dyspnea because the accumulation of secretions increases airway obstruction.

Cough may be absent or inconspicuous during the early stages, but in most patients, cough is present for 15 to 25 years before the onset of dypsnea. The severity of the cough is frequently out of proportion to the amount of expectoration. Sooner or later, however, defective drainage is followed by infection and the production of mucoid or purulent sputum, and utimately there may be profuse expectoration. At this stage the condition may resemble bronchiectasis, and indeed, bronchiectasis may finally supervene as a consequence of frequent attacks of pneumonitis.

General nourishment is usually below normal, and weight loss is common. Occasionally the weight loss may be so rapid that a neoplasm may be suspected.

Clubbing of the digits does not occur in emphysema. When it is present, an associated **bronchogenic carcinoma** or complicating septic condition should be considered to be present until proven otherwise.

In advanced disease, the chest is hyperinflated and the diaphragm is depressed. Movement of the chest cage is noticeably diminished but equal bilaterally, often with inspiratory in-drawing, particularly in the areas overlying the insertions of the diaphragm. There is excessive use of the accessory muscles of respiration, particularly the pectoral muscles, which raise the anterior part of the chest cage in a "heaving" manner. Since the ratio of air-containing tissue to solid tissue is increased, tactile and auditory fremitus are diminished and the percussion note is hyperresonant. The breath sounds are distant, especially at the bases of the lungs, and in the late stages the lungs may become so silent as to suggest a pneumothorax. The expiratory breath sounds are prolonged because of the airflow limitation. Wheezes may not be detected during ordinary breathing, but extremely high-pitched sibilant wheezes can frequently be elicited during the late phase of a forced and prolonged expiration.

The heart sounds are often inaudible or heard very faintly at the apex, although they are usually easily detected in the epigastrium. If pulmonary hypertension has developed, the pulmonic second sound will be accentuated, and it may not split normally during inspiration.

The most serious threat to the life of the patient suffering from emphysema is an increase in hypoxemia and respiratory acidosis (hypercapnia), which is usually precipitated by an acute infection, pneumothorax, or pulmonary embolism. The deterioration in gas exchange further increases the pulmonary vascular resistance, with elevation of the pulmonary artery pressure and often acute right ventricular failure. In the late stages of the disease, chronic right-sided heart failure may develop; it is manifested by cardiac enlargement, an elevated venous pressure, hepatomegaly and edema.

Radiologic Manifestations

Roentgenograms are usually not helpful in establishing the diagnosis of emphysema when the condition is mild. The roentgenologic appearance of emphysema is usually no different from the hyperinflation seen in chronic bronchitis or asthma. On the posteroanterior roentgenogram the lungs are usually hyperlucent bilaterally, although only one or more lobes may be involved. In alpha-1-antitrypsin deficiency, the overinflation is usually predominant in the lower lung zones. In the lateral projection, the retrosternal space is abnormally increased and translucent. The diaphragm is usually depressed and flat, and the thoracic contour may be altered, the ribs running in a more horizontal direction, especially in the upper half of the chest. The peripheral vascular markings often taper rapidly and they may be very sparse. Conversely, the markings may be increased in size and more numerous peripherally, particularly in patients with pulmonary hypertension and cor pulmonale.

The heart is usually long and narrow, having been drawn downward by the descending diaphragm. In the later stages, there may be evidence of hypertrophy of the right ventricle, with an increase in cardiac size, prominence of the main pulmonary artery segment and enlargement of the hilar pulmonary arteries.

Functional Manifestations

Because of the loss of lung elastic recoil, the total lung capacity is usually considerably greater than normal, as are the functional residual capacity and residual volume. The vital capacity may be nearly normal in size, or it may be reduced because of the hyperinflation and increased residual volume. As we have seen in Figure 15, the pressure-volume curve of the lungs is shifted upward (lung volume is greater) and to the left (pressure is less), the slope of the curve being increased (compliance is increased). Airflow limitation is marked, particularly during expiration, because of both increased airway resistance and the loss of lung elastic recoil, so that the FEV_1, the FEF_{25-75} and $\dot{V}_{max}$ at all lung volumes are reduced.

Because the changes in lung elastic recoil and flow resistance are nonuniformly distributed in the lung, the inspired air is distributed unequally, and there is gross mismatching of ventilation and perfusion throughout the lung. Some alveoli with little perfusion are relatively overventilated, so that the physiologic dead space is increased. The blood perfusing these alveoli is fully oxygenated and excessively depleted of carbon dioxide. In addition, there is excessive perfusion of poorly ventilated alveoli, i.e., venous-admixture–like perfusion, and this results in arterial hypoxemia and a tendency toward carbon dioxide retention. Carbon dioxide retention does not occur as long as there is sufficient hyperventilation of the remaining well-ventilated, well-perfused alveoli. In advanced disease, however, particularly when bronchitis is associated, hypercapnia may develop, even at rest, because the alveolar ventilation is insufficient to cope with the carbon dioxide production.

The diffusing capacity of the lungs is reduced in this condition, particularly in the later stages, predominantly because of the marked mismatching of blood and gas distribution, although the reduced pulmonary vascular bed likely also contributes. Because of obliteration of the pulmonary capillaries, pulmonary vasoconstriction due to hypoxemia and, in some cases, acidemia, the pulmonary vascular resistance is frequently elevated, even at rest, and it may rise considerably during exercise. This imposes a heavy load on the right ventricle, so that it eventually hypertrophies and may even fail, producing the clinical picture of cor pulmonale.

The presence of hypercapnia and a diminished ventilatory response to inhaled CO_2, suggests a reduced sensitivity of the respiratory center, although, as pointed out earlier, these findings are at least partially the result of the mechanical difficulty in ventilating the lungs. Nevertheless, when the ventilatory response to carbon dioxide is diminished, the peripheral chemoreceptors may become the principal regulators of the respiratory drive, and hypoxemia the prime stimulus—a factor that is extremely important when oxygen therapy is considered.

BRONCHIECTASIS

The term *"bronchiectasis"* is derived from the Greek words "bronchos," meaning "windpipe," and "ektasis," meaning "extension," and is applied to a disease characterized by permanent abnormal dilatation and distortion of either the bronchi, the bronchioles, or both. This condition can develop when the bronchial walls are weakened by chronic inflammatory changes involving the bronchial mucosa, submucosa and the muscular coat.

Pathogenesis

The many theories that have been advanced to explain the pathogenesis of bronchiectasis include congenital or developmental defects, distension of the bronchi by cough, destruction of the bronchial wall by necrotizing inflammation, obstruction, atelectasis and fibrous retraction. Congenital forms do exist, and the condition may be associated with sinusitis and dextrocardia as well as an alteration of ciliary activity (*Kartagener's syndrome*). There is also a rare form of bronchiectasis caused by maldevelopment of the bronchi, which can simulate the acquired form of the disease both clinically and radiologically. The origin of the congenital variety is similar to that of congenital cystic disease of the lungs, except that the bronchial sacculations probably develop from an outgrowth of bronchial tissue rather than from pinched-off bronchial buds.

The majority of cases of bronchiectasis develop following an atelectasis. Any condition that leads to narrowing of a bronchial lumen, be it extramural, intramural or intraluminal, may produce bronchiectasis distal to the obstruction. Certain pulmonary infections, such as *tuberculosis, adenovirus infection,* or *pneumonia* complicating *measles, pertussis* and *influenza*, are more liable to be followed by bronchiectasis.

The bronchi presumably dilate because of an increased pull on the bronchial walls by the high intrathoracic pressure required to overcome the increased elastic resistance of atelectatic lung tissue. If the bronchial obstruction has been prolonged, secondary infection inevitably supervenes, and this leads to destruction of the bronchial walls and dilatation of the bronchi. The consequent reparative laying down of fibrous tissue further increases the traction on the bronchi and leads to still greater distortion. The degree of bronchial dilatation depends on the site and size of the bronchus affected. A large bronchus with cartilaginous rings does not dilate as readily as the

more muscular medium-sized or smaller bronchi. Relief of bronchial obstruction before chronic infection develops allows the bronchi to return to their
normal caliber slowly as the atelectatic area re-expands. This may explain
the cases of dilated bronchi demonstrated after pneumonia that return to a
normal size later (the so-called ***reversible bronchiectasis***).

Bronchiectasis is usually localized to a lobe or a segment, and the lower
lobes, particularly that of the left lung, are most commonly involved. Fresh
areas of bronchiectasis may develop subsequently in other parts of the same
lung, but they are usually associated with a fresh bronchial obstruction. In
fully established bronchiectasis, the bronchial arteries tend to enlarge, often
reaching the size of the pulmonary arteries at the same level, and they may
anastomose freely with the pulmonary vessels. It has been postulated that
transmission of the high bronchial artery pressure to the pulmonary arterioles
through the anastomoses results in the shunting away of poorly oxygenated
blood from diseased portions of lung to other, healthy areas, where the
pulmonary vascular resistance is lower.

Clinical Manifestations

Cough and phlegm are the predominant symptoms in bronchiectasis. In
many patients there may be no symptoms except during periods of acute
infection, when cough and expectoration of purulent sputum develop. There
may be a nonproductive cough (so-called ***dry bronchiectasis***), small quantities
of mucopurulent sputum or large quantities of purulent sputum, depending
on the size of the bronchiectatic cavities, their location and the organisms
involved. Bronchiectasis in the upper lobes, which is usually secondary to
arrested pulmonary tuberculosis, may be relatively asymptomatic, because
the upper lobes drain effectively in the erect position. In some cases, the
diseased bronchi may be insensitive and ciliary activity diminished or absent,
so that cough and expectoration of purulent material may be induced only
after a change in posture results in movement of secretions into the larger
bronchi, which have normal respiratory epithelium.

The expectorated material usually separates into three layers if left
standing: an upper, frothy, watery layer; a middle, turbid, mucopurulent
layer; and a lower, opaque, purulent layer. The purulent layer may contain
collections of small dirty-white or yellowish masses, known as ***Dittrich's
plugs***, or bits of elastic fibers if lung tissue has been destroyed. Blood
streaking and frank hemoptysis are common and presumably result from
necrosis of the bronchial epithelium as well as the bronchopulmonary
anastomoses.

As with other chronic airway disease, a large proportion of patients
with suppurative bronchiectasis also have chronic upper respiratory tract
infection, and acute exacerbations of sinusitis may mask the lower respiratory
tract symptoms. The causal relationship between upper and lower respiratory
tract infection is debatable, but it is suggested that the sinuses may become
secondarily infected by sprays of purulent sputum during paroxysms of

coughing. Conversely, chronic upper respiratory tract infection, with constant drainage of purulent secretion into the tracheobronchial tree, may lead to bronchial obstruction and to sepsis.

Although not a usual feature of bronchiectasis, breathlessness may become a distressing symptom if both lungs are extensively involved, particularly if fibrosis develops. Constitutional symptoms are not ordinarily present unless an acute pneumonic infection has developed or there is extensive suppurative disease. Under these circumstances, the patient may complain of undue fatigability, weight loss, profuse night sweats, anorexia and vague abdominal discomfort. Clubbing of the digits may develop, particularly when there is extensive suppuration, and if severe enough, it may progress to the stage of hypertrophic pulmonary osteoarthropathy. However, the development of digital clubbing does not appear to be related to either the duration or the extent of the disease.

The physical signs depend on the degree of bronchiectasis, its location and the extent of pulmonary involvement. In many cases, the physical findings are similar to those found in atelectasis, pulmonary consolidation or fibrosis and bear no relationship to the bronchiectasis. The extent of bronchial involvement can be determined only from the adventitious sounds that may be heard. Coarse, low-pitched crackles during the initial third of inspiration are thought to be produced by secretions in the larger bronchi; medium-pitched crackles, during the middle third of the inspiration by secretions in the smaller bronchi; and fine, high-pitched crackles, during the final third of inspiration by exudate within the airless, collapsed surrounding alveoli. The crackles heard during the initial and middle thirds of inspiration usually disappear if the patient coughs vigorously, but those in the final third usually persist. Expiratory wheezes, whose pitch depends on the caliber of the bronchi involved, may be produced by an inflamed swollen mucosa, bronchospasm and secretions.

Radiologic Manifestations

Dilated bronchi do not cast a roentgenologic shadow, so that bronchiectasis is not excluded by a normal posteroanterior and lateral roentgenograms of the chest. However, there are a number of radiographic abnormalities that are suggestive although not diagnostic of the presence of bronchiectasis. There may be linear radiotranslucencies, heavy basal markings and irregular dense strands due to peribronchial fibrosis radiating downward and outward from the hilum. Occasionally, the dilated bronchi may appear as thin-walled, translucent spaces, occasionally with cystic spaces, that may contain a fluid level. Vascular markings are often increased, but they are often crowded together, indicating a loss of volume of the affected region. Atelectasis or fibrosis may develop in severe bronchiectasis, and uninvolved lobes or an entire lung may undergo compensatory overinflation. Bronchography, in which the lumen of the tracheobronchial tree is outlined with radiopaque material (provided they are patent), is the only satisfactory method of establishing the diagnosis, but this special investigation is usually performed only if surgical intervention is being contemplated.

Functional Manifestations

The alterations of pulmonary function in bronchiectasis are extremely variable and depend upon the number of bronchi involved as well as the associated parenchymal disease. Minimal bronchiectasis does not appear to have a significant effect on ventilatory function. In more advanced disease, lung volume may be increased or decreased, whereas airflow resistance is often mildly increased, so that the FEV_1, FEF_{25-75} and $\dot{V}_{max}$ at any lung volume are reduced. Even in mild disease the distribution of the inspired gas is impaired, and hypoxemia may be present because of perfusion of poorly ventilated areas of lung, whereas hyperventilation of the uninvolved portions of the lung helps to maintain a normal or slightly lowered arterial carbon dioxide tension. When there is diffuse disease, there may be gross mismatching of ventilation and perfusion, and the work of breathing may be so great that alveolar hypoventilation with consequent severe hypoxemia and hypercapnia may develop.

CYSTIC FIBROSIS

Cystic fibrosis, also known as *fibrocystic disease of the pancreas* and *mucoviscidosis*, is a disease that is inherited as an autosomal recessive disorder. It involves the exocrine glands of the body and possibly other organs as well. However, 90 per cent of the morbidity and mortality associated with the disease is due to involvement of the respiratory tract. This disorder is a major cause of chronic pulmonary disease in childhood. It occurs in approximately 1 out of 2000 live births in the Caucasian race, but is rare in the Negro, Eskimo, Indian and Asian populations. It has been estimated that about five per cent of the Caucasian populations are carriers (heterozygotes) of the gene. This disease is also becoming a major consideration in adult patients with bronchiectasis, because improved treatment has reduced the mortality and improved prognosis so that many patients now reach adulthood.

Pathogenesis

Although the precise etiology of this disorder has not been elucidated, a generalized inborn error of metabolism, whose precise nature is not known, has been implicated. The major manifestations result from obstruction due to abnormal secretions in the respiratory tract, sweat glands, mucosal glands of the small intestine, the pancreas and bile ducts of the liver.

Respiratory Tract. Pulmonary involvement occurs in more than 98 per cent of patients suffering from *cystic fibrosis*, but the amount of involvement is quite variable. The size of the bronchial glands is apparently normal at birth, but hypertrophy of the bronchial glands and hypersecretion develop rapidly thereafter. The initial insult that leads to the hypersecretion is not known, but the thick, tenacious mucus results in obstruction of small bronchi and bronchioles and impairment of mucociliary clearance in the bronchial tree.

The stagnant mucus serves as an excellent culture media for bacteria, particularly *Staphylococcus aureus* and *Pseudomonas aeruginosa*. Mucoid strains of pseudomonas are commonly seen, and *Hemophilus influenzae, Escherichia coli,* and *Klebsiella* may also be found. *Candida* and *Aspergillus* are also commonly found in the sputum, but they do not seem to be associated with disseminated infection. Although specific IgE to *Aspergillus*, along with a positive skin reaction and serum precipitins, is present in 50 per cent of children with cystic fibrosis, only a few patients actually develop clinical aspergillus infection. The tracheobronchial infection further increases mucus production and the interference with the clearance of secretions, so that a vicious circle is set up. Progression of the disease results in a chronic suppurative bronchitis with destruction of the normal ciliated epithelium as well as squamous metaplasia. As a result, cylindrical and saccular bronchiolectasis, peribronchial fibrosis, pneumonitis and multiple abscesses may develop. The lungs become hyperinflated, but alveolar wall destruction occurs only occasionally. With further progression, marked hypoxemia and hypercapnia develop, followed by pulmonary hypertension, which leads to right-sided heart failure.

The upper respiratory tract is frequently affected, and chronic sinusitis is usually present. Nasal polyps are found frequently and may appear as early as 3 years of age. Multiple, bilateral nasal polyps are found in 10 per cent of patients older than 10 years of age.

Salivary and Sweat Glands. Although the rate of sweating and water reabsorption in the excretory ducts is normal, reabsorption of both sodium and chloride is diminished in patients with cystic fibrosis. The high concentration of sodium, chloride and potassium in the sweat and the saliva forms the basis of the most reliable diagnostic test for this disease. The sweat chloride concentration is markedly elevated in 98 per cent of patients with cystic fibrosis, and a concentration greater than 60 mEq/l. is considered to be diagnostic of this disease.

Gastrointestinal Tract. The mucosal glands of the small intestine are involved early in about 10 per cent of newborn infants with cystic fibrosis. A homogeneous, acidophilic secretion accumulates within the mucous glands, and the meconium is tarry and extremely viscid. The terminal ileum is the commonest site of obstruction, and perforation, with meconium peritonitis, volvulus or secondary atresia may occur.

Pancreas. Eighty per cent of the patients with cystic fibrosis suffer from pancreatic insufficiency because there is secretion of a reduced volume of highly viscous fluid, whose enzyme content may or may not be decreased, depending on the extent of pancreatic involvement. As a result, steatorrhea and azotorrhea along with fat malabsorption predominate, hypoproteinemia develops, and there is a failure to grow and develop normally.

Liver. The basic lesion in the liver is similar to that seen in the pancreas. Bile-containing mucous plugs produce focal obstructive lesions, which result in cell atrophy, fatty metamorphosis, periportal fibrosis and proliferation of the bile ducts. Adjacent to the areas of proliferation are bile ducts with dilated obstructed lumens. Focal lesions of this nature are seen at autopsy in about 20 per cent of patients with cystic fibrosis; in 5 per cent of patients, there is more diffuse involvement leading to biliary cirrhosis, which is occasionally associated with portal hypertension.

Clinical Manifestations

As has already been indicated, the clinical manifestations of this condition are variable and depend upon the degree of involvement of the various organ systems. Meconium ileus is the earliest manifestation of the disease and should be strongly suspected in the newborn infant who presents with abdominal distention and has not passed meconium within 12 hours after birth. A positive family history of cystic fibrosis is helpful in making the diagnosis.

After the newborn period, most of the early manifestations of the disease are due to pancreatic insufficiency or pulmonary involvement. The earliest pulmonary symptom is a dry, hacking cough, which develops during the first few months of life. This usually progresses to paroxysmal coughing spells that sound productive. Fever is not a frequent manifestation, although acute febrile respiratory illnesses may initiate flare-ups of cough and phlegm. Other symptoms and signs include tachypnea, easy fatiguability, decreased exercise tolerance, irritability and occasionally cyanosis during crying spells.

In hot climates, the excessive loss of sodium and chloride in the sweat may lead to *"heat stroke,"* and this may be the initial presentation. It is for this reason that additional salt must be given to patients with cystic fibrosis who live in hot climates.

With advanced pulmonary involvement the anteroposterior diameter of the chest is increased, there is hyperresonance on percussion, decreased breath sounds with prolonged expiration, and wheezes, along with localized or generalized crackles. With severe involvement, pigeon breast, costal flaring and intercostal retractions, cyanosis at rest or during exercise and severe clubbing of the fingers and toes may be present.

Radiologic Manifestations

The pulmonary roentgenologic changes depend on the degree of involvement. Early, there may be minimal bronchial wall thickening, increased perihilar markings or scattered infiltrates and mild hyperinflation; later, abnormal densities radiating out from the hilum and along the blood vessels, as well as generalized hyperinflation, become evident. Bronchi seen end-on have markedly thickened walls because of the inflammatory reaction in and around these structures. Rounded densities in the periphery represent secretions within airways, and lobular or lobar atelectasis and abscesses, cysts, and bullae may develop. Prominence of the pulmonary artery and enlargement of the heart indicate the onset of cor pulmonale.

Functional Manifestations

The earliest abnormalities in pulmonary function are obstruction of the peripheral airways (with an increase in residual volume and functional residual capacity and, to a lesser extent, of the total lung capacity). With progression, the airflow limitation increases, and the FEV_1, FEF_{25-75} and $\dot{V}_{max}$ at all lung volumes decrease.

There is gross mismatching of blood and gas within the lung, as evidenced by an increase in the physiologic dead space, impaired gas distribution, an elevated $P_{(A-a)}O_2$ and hypoxemia. In severe disease, there may be right-to-left shunting that is not corrected by breathing 100 per cent oxygen. With acute infection or accumulation of secretions, the hypoxemia increases, and when the work of breathing becomes excessive, hypercapnia and respiratory acidosis develop. Progression of the disease can lead to severe pulmonary hypertension and cor pulmonale.

15

LUNG PARENCHYMAL DISEASE

As discussed earlier, the lung remains amazingly healthy despite its continued exposure to the environment and all of its foreign material. If the mucociliary system or the cough reflex is altered, microorganisms that are normally resident in the healthy upper respiratory tract can enter the lower respiratory tract, where they may propagate and invade the lung parenchyma. Even with healthy defenses, aspiration of irritating substances can set up severe inflammatory reactions in the lung parenchyma. Postnasal mucus or inflammatory exudate may be aspirated into the tracheobronchial tree, particularly during sleep. Similarly, lipid substances such as mineral oil or oily nose drops, which tend to adhere to the posterior pharyngeal wall, can be aspirated into the lungs during sleep, cause damage to the lung parenchyma and produce a "lipid" pneumonia. Pneumonia may follow the aspiration of substances such as water or particulate matter in cases of drowning; vomitus in comatose or anesthetized patients; or regurgitated food in patients with esophageal obstruction. Accidental inhalation of irritating gases such as nitrogen dioxide, which may be present in silos, or sulphur dioxide, which occasionally occurs in underground mine explosions, may lead to an inflammatory reaction of the lung parenchyma. Severe, acute parenchymal inflammation can also develop following the inhalation of the fumes of toxic substance such as cadmium, beryllium and mercury. All of these factors may cause inflammation of the lung parenchyma and may favor the spread of bacteria or lead to the development of interstitial fibrosis.

PNEUMONIA

When a pneumonia is the presenting illness, it is usually a primary infection of viral, bacterial or mycoplasmal origin, but it may also develop secondarily as a complication of a preceding nonrespiratory illness. Most

299

acute pneumonias are viral in origin, but because the majority of these infections are mild, they frequently remain undiagnosed. Bacterial pneumonia is often preceded by a viral infection of the respiratory tract, which injures the ciliated epithelial cells lining the tracheobronchial tree. This impairs mucociliary clearance so that bacteria multiply in the lower respiratory tract, and a pneumonia may develop. Although bacterial pneumonias account for less than one-third of the acute infections of the lower respiratory tract, they are much more serious in nature and are, therefore, most frequently seen in hospitals.

BACTERIAL INFECTION
Gram-positive Cocci

Gram-positive microorganisms are responsible for the majority of bacillary pneumonias, and **Diplococcus pneumoniae** is by far the most frequent and important microorganism involved. **Pneumococcal pneumonia** is usually preceded by the symptoms of a common cold and is heralded by the onset of violent shaking chills, chest pain, a rapidly mounting fever and cough, with expectoration of tenacious rusty-colored sputum, dyspnea and cyanosis. Consolidation, a pathologic process in which the air within the alveolar spaces is replaced by cellular exudate, may involve the whole or part of a lobe. The condition may be complicated by bacteremia, empyema or meningitis.

Staphylococcus aureus infection usually produces a lobular consolidation that tends to involve adjacent areas. It most often develops secondarily in patients who have a **bacteremia** due to distant infected sites or in debilitated patients and those suffering from chronic disease. Occasionally it develops following **measles** or **influenza.** The onset is usually gradual with a progressive, increasingly severe cough and purulent sputum, a high, swinging temperature, shaking chills and often a pleuritic type of chest pain. In infants and children the disease is more acute and fulminating. The illness is frequently prolonged and often leaves the patient with permanent lung damage. A **staphylococcal pneumonia** frequently breaks down into a necrotic abscess, and this may spread to the pleura and produce an **empyema** or a **bronchopleural fistula** and **pyopneumothorax. Bacteremia** is a serious complication, for it can result in widely disseminated metastatic abscesses involving such organs as the brain, liver, bones and kidneys.

Streptococcus pyogenes, once a very frequent cause of secondary pneumonia, also tends to produce a lobular type of consolidation. It is now relatively infrequent, but it may still complicate many of the common childhood infectious diseases, such as **measles.** It usually begins insidiously, severe bronchitis being the prominent feature. Suppurative complications similar to those caused by the pneumococcus, particularly **empyema** and rarely **pericarditis** and **mediastinitis,** may occur.

Gram-negative Bacilli

The number of cases of pneumonia due to gram-negative bacilli is low when compared with those produced by the gram-positive cocci, but the prevalence has risen considerably of late, particularly in critically ill patients.

Klebsiella pneumoniae, which is responsible for *Friedlander's pneumonia,* occurs in alcoholics or elderly, debilitated persons who are suffering from some chronic disease, such as *diabetes.* The pneumonia generally begins abruptly, without preceding upper respiratory symptoms. There is a high temperature, shaking chills and a severe cough, with the expectoration of thick, tenacious, jelly-like, purulent sputum, which is frequently blood stained. Because this type of pneumonia produces suppuration and destruction of lung parenchyma, a *lung abscess* is a common complication, and frank blood is frequently expectorated. A serious and often fatal complication is a gram-negative *bacteremia,* which may result in an acute cardiovascular collapse.

Pseudomonas aeruginosa is a frequent cause of infection in patients who are in intensive care units, as well as in individuals suffering from cystic fibrosis. It is possible that many cases are related to the use of poorly cleaned inhalation therapy equipment.

An outbreak of severe pneumonia following a convention of the American Legion has led to the identification of a gram-negative bacillus named *Legionella pneumophila.* This organism can cause multisystem illness involving the gastrointestinal tract, kidney and central nervous system in addition to the lungs. Several epidemics have been described in association with contamination of aerosols from cooling towers and evaporative condensers, with dusts from landscaping and with construction requiring the excavation of soil. In addition, the organism has been cultured from shower heads in hospitals and hotels that have had cases of *legionnaire's disease.*

Anaerobic Bacilli

Patients with carious teeth and gingival disease, or those who have aspirated oropharyngeal contents, are predisposed to develop a necrotizing pneumonia. This is due to a mixture of aerobic and anaerobic bacteria, such as *bacteroides* and *fusobacterium. Lung abscess* and *empyema* are the main complications of this condition.

Gram-positive Bacilli

Actinomyces israelii are pleomorphic gram-positive rods. They are anaerobic and cause chronic inflammation, sinuses and fistulas if they penetrate mucosal barriers or gain access to necrotic tissue. They frequently form sulfur granules that have a sunburst or a *"ray fungus"* appearance on microscopic examination. Pneumonia caused by this organism may spread to the pleural space and produce *empyema* and then *pleurocutaneous sinuses.*

Nocardia asteroides is an aerobic organism that is often weakly acid-fast and that may produce a pneumonitis if inhaled. It may also spread to the pleural space and involve the chest wall. *Nocardiosis* usually develops in patients with other diseases, especially in those suffering from immuno-deficiency or immunosuppression in association with an organ transplant.

Acid-fast Bacilli

Tuberculosis. Of all the acid-fast bacilli, the one that causes the most common, most serious and most contagious disease is *Mycobacterium tuberculosis. Tuberculosis* can be produced by several strains of this orga-nism, but the human type is the commonest and most important cause. The bovine type, which is responsible for intra-abdominal and bone disease, has been fairly well eradicated.

The initial, or primary, tuberculous infection results from the inhalation of mycobacteria into the respiratory tract; the extent of the infection depends on the size of the infecting dose and the resistance of the patient. The inhaled bacilli are ingested by alveolar macrophages but, unlike other bacteria, they are not destroyed, and instead appear to multiply. Soon after inhalation, the mycobacteria sensitize T-lymphocytes to the tuberculoprotein, so that one develops a delayed hypersensitivity to the bacilli and its products. The "primary lesion," the tubercle or *"Ghon focus,"* which is composed predominantly of macrophages and T-lymphocytes, develops approximately 6 weeks after the initial infection, coincident with the development of a positive skin reaction to tuberculin. In the majority of patients there is a mild, short-lived illness; after the development of hypersensitivity, the lesion usually heals and calcification occurs in the nodes and the lung lesion, which then constitutes the *"Ghon complex."*

Invasion of pulmonary tissue by the tubercle bacillus produces a gran-ulomatous reaction and results in a pneumonic consolidation with a lobular distribution. As the granuloma infiltrates the surrounding tissue, the central portion may undergo necrosis and form a cavity containing caseous material. Organisms that lodge in the subpleural areas may cause a serous pleural effusion after the initial infection. The infection in the lung spreads by way of the lymphatics to involve the draining lymph nodes in the hilum. If there has been massive infection by virulent organisms, the disease process may erode into a pulmonary vessel and the caseous material may be discharged into the blood stream; this may result in miliary tuberculosis and tuberculous meningitis. Indeed, it has been suggested that there is always a bacteremia between the initial infection and the development of the immune reaction and that when the immune response takes place, organisms circulating in the blood stream are trapped in various organs, where they may lie dormant for years. Later in life, these trapped organisms may propagate and produce active disease in such organs as the lung, kidney or bone.

The usual site of reactivation of the disease is in the apex of the lung.

This "adult" form of the disease is usually subacute or chronic and generally develops insidiously with a low-grade fever, slight cough and the expectoration of a scanty amount of mucoid sputum. Cavitation is a common feature that develops as the disease progresses, with expectoration of purulent sputum, blood or blood-stained sputum. Frequently, the patient has excessive sweating that has soaked his nightclothes, the so-called night sweats.

In the early stages of the disease, physical examination of the lungs often reveals no abnormality, the disease being apparent only on roentgenologic examination. In more extensive disease, the physical signs are those of a consolidation, most commonly affecting the posterior segment of the upper lobe. Often there are crackles, and occasionally there is bronchial breathing, especially if there is cavitation.

Nontuberculous Mycobacteria. The majority of the nontuberculous mycobacteria are common contaminants in nature. They can be found in sewage and tap water as well as in the gastric contents of humans. There is, however, a small heterogeneous group of these acid-fast mycobacteria that are capable of producing disease in man. It has been suggested that these forms of mycobacteria are saprophytes that become pathogenic because of heavy colonization that enables them to invade tissue already affected by a disease process. In contrast to the tubercle bacillus, nontuberculous mycobacteria have never been shown to cause a contagious disease.

The nontuberculous mycobacteria have been classified into four major groups on the basis of their rate of growth and the color of their cultures.

Cultures of group I organisms *(photochromogens)* are characterized by nonpigmented colonies that turn yellow when exposed to the light. Of these, *Mycobacterium kansasii* has the greatest potential for disease production in the human, causing pulmonary and lymph node disease similar to tuberculosis. Extrapulmonary infection and generalized disseminated infection are rare.

The group II organisms *(scotochromogens)* are a heterogeneous group consisting of many strains that are often recovered from the sputum and gastric contents of healthy people as well as from tap water. Their colonies develop a yellow-orange pigment when grown in the dark. These organisms rarely infect the lung, but **M. scrofulaceum** can cause **cervical lymphadenitis,** especially in children.

The group III organisms *(nonphotochromogens)* produce no pigment whether grown in the dark or light. **M. intracellulare,** which is frequently isolated from throat swabs of healthy people, produces a disease that is clinically identical to tuberculosis. A large majority of cases arise in individuals with other lung disorders, especially **chronic bronchitis** or **bronchiectasis.** **M. intracellulare** can cause a disseminated disease, especially in patients with alterations of the immune system or carcinoma.

The group IV organisms, the **rapid growers** in culture, also have no pigment, but their cultures grow in a matter of days; the other nontuberculous mycobacteria require weeks. **M. fortuitum** can result in a progressive pulmonary infection, particularly in patients with chronic pulmonary disease, such as *chronic bronchitis,* or in patients with *ankylosing spondylitis.*

MYCOPLASMAL INFECTION

Mycoplasma pneumoniae, the most frequent cause of nonbacterial pneumonia in the civilian population, is usually endemic and occurs throughout the year. This organism shares both viral and bacterial characteristics; its particle size is similar to that of viruses, but its enzyme systems are similar to those of bacteria. Mycoplasmal and viral pneumonias present with strikingly similar clinical features. Constitutional symptoms predominate initially, and feverishness, generalized aches and pains and a severe headache are usually associated with a watery nasal discharge and a severe sore throat. These are then followed by substernal soreness due to acute tracheobronchitis, a paroxysmal cough and a scanty amount of mucoid sputum. In somewhat less than half of the patients, the diagnosis is indicated in the early stages by the development of cold-hemagglutinating macroglobulin antibodies to the organism. In addition, the serologic complement fixation level rises in 80 to 90 per cent of cases.

VIRAL INFECTION

Pneumonias due to *influenza A and B* viruses are the most frequent cause of epidemics. The serologic complement fixation test, particularly if monitored in the convalescent phase, is usually indicative of influenzal infection. Other viruses causing pneumonia are the *respiratory syncytial virus,* which has a predilection for children, and *adenoviruses 4 and 7,* which can cause *pharyngitis, tracheobronchitis* and pneumonia. *Parainfluenza 3 virus* causes *bronchiolitis* and pneumonia, and *parainfluenza 1 and 2* usually cause *laryngotracheobronchitis.* In 80 to 90 per cent of parainfluenzal and respiratory syncytial virus infections the complement fixation test is positive.

Characteristically, the radiologic opacities in viral pneumonia are much more extensive than is suggested by the clinical examination. The consolidation is usually lobular in distribution and may affect one or both lungs. Aside from epidemics in which a specific viral agent is identified, an etiologic diagnosis in the sporadic case based on clinical grounds alone is virtually impossible.

CHLAMYDIAL INFECTION

Psittacosis is an infectious disease due to *Chlamydia psittaci,* which may affect any member of the bird family and can be transmitted to humans. This intracellular parasite, which resembles a virus but has bacteria-like properties, is present in the excrement of birds suffering from this disease. When it is inhaled by humans, the disease closely resembles the pneumonia produced by a viral infection. Constitutional symptoms, with a high fever, generalized myalgia and severe headache, predominate, and a dry, hacking, usually nonproductive cough is often present. Once again a lobular consolidation is more prominent radiologically than on clinical examination. Here, too, the diagnosis is confirmed by a significant rise in complement-fixing antibody titers.

RICKETTSIAL INFECTION

Rickettsial microorganisms, which are intracellular parasites, are the size of bacteria and are readily visible by light microscopy. They are responsible for a variety of acute, self-limiting, infectious diseases, such as *typhus, Rocky Mountain spotted fever* and *Q fever.* Of these, *Q fever,* which is due to *Coxiella burneti,* is the only one commonly associated with a pneumonia. It is lobular in character and tends to be confined to a portion of a lobe. As in viral pneumonia, fever, chills, headache and myalgia predominate, mild respiratory symptoms developing only several days later. Infected sheep, goats and cattle, whose excreta can contaminate the area where they are housed, are the source of infection. The diagnosis can also be established by a rise in specific complement-fixing antibody titers.

FUNGAL INFECTION

Although much less frequent than other infectious agents, the possibility of fungal infection must be considered in any case of pneumonia that runs an atypical or complicated course. Fungi are frequently secondary invaders of the lung, particularly when there is a pre-existing bronchopulmonary disease, such as *bronchiectasis, lung abscess* or *bronchogenic carcinoma.* Less frequently they are the primary and sole cause of the pulmonary lesion. A fungal pneumonia is generally characterized by necrosis and suppuration, resulting from either the liberation of toxin by the fungi or hypersensitivity of the host to either the fungi or their breakdown products. Fungal pneumonias produce no characteristic symptoms or signs. Increasing fatigability, progressive weight loss, general malaise, profuse slumber sweats, cough and the expectoration of purulent sputum are all features of these diseases.

Some fungal infections, such as *moniliasis* and *cryptococcosis,* are endogenous and occur in any part of the world with no regard to climate or social status. All of the other fungal infections in man are exogenous and result from the inhalation of airborne spores. The majority of these organisms have been isolated from the soil; their prevalence is higher among certain occupations, such as farming.

Some fungal infections have a fixed geographic distribution. *Histoplasmosis,* an extremely common disorder that is caused by *Histoplasma capsulatum,* occurs in the valleys of great rivers, such as the Mississippi, the Ohio and the St. Lawrence. When inhaled into the lungs, the organisms are phagocytosed by alveolar macrophages, and a granulomatous reaction develops in the interalveolar septa and around the bronchioles. Most infections with this organism are asymptomatic. Dissemination occurs occasionally, and caseating granulomas, which heal and calcify, are found in the organs involved, particularly the lungs, lymph nodes, liver and spleen.

Coccidioidomycosis, which is caused by *Coccidioides immitis,* is endemic in the deserts of North America and southern and northern Mexico. It, too, appears to be particularly prevalent in individuals who have been in contact with freshly turned soil or exposed to excessive dust during storms. The disorder can be asymptomatic. It may be mild and self-limited, or it may disseminate and involve the bones and the meninges. Pulmonary consolidation is common, and there is an associated hilar node enlargement. The consolidation usually clears, but occasionally a cavity may develop in a granulomatous area. Precipitins appear early in this disorder, and complement-fixing antibodies develop later.

Blastomycosis is a systemic fungal disease caused by *Blastomyces dermatitidis.* It has an endemic area quite similar to that of histoplasmosis, and is also found most frequently in individuals whose occupations bring them into intimate contact with the soil. There may be a mild self-limited form of pulmonary infection, a local bronchopneumonia, a miliary picture, or an acute and fulminating process. The condition can become indolent, often with dissemination to the skin, subcutaneous tissue, genitourinary tract, bones, and central nervous system. The fungus can be demonstrated as double-walled light refractile bodies in fresh sputum when a 10 to 15 per cent potassium hydroxide solution is added.

Cryptococcosis is caused by the entry of *Cryptococcus neoformans* into the lungs, where it proliferates. Consolidation may occur, or there may be miliary lesions as granulomas develop. Dissemination is common particularly to the brain, skin and bones. The fungus can be isolated in sputum, and, in patients with meningitis, wet mounts of cerebrospinal fluid with India ink will demonstrate the presence of cryptococci.

Aspergillus fumigatus generally affects the lungs secondarily and can cause a mycetoma or fungus ball in a cavity or a cystic space. Hypersensitivity pneumonitis and bronchopulmonary aspergillosis complicating asthma are also seen frequently. Aspergilli can be cultured in the sputum of patients with bronchopulmonary aspergillosis, and serum precipitins to Aspergillus can be found.

PROTOZOAL INFECTION

Toxoplasmosis, which is caused by the protozoa *Toxoplasma gondii,* is a rare cause of lung disease. Serologic studies have shown that subclinical infection by this protozoa is widespread among the general population throughout the world. An interstitial pneumonitis is a feature in the acquired disease, and the illness resembles that of the viral pneumonias. The central nervous system is frequently involved, especially in compromised hosts. In the congenital form of the disease, in which the fetus is infected by the diseased mother through the placenta, the central nervous system is also chiefly affected.

Although most commonly seen in debilitated and premature infants, *Pneumocystis carinii* infection also produces extensive diffuse lobular opacities in adults suffering from diseases of the reticuloendothelial system, such as *Hodgkin's disease* and *lymphosarcoma,* and particularly in those being treated with cytotoxic agents, irradiation or corticosteroids. Sputum production is minimal in this condition, and the organisms are rarely found in the sputum. However, groups of erupted organisms can be demonstrated in lung tissue by performing a methenamine silver stain. Recently, this form of pulmonary infection has been found in homosexuals, and an *acquired immune deficiency syndrome* has been described.

CLINICAL MANIFESTATIONS

Certain clinical features enable the examiner to distinguish between bacterial, viral and mycoplasmal pneumonias. Cough and purulent sputum at the onset of the disease suggest a bacterial pneumonia, whereas cough, often nonproductive, is usually a late feature in viral and mycoplasmal pneumonia. In these latter conditions, sputum, when it does develop, is scanty and mucoid in character, although it may later become purulent because of a secondary bacterial infection. Blood-stained sputum is also a feature of bacterial pneumonia and is extremely uncommon in a viral pneumonia. In bacterial pneumonias, the administration of the appropriate antibiotic, i.e., one based on identification of the offending organism and its sensitivity, usually results in a prompt improvement in the patient's illness. On the other hand, a viral infection runs its course of fever for a period of 5 to 6 days despite the administration of antibiotics, before the temperature finally subsides by lysis.

The abnormal physical findings in pneumonia depend upon the amount of parenchymal tissue involved and are clearly more distinctive when the consolidation involves a lobe than when patchy areas are involved. Because the alveolar air is replaced by exudate, distensibility is reduced and the density of the lung is increased. The trachea and the apex beat of the heart are not displaced from their normal position, but movement of the chest cage over the affected area is restricted, there is dullness on percussion and bronchial breath sounds and whispering pectoriloquy are present.

RADIOLOGIC MANIFESTATIONS

A consolidation appears radiologically as an opacification of the affected area of the lung. This may be evident in one or more segments of a lobe, or it may involve several lobes. If the pneumonia has a lobular distribution, the consolidated lobules may present as scattered, poorly outlined patchy opacities, although several of these may coalesce to involve a few segments or even an entire lobe. Frequently the bronchi can be visualized in the opacity (*air bronchogram*). Another important point to be noted is that the mediastinum occupies its normal midline position (Fig. 98).

With resolution the radiologic opacities lose their homogeneity and become streaky and weblike, finally disappearing completely. Pneumonias caused by *E. coli, Bacteroides* and *Pseudomonas* usually affect the lower

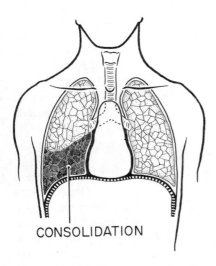

Figure 98. Consolidation of the right lower lobe.

CONSOLIDATION

lobes and may be associated with a large *empyema; B. proteus* and the *Klebsiella-Aerobacter* group usually cause dense infiltrates involving the upper lobes.

Occasionally, areas of translucency may develop within the radiologic opacities. Although these may be cavities, they actually may represent re-aeration of the consolidated lung tissue during the process of healing. *Pneumatoceles,* air-containing cysts possessing smooth, thin walls, are tension cavities produced by a check-valve obstruction and are a common feature of acute *staphylococcal pneumonia,* particularly in young children.

FUNCTIONAL MANIFESTATIONS

The degree of disturbance in pulmonary function that occurs in pneumonic consolidation depends on the extent of the disease process. Ventilatory function may be impaired, but the major impact is on gas exchange. Hypoxemia results from continued perfusion of consolidated and nonventilated areas of the lung. The arterial carbon dioxide tension is frequently lower than normal because of the hyperpnea induced by the hypoxemia.

PULMONARY ABSCESS AND CAVITATION

A pulmonary abscess is a collection of pus within the substance of the lung. It is not a distinct entity in itself, nor is it ever a primary condition. It is a pathologic process that develops during the course of any number of inflammatory conditions of the lung and is caused by a combination of suppuration and necrosis of lung tissue. The more chronic an abscess, the more thickened its wall and putrid its contents.

Through long usage, a chronic tuberculous abscess is generally called a *"cavity,"* whereas the term *"abscess"* is applied to a wide variety of other suppurative diseases of the lung. However, there is no difference between the lung excavation that follows the discharge of tuberculous caseous material and that which follows the evacuation of purulent material of a suppurative pneumonia. Both are abscess cavities, the only difference being the etiologic agent.

PATHOGENESIS

A pulmonary abscess develops most commonly following the aspiration of infected or foreign material, but it may also complicate a primary *pneumonia,* an infected *embolus* or a *pulmonary infarct.* Abscess formation rarely complicates primary *pneumococcal* or *streptococcal pneumonia,* except in infancy or debilitation, but it frequently is caused by *staphylococci, Friedlander's bacilli, tubercle bacilli* and certain fungal infections, such as *blastomycosis.* An abscess cavity may occasionally develop within the substance of a pulmonary neoplasm, whether primary or secondary, most frequently in *squamous cell carcinoma.* A pyogenic abscess is generally smooth and round, whereas a malignant cavity characteristically has a thick wall with a shaggy, irregular appearance.

In the normal course of events, the bronchial defenses are able to deal adequately with nasopharyngeal and oral secretions that may be aspirated into the tracheobronchial tree during sleep. During anesthesia, alcoholic stupor, traumatic shock, coma or the postoperative state, these defenses are seriously impaired. In addition, the aspiration of thick tenacious sputum or the presence of clotted blood may impair ciliary activity. Aspiration of a large quantity of irritant fluid, such as vomitus, usually results in a diffuse lobular pneumonia with multiple abscesses, whereas solid matter, such as a piece of a tooth, usually causes a localized abscess.

The site of development of an aspiration abscess depends on the force of gravity as well as the posture of the patient during aspiration. Aspirated material tends to lodge in the most dependent bronchus, so that if the patient was supine the superior segment of the lower lobe is usually affected. If lying on one side, the most likely site is the upper lobe, and if upright, such as during a dental extraction, the lower lobes are most likely to be affected.

As long as it is in communication with a patent bronchus, a pulmonary cavity always contains air, either alone or in association with fluid. The abscess is generally spherical in shape. This is because of the pull of the surrounding healthy elastic lung parenchyma, as would be seen in a thin elastic sheet in which small, irregular holes have been burned. When stretched taut, the irregularly shaped holes assume a perfectly round shape.

CLINICAL MANIFESTATIONS

The symptoms and clinical course of a pulmonary abscess depend on the cause of the abscess, its size and progression and the presence of complications, such as *empyema.* Often the clinical picture is dominated by the underlying pulmonary disease, the abscess frequently being discovered only by roentgenography. Nevertheless, a lung abscess should be suspected if a febrile respiratory illness develops suddenly in a patient who has recently undergone a surgical procedure, particularly involving the mouth, nose or throat. It should also be considered in a patient who has had an unconscious episode, or a sudden choking spell while eating.

Rupture of an abscess into a bronchus is heralded by the sudden expectoration of a large quantity of sputum. The sputum is frequently green or brown, may be mixed with blood and often has a very offensive odor. Large quantities of purulent sputum may continue to be expectorated daily, especially when the patient changes position suddenly. If the abscess should persist, low-grade constitutional symptoms continue, and acute exacerbations may alternate with periods of relatively good health.

The physical signs depend on the size of the abscess cavity, the degree of surrounding pneumonitis, and the distance from the chest wall. If the cavity is comparatively empty of secretions and in communication with a patent bronchus, a loud, hollow-sounding form of bronchial breathing known as "amphoric breath sounds" may be heard. Coarse crackles may be present over the affected area of the lung during the middle and late phases of inspiration. Digital clubbing is frequently present and may progress to *hypertrophic pulmonary osteoarthropathy.* This condition rapidly regresses when the abscess heals.

RADIOLOGIC MANIFESTATIONS

An abscess can generally be recognized on the chest roentgenogram by its radiolucent circular shadow. The thickness of its border depends on the extent of involvement of the surrounding parenchyma. The most distinguishing feature of an abscess is the presence of a fluid level that can be recognized by its straight horizontal upper border. The radiologic opacity that is produced by the surrounding pneumonitis may be so dense as to obscure the abscess cavity on the standard film, but it can often then be demonstrated with tomography.

CYSTS OF THE LUNG

In cystic disease of the lungs, whether congenital or acquired, the continuity of the lung parenchyma is interrupted by thin-walled, sharply defined, open spaces that contain either fluid or air, and often both. These may occur singly, or there may be many in one or both lungs. Several small cysts may coalesce into a solitary cyst. Multiple cysts may be confined to a segment, a lobe or an entire lung, or both lungs may be riddled with small cysts, giving the involved tissue a honeycombed or spongy appearance.

Congenital cystic disease is not as uncommon as was formerly thought, and a large number of cases are being diagnosed by surgical excision. They are frequently associated with other congenital abnormalities, and there appears to be a familial tendency. It is generally agreed that the cysts arise during fetal lung development by separation of a fragment from the main bronchial buds or their derivatives, which are the forerunners of the bronchi. If only one bronchial bud is involved, a solitary cyst is formed; if many bronchial buds are affected, multiple cysts develop.

The structure of the cyst wall varies considerably and may contain tissues resembling those of bronchi, bronchioles or alveoli. They may be lined with ciliated, columnar or cuboidal epithelium, and they may contain muscle fibers, elastic tissue and cartilage. The cyst may be filled with air or fluid, which is usually clear and watery in consistency. Since the lungs are normally sterile, these cysts rarely become infected, but when they do the fluid may be viscid or purulent and foul smelling.

PULMONARY FIBROSIS

The term "fibrosis" implies an excessive amount of connective tissue in the whole or part of an organ. It is a method of tissue repair that follows any disease process that produces inflammation or necrosis of tissue. In the lung, the reconstruction of an injured site by fibrosis can result in marked disturbances in function. Thus fibrosis of the lung represents an example of repair that induces a deleterious effect.

PATHOGENESIS

Clearly, the deposition of excess fibrous tissue in the lungs can be a sequel to a variety of disorders. The distribution of the fibrous tissue in the lungs varies in different disease processes, and the resulting scar tissue may be confined to a small segment of lung parenchyma, a lobe, a lung or both lungs.

Unilateral Fibrosis

A localized area of the lung is the commonest type of pulmonary fibrosis encountered clinically. This is usually the consequence of tissue necrosis, such as may follow a *suppurative pneumonitis,* a *lung abscess* or *tuberculous caseation.* A similar but more widespread type of fibrosis of one lung may be produced by repeated irradiation of the lung, such as is administered after surgery for *carcinoma of the breast,* or by the aspiration of irritating substances, such as vomitus, oily nose drops or liquid paraffin.

Diffuse Pulmonary Fibrosis

A generalized form of pulmonary interstitial fibrosis, involving both lungs diffusely, may follow a widespread pulmonary infection or the inhalation of organic dusts or noxious fumes. Prolonged exposure to inorganic dusts containing minute particles of irritating inorganic chemicals such as silicon dioxide, silicates or asbestos frequently leads to extensive pulmonary fibrosis, which is known as ***pneumoconiosis.*** Extensive fibrosis may also develop in certain types of noncavitating granulomatous diseases, such as ***sarcoidosis,*** or in collagen diseases, such as ***scleroderma.***

IDIOPATHIC PULMONARY FIBROSIS

In recent years, the number of patients in whom the etiology of diffuse pulmonary fibrosis cannot be determined, the so-called ***idiopathic pulmonary fibrosis,*** has increased considerably. Although there is probably a multiplicity of causes of this condition, no external causal agents have been identified. Characteristically, the disease process is extremely heterogeneous, and there is marked distortion of the pulmonary architecture with an increased amount of fibrous tissue in the alveolar and interlobular septae. The bronchioles are also involved, and there is peribronchiolar fibrous tissue or mononuclear inflammatory cells or both. In addition, there is much cellular debris or mucus in the airways, and numerous airways are narrowed.

Where the alveolar septum is thickened, there is loss of type I cells and proliferation of type II cells. Inflammatory cells, mainly lymphocytes, macrophages and plasma cells, are always seen in the areas of increased fibrous tissue, often along with eosinophils and neutrophils. The extent of neutrophil infiltration in the interstitium and of desquamated cells in the alveoli varies considerably, presumably depending on the stage of the disease when the tissue is examined. Cells are numerous in the early stage, when an alveolitis with inflammatory cells and desquamation may be present, whereas alveolar septal fibrosis predominates at a later stage.

Although the mechanism of production of the lung lesions is unknown, the consistent presence of mononuclear inflammatory cells in the lesions suggests that inflammatory or immunologic mediators may be involved. Circulating autoantibodies to nuclear and cytoplasmic constituents and to denatured gamma globulin have been described. In addition, circulating immune complexes, along with granular deposition of IgG and complement along the alveolar walls and capillaries, may be present during the active cellular phase of the disorder. The immune complexes have not been characterized further, and the nature of the offending antigen, i.e., whether it is an inciting agent or an altered lung tissue component, it not known. A theory that has been advocated proposes that complement and immune complexes in the pulmonary parenchyma induce the release of chemotactic factors, which attract granulocytes into the lungs. The immune complexes are also thought to interact with alveolar macrophages, which in turn initiate a number of events. They stimulate fibroblasts to replicate and produce collagen, and they also release a chemotactic factor for neutrophils, which are attracted into the alveoli. These neutrophils injure the lung cells and release collagenase, which destroys type I collagen, and myeloperoxidase, which, in the presence of other mediators, causes oxidant injury to the lung parenchymal cells.

Much of the current thinking about interstitial lung disease emanates from analysis of the constituents of bronchoalveolar lavage fluid (BALF). In healthy individuals the majority of cells (90% or more) in the lavage fluid are alveolar macrophages, and only about one per cent of the cells are neutrophils. It has been suggested that the inflammatory and immune-effector cells are increased in *idiopathic pulmonary fibrosis.* Some investigators have reported that the neutrophils in the bronchoalveolar lavage fluid are increased in patients with *idiopathic pulmonary fibrosis.* BALF neutrophils are also elevated to about 5 to 10 per cent in many of the interstitial lung diseases associated with *collagen vascular disorders* and in *asbestosis.* The eosinophils may be increased in individuals with early acute disease, whereas in *sarcoidosis,* it is the lymphocytes that are frequently increased. It has been hypothesized that the number of neutrophils present is a reflection of the alveolitis stage of the disorder. It has been proposed that the neutrophils in the lungs produce *collagenase* and *elastase,* which selectively attack and degrade *type I collagen* and cleave *type III collagen,* respectively, and that the lung interstitial connective tissue becomes deranged as a result. Repair of the mesenchyma is apparently directed by the alveolar macrophage, which attracts fibroblasts and stimulates them to replicate and produce collagen.

SARCOIDOSIS

Sarcoidosis is a granulomatous disease in which cellular immune processes appear to be enhanced. It is thought to develop as an intense mononuclear cell alveolitis, which progresses to granuloma formation. It has been reported that the helper T-lymphocytes are increased, whereas the suppressor T-lymphocytes are decreased in the bronchoalveolar lavage fluid in this condition. It is further thought that the T-lymphocytes release monocyte chemotactic factor, which attracts monocytes from the blood, and that these are the basis of the granuloma formation.

HYPERSENSITIVITY LUNG DISEASES

Parenchymal fibrosis may also develop following the repeated inhalation of organic antigens. The "hypersensitivity" disorder is mediated either by humoral immune mechanisms involving antibodies or by cellular immune mechanisms involving sensitized T-lymphocytes. *Wegener's granulomatosis* and pulmonary reactions to drugs like *nitrofurantoin* or *busulfan* are believed to involve hypersensitivity mechanisms, but the exact pathogenetic mechanisms of these conditions are still to be elucidated.

Goodpasture's syndrome is an example of complement mediation of a reaction between tissue and cell-surface antigen and the corresponding autoimmune antibodies. In this condition, there is interstitial and alveolar hemorrhage, along with glomerular nephritis, the pulmonary and renal lesions being associated with anti–basement membrane antibodies, which are detectable along the glomerular and pulmonary alveolar basement membranes and in the circulation. On pathologic examination of the lungs, intra-alveolar hemorrhage, with numerous hemosiderin-containing macrophages, is prevalent. Early glomerular lesions show fibrinoid necrosis in the capillary tuft, focal epithelial and occasionally endothelial proliferation. In more severe cases, epithelial crescents, fibrosis of glomeruli and interstitial inflammation are seen.

In *farmer's lung* or *bird fancier's disease,* conditions that have also been called *"extrinsic allergic alveolitis,"* complement activation is apparently mediated by soluble antigen-antibody complexes. In these conditions, exposure to a particular allergen, such as the spores of the thermophilic actinomycete *Micropolyspora faeni,* which causes *farmer's lung,* or the protein in pigeon or budgerigar droppings, which causes *bird fancier's disease,* may sensitize some persons to the specific allergen and produce the precipitins against it.

Examination of the lung biopsies in early cases of the condition demonstrates infiltration of the alveolar walls and peribronchiolar tissue, mainly with lymphocytes; mononuclear and plasma cells and epithelioid cell granulomata are seen later. Fibrotic changes occur in areas of inflammatory cellular infiltration, and organizing endobronchial exudates, bronchiolitis obliterans and acute vasculitis of the alveolar capillaries are also seen. Indeed, the end-stage is often indistinguishable from that of *idiopathic pulmonary fibrosis.* The histologic findings, i.e., the granulomas and lymphocyte infiltration and the presence of T-lymphocytes in bronchoalveolar lavage fluid, suggest that cell-mediated immunity may also be involved. The dominant effector cells are likely macrophages, which activate lymphocytes.

CLINICAL MANIFESTATIONS

The severity of the symptoms present in pulmonary fibrosis is related not so much to the extent of the fibrosis but rather to its pattern of distribution. There may be no symptoms in a case of long-standing localized pulmonary fibrosis, even when there is gross shrinkage of a lung.

In interstitial pulmonary fibrosis, the primary symptom is dyspnea on exertion, which is often first noted following a viral illness, the degree depending on the extent of the fibrosis. Few abnormal physical signs are usually found, but one can often hear bilateral crackles or dry, interrupted, creaky "Velcro-like" sounds throughout inspiration and expiration in both lung bases. Clubbing of the digits is moderately common.

In extrinsic allergic alveolitis, the classic story is one of repeated attacks of fever, cough, dyspnea, malaise and generalized aches and pains that begin 6 to 12 hours after exposure to a specific allergen and last 24 to 48 hours. In some patients who are exposed to lesser concentrations of allergen over a prolonged period, the disease may develop insidiously without the characteristic attacks.

RADIOLOGIC MANIFESTATIONS

The radiologic appearance of a localized pulmonary fibrosis is similar to that of an *atelectasis* (Fig. 99). Because the size of the lobe is decreased, the fissure that forms its boundary is usually displaced. The mediastinal structures are shifted to the affected side, and the ribs over the fibrotic area are drawn closer together. The diaphragm is elevated and often irregular because of pleural adhesions.

In diffuse pulmonary fibrosis, there are bilateral, coarse linear interstitial strands, or reticular nodular infiltrates are visible throughout both lungs, and the mediastinum is usually not displaced from its midline position. The upper lobes are often predominantly involved in *extrinsic allergic alveolitis,* whereas the lower lobes are predominantly affected in *idiopathic pulmonary fibrosis.* Multiple small, thin-walled cysts or *honeycombing,* which is a late manifestation of fibrosis, may be present throughout both lung fields.

Radioactive gallium scanning of the lungs has been advocated as a means of evaluating the extent of cellular inflammation of the alveolar structures, and this may be particularly useful in *sarcoidosis.* This technique may also be useful for localizing inflammatory disease and activity in other parts of the body.

FUNCTIONAL MANIFESTATIONS

The disturbances of pulmonary function in pulmonary fibrosis depend upon the extent of the fibrosis as well as the pattern of its distribution. The distensibility of the lung is diminished, and the total lung capacity and its subdivisions are reduced, the extent of reduction also depending on the amount of fibrosis. The static pressure–volume curve of the lung is shifted downward and to the right (i.e., an increased pressure at any lung volume). There is usually no measurable increase in flow resistance using the standard indices of airflow resistance. On the other hand, the maximal expiratory flow rates may be low, because of the reduced lung volume, and the *"upstream resistance"* to airflow may be increased, depending on the stage of the disorder when studies are carried out. Since the ventilation-perfusion ratios are altered considerably, the $P_{A\text{-}a}O_2$ is elevated and the arterial Po_2 is

Figure 99. Localized pulmonary fibrosis involving the right lower lobe.

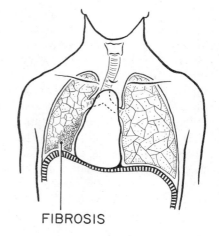

FIBROSIS

low. Because of the increased ventilation induced by the hypoxemia, the arterial carbon dioxide tension is frequently lower than normal.

HYALINE MEMBRANE DISEASE

Hyaline membrane disease (infant respiratory distress syndrome) is a restrictive lung disorder due to a diffuse atelectasis, which develops because of a deficiency of pulmonary surfactant. The condition is a manifestation of insufficient development of the lungs for normal postnatal gas exchange, so that it principally affects the preterm infant (i.e., less than 37 weeks of gestation).

PATHOGENESIS

The condition is worldwide, affecting all races and occurring in males more often than in females. It accounts for about 40 per cent of the deaths of premature infants. Aside from a low birth weight and gestational age, the risk of developing hyaline membrane disease appears to be enhanced by antepartum hemorrhage, cesarean section (particularly when associated with maternal hemorrhage), a history of a previous child with respiratory distress, and signs of fetal or perinatal asphyxia.

In this disorder there is a deficiency of the phospholipid, i.e., *surfactant*, which lines the alveoli at the air-alveolar membrane interface in the lungs, perhaps because the alveolar type II cells, which are responsible for surfactant production, are immature and fail to produce sufficient surfactant to prevent atelectasis. The disease may also be the result of an ischemic insult to the lungs, either while the fetus is *in utero* or during the time of delivery. Since the fetal pulmonary vasculature is exquisitely sensitive to hypoxia and acidosis, an asphyxial insult around the time of birth may produce ischemia of the lungs and result in insufficient surfactant production for normal pulmonary function. This would explain the association between perinatal asphyxia and the high incidence of the disease.

Whatever the precise mechanism for the deficiency of surfactant, extracts of the lung of such infants studied in postmortem examinations exhibit an elevated surface tension. *In vivo* this will result in poor distention of the lung during inspiration and a marked propensity toward alveolar collapse during expiration. Indeed, at postmortem examination the lungs are completely atelectatic and have the consistency and color (red-purple) of the liver. On histologic examination, atelectasis is interspersed with areas of overdistended terminal bronchioles and alveolar ducts, producing the so-called Swiss cheese appearance. Eosinophilic, refractile hyaline ("glossy") membranes, from whence the name of the disease is derived, line the aerated portions of lung. The membrane is not unique to this condition, since it may be found in the lungs of patients dying from a number of other causes, including viral pneumonia and radiation pneumonitis. Indeed, a hyaline membrane is rarely present in those infants who live less than a few hours, a fact that supports the view that the cardinal feature of the disease is atelectasis secondary to surfactant deficiency.

CLINICAL MANIFESTATIONS

The high incidence of this disease in preterm infants and in those suffering from perinatal asphyxia has already been noted. Most infants who eventually die from this disease are in fair to poor condition from birth and have a low Apgar score at one minute of age.

The disorder is characterized by the onset of respiratory difficulty at or within two hours of delivery. The respiratory rate is usually between 70 and 100 but may be as high as 120 breaths per minute. Since the chest wall of the preterm infant is very compliant, there is retraction of the intercostal and subcostal muscles, the extent depending on the severity of the disease. In severe disease, the lower portion of the sternum is markedly retracted during inspiration, and indeed the entire sternum may remain depressed during expiration so that the upper chest appears overinflated. The abdomen may protrude in a sort of "seesaw" pattern with respect to the chest during inspiration.

In the mildly ill baby, the inspiratory breath sounds are harsh, and frequently there are fine crackles in the terminal phase of inspiration. With severe disease, the breath sounds may be markedly diminished or even absent. An expiratory grunt may be heard with the stethoscope, or it may be loud enough to be audible with the naked ear. The respiratory rate continues to be rapid for 36 to 72 hours. Although cyanosis may not be recognized while the baby is breathing room air, arterial hypoxemia can be severe, and the infant with this disorder will require elevated inspired oxygen concentrations. In many cases, a diuresis occurs on the second or third day, and the respiratory rate gradually slows, the infants becoming more alert as they improve.

The severely ill infant continues to grunt loudly, and deep retractions persist for several days. Cyanosis is always present in severe disease, and progressive cyanosis despite oxygen therapy is a grave prognostic sign. During the second day of life the respiratory rate may fall as the baby becomes physically exhausted. Irregular respirations may be followed by periods of apnea, bradycardia and ashen cyanosis. Systemic hypotension and poor peripheral circulation are also features of severe disease. Death may occur if ventilatory assistance is not provided.

A variety of complications may alter the clinical picture and the course of the disease. Pneumothorax, pneumomediastinum or pneumopericardium are the commonest complications encountered. Severe hypoxemia may be associated with intracranial hemorrhage and the sudden onset of apnea. Patent ductus arteriosus is not uncommon. Other complications may be the result of therapy: bronchopulmonary dysplasia, fibrosis of the lungs, retrolental fibroplasia, and cerebral palsy may occur in about 10 per cent of infants surviving ventilator therapy.

TABLE 15. Some Causes of Respiratory Distress in the Neonatal Period

1. *Congenital Malformations*
   Choanal atresia
   Laryngeal webs or clefts
   Tracheal or bronchostenosis
   Cysts
       Bronchogenic
       Solitary or loculated in parenchyma
       Cystic adenomatoid malformation
   Lobar emphysema
   Hypoplasia or agenesis
   Accessory or sequestered lobes
   Tracheoesophageal fistula

2. *Trauma*
   Pneumothorax (spontaneous or iatrogenic)
   Phrenic nerve palsy (Erbs)
   Fractured clavicle or ribs

3. *Aspiration Syndromes*
   Aspirated meconium, squames, thick mucous from amniotic
       fluid, gastric contents
   Transient pharyngeal incoordination
   Vocal cord paralysis

4. *Immaturity*
   Hyaline membrane disease (idiopathic respiratory distress
       syndrome or IRDS)
   Pulmonary hemorrhage

5. *Disorders in Other Systems*
   Hypoventilation from CNS depression
   Airway compression from aberrant vessels
   Pulmonary edema

6. *Delayed Physiologic Adjustments at Birth*
   Transient tachypnea of newborn
   Persistent fetal circulatory pathways

7. *Toxic*
   Salicylates
   Reserpine
   NH_4Cl

8. *Infection*
   A. Transplacental
       Cytomegalic inclusion disease
       Rubella
       Coxsackie
       Syphilis
       Tuberculosis
       Toxoplasmosis
   B. Retrograde (intrauterine)
       E. coli, Staphylococcus, Streptococcus
   C. Postnatal (acquired)
       Chiefly gram-negative bacilli
       Pneumocystis carinii

It should be pointed out that the clinical signs and course, which have been described, are not pathognomonic of this disease and that a wide variety of diseases may cause respiratory difficulty in the immediate neonatal period (Table 15).

RADIOLOGIC MANIFESTATIONS

Uniform, minute reticulogranular densities, which probably represent groups of atelectatic alveoli, are usually distributed evenly throughout both lung fields. Marked reticulogranularity or even solid lung fields are found in very severe disease, and this finding is associated with a poor prognosis. Air-filled bronchi, i.e., an "air bronchogram" may be seen in relief against the opacified peripheral areas. The lateral view may show an increased convexity of the upper thorax and retraction of the lower sternum.

FUNCTIONAL MANIFESTATIONS

Despite uncertainty as to the precise etiology of hyaline membrane disease, a high surface tension of lung extracts and a relative deficiency of pulmonary surfactant have been well documented. The resultant increase in the retractive force of the lung on deflation leads to atelectasis. Lung compliance, functional residual capacity and total lung capacity are decreased, indicative of a restrictive lung disorder. The severe retractions of the chest wall are the result of the markedly increased transpulmonary pressure required to produce a tidal volume.

The pulmonary vascular resistance is markedly increased, and marked ventilation-perfusion abnormalities are present; areas of lung are overventilated in relationship to their blood flow, and the physiologic dead space may be as much as 75 per cent of the tidal volume. Other areas of lung are markedly underventilated in relation to their blood flow; a right-to-left shunt of as much as 70 per cent of the cardiac output may be present, about three-quarters of the shunt being due to continued blood flow through areas of the lung that are not ventilated. As a result, hypoxemia is severe.

The prognosis of this condition is relatively good in those infants whose arterial oxygen tension rises above 100 mm. Hg while breathing 100 per cent oxygen within 10 hours of birth. It is poor in those whose arterial oxygen tension does not rise to 100 mm. Hg and in whom the arterial pH is below 7.20. The shunt increases during the first 36 to 48 hours in severe disease and then may begin to decrease if the infant is going to recover. The hypoxemia is often not reversed, even by the administration of high concentrations of oxygen. The severe hypoxemia interferes with aerobic metabolism, so that lactic acid accumulates and a metabolic acidemia is present. As the disease worsens, there may be a gradual rise in the arterial P_{CO_2} so that a respiratory acidosis is added to the metabolic acidosis.

PULMONARY VASCULAR DISEASE

Like the liver, the lungs have a double supply of blood. One comes from the right ventricle via the pulmonary circulation, and the other from the left ventricle through the bronchial circulation. The major portion of the blood supply to the lungs comes in the pulmonary arteries; the bronchial arteries normally provide only about 1 per cent of the blood supply. Although anastomoses have been demonstrated between the bronchial and pulmonary arteries, these have never been shown to function in normal lungs. In diseased lungs, however, these anastomoses dilate, and the bronchial arteries may contribute a considerable proportion of the pulmonary circulation.

THE PULMONARY CIRCULATION

The pulmonary trunk and the large pulmonary arteries are elastic arteries whose media consist predominantly of elastic tissue; histologically, they resemble the aorta fairly closely. In each pulmonary artery the media is composed of smooth muscle fibers bounded by internal and external elastic laminae. The anatomy of the pulmonary arteries that lie close to the bronchioles, respiratory bronchioles and alveolar ducts is similar to that of systemic vessels, such as the femoral and brachial arteries. However, the pulmonary arteries are very much smaller (0.1 to 1.0 mm. diameter) and have much thinner walls than the muscular arteries of the systemic circulation. The walls of the pulmonary arterioles, whose diameter is less than 0.1 mm., consist of an endothelial lining, a single elastic lamina with no smooth muscle and virtually no adventitia. Thus the pulmonary circulation does not contain any vessels corresponding to the muscular arterioles of the systemic circulation.

The pulmonary blood vessels derive their nerve supply from both the sympathetic and parasympathetic nervous systems. Both afferent and efferent fibers of each system are present. The nerve supply is less abundant than that of either the systemic arteries or the bronchial arteries.

PULMONARY BLOOD VOLUME

The pulmonary circulation constitutes a distensible reservoir that is situated between the right and left ventricles. Normally about 10 per cent of the total circulating blood volume is in the lungs. Of this, about 30 per cent is in the arteries, 60 per cent in the veins, and 10 per cent in the pulmonary capillaries. The pulmonary capillary blood volume while at rest has been estimated to vary between 75 and 100 ml., depending on the size of the lung. Although this seems small, the surface area of the capillaries necessary to contain this volume of blood is about 70 square meters.

The major portion of the pulmonary vasculature is surrounded by a pressure that is less than atmospheric. The pulmonary arteries and veins are exposed to the pleural pressure, but the capillaries that surround the alveoli are exposed to alveolar pressure, which varies above and below atmospheric pressure during breathing. The pulmonary blood flow and blood volume are not constant. For instance, they are influenced by respiration, increasing during inspiration and decreasing during expiration, largely as a result of changes in the intrathoracic pressure, which in turn causes variations in the venous return to the right side of the heart. In addition, not all of the pulmonary capillaries are open at rest, and new capillaries are recruited when the blood flow increases. The pulmonary capillary blood volume has been estimated to increase by 60 to 90 ml. during exercise, presumably because of the opening of these previously closed capillaries. The pulmonary capillary blood volume is also influenced by disease. For example, in congestive heart failure, the pulmonary capillary blood volume is increased, and in other conditions, such as pulmonary fibrosis, it is reduced.

PULMONARY BLOOD PRESSURE AND FLOW

The blood pressure in the pulmonary blood vessels is less than 15 per cent of that in the peripheral circulation, and the drop in pressure from the main pulmonary artery to the left atrium is about 10 per cent of that between the aorta and the right atrium. In a normal person who is breathing quietly, the systolic and diastolic pressures in the pulmonary artery are approximately 23 and 8 mm. Hg, with a mean pressure of about 14 mm. Hg. The pressure in the pulmonary capillaries is somewhere between 14 mm. Hg and the pressure in the pulmonary veins (about 5 mm. Hg), and is likely about 8 mm. Hg.

Pulmonary blood flow has been shown to be pulsatile. In the basal state, the rate of pulmonary blood flow is very stable, averaging about 3.0 liters per minute per square meter of body surface area. Despite considerable increases in blood flow, the pulmonary artery pressure barely rises. In fact, it does not rise appreciably until the blood flow increases three- to four-fold. Clearly then, since flow increases appreciably during exercise, the pulmonary arteriolar resistance must fall until the pressure rises.

As was pointed out in Chapter 2, the amount of blood flow in any part of the lung depends on the relationship between the arterial, capillary, venous and extravascular pressures as well as the state of contraction of the vascular smooth muscles. In the upright individual, the amount of blood flow at the apex of the lung is less than at the base, and this is because of the effect of gravity. During exercise, blood flow at the apex of the lung increases more than at the base, although there is still a gradient in blood flow down the lung.

When hypoxemia develops as a result of respiratory disease, or if there is a reduction in the inspired oxygen concentration as occurs at high altitudes, the pulmonary blood vessels constrict, and this results in an elevated pulmonary vascular resistance and a rise in pulmonary artery pressure. Such vasoconstriction, which probably involves both the precapillary and postcapillary vessels, is particularly important, because it causes blood to be shunted away from poorly ventilated areas of the lung toward better ventilated regions.

Mild increases in the concentration of carbon dioxide in the inspired air do not appear to affect the pulmonary circulation in healthy individuals, but high concentrations of carbon dioxide increase the pulmonary vascular resistance, presumably because of the acidemia they produce. When acidemia is present in patients with respiratory disease, the pulmonary vascular resistance increases. When hypoxemia and acidemia are combined, the pulmonary vascular resistance rises markedly; this has important implications in the management of patients with severe cardiopulmonary insufficiency.

Certain pharmacologic preparations also affect the pulmonary circulation. The injection of a small dose of acetylcholine into the pulmonary artery of a patient suffering from hypoxemia and pulmonary hypertension leads to a transient fall in the pulmonary artery pressure. On the other hand, epinephrine produces a transient vasoconstriction of the pulmonary arterioles and a slight rise in the pulmonary artery pressure, and histamine, norepinephrine and serotonin also appear to be potent pulmonary vasoconstrictors. The role of any of these substances in the development of pulmonary hypertension, however, is not clear.

THE BRONCHIAL CIRCULATION

In humans, the bronchial arteries usually arise from the proximal portion of the thoracic aorta or one of the first two intercostal arteries. Each lung possesses at least one bronchial artery. These vessels follow the course of the bronchial tree into the lung parenchyma, where they branch elaborately and rejoin to form plexuses around the bronchi and in the bronchial submucosa. The bronchial arteries are nutrient arteries, and they deliver oxygenated blood to the walls of the tracheobronchial tree and to the tissues of the pulmonary arteries and veins. They supply the lower part of the trachea, the bronchi as far as the respiratory bronchioles, and the visceral pleura. Through anastomoses with numerous other vessels, they also supply the vasa vasorum of the pulmonary artery and vein, the vagi, the tracheo-bronchial lymph nodes, and the mediastinal structures, particularly the pericardium.

In a healthy person, blood brought to the lungs via the bronchial arteries may follow one of two courses in returning to the heart. In the proximal part of the major bronchi, some of the blood is carried via the bronchial veins into the azygos veins and then to the right atrium. More distally, the venous drainage enters into the pulmonary veins. Thus, it can be seen that the pulmonary veins normally carry small amounts of poorly oxygenated blood. Although there have been numerous attempts to measure the bron-chial arterial blood flow in humans, it is too small in the healthy individual to be measured by the indirect techniques that have been utilized.

BRONCHOPULMONARY ANASTOMOSES

At the capillary level and the precapillary connections between the pulmonary and the bronchial arterial systems in the normal lung, there are extensive microscopic vascular connections. These shunts are located in the lobular subdivisions of the bronchopulmonary segments as well as in the pleura.

When the pulmonary capillary bed is reduced by disease, the lumina of the peripheral bronchial arteries frequently enlarge, often reaching the size of the pulmonary artery at the same level. Many plexuses of collateral arterial vessels may develop, and there is often conspicuous dilatation of the bronchial veins in such conditions as *pulmonary embolism* with infarction, *lung abscess* and certain forms of *congenital heart disease.* The most striking changes are seen in severe chronic cases of *bronchiectasis,* where the bronchial arteries often form a dense plexus of thick-walled, large-lumened channels. Their anastomoses with the pulmonary artery are situated distally in the walls of the bronchiectatic sacs and may be as large as 2 mm. in diameter. The burden of this collateral circulation must fall on the left side of the heart, for the blood is brought to the lung from the aorta and then returned to the left atrium, principally by means of the pulmonary veins. In other words, the collateral circulation represents a shunt between the aorta and the left atrium. The added work load on the left side of the heart may lead to the development of left-sided heart failure, and it may also account for the left ventricular hypertrophy that is occasionally observed in cases of right-sided heart failure or *cor pulmonale.* Conversely, blood shunted into the pulmonary arteries by way of these bronchial anastomotic channels tends to elevate the pressure within the lesser circulation, thereby increasing the work of the right side of the heart and thus predisposing the individual to cor pulmonale. In addition to the local vasoconstriction that is brought about by hypoxemia, it is thought that propagation of the high pressure in the bronchial arterial system to the pulmonary circulation through the broncho-pulmonary anastomoses prevents the flow of poorly oxygenated pulmonary arterial blood into the diseased portions of the lung, and thus diverts it to more normal areas of lung. Thus, in patients with extensive disease of one lung, there may be only slight desaturation of the systemic arterial blood.

The large pulmonary arterial vessels containing blood under systemic pressure are often situated superficially within the lamina propria of the bronchi, and any ulceration may easily rupture them. This may account for the pulmonary hemorrhages that occur in *bronchiectasis* or other chronic pulmonary diseases, where the bleeding may be massive and may consist of obviously oxygenated, bright red blood.

PULMONARY VASCULAR RESISTANCE

The pulmonary vascular resistance is determined from the following formula:

$$\text{Resistance (R)} = \frac{\text{Pressure gradient}}{\text{Flow}}$$

The pressure gradient is that across the lung vasculature, i.e., between the pulmonary artery and the left atrium. Thus:

$$R = \frac{\text{Pulmonary artery pressure—Left atrial pressure}}{\text{Pulmonary blood flow}}$$

Pulmonary vascular resistance is usually expressed in units of force. Pressures in mm. Hg are converted to dynes/square centimeter and flow (liters/minute) is converted to milliliters/second. The normal gradient between the pulmonary artery and the left atrium is about 8 to 12 mm. Hg, and the pulmonary vascular resistance is about 80 to 160 dynes/sec./cm^5.

PULMONARY HYPERTENSION

As we have seen, there is a large pulmonary vascular reserve in a healthy person, and the pulmonary artery pressure does not rise appreciably during exercise until there is a greater than three- or four-fold increase in pulmonary blood flow. This indicates a decrease in total pulmonary vascular resistance during the exercise, most likely due to an increase in the size of the pulmonary vascular bed because new vessels open up. However, a greater increase in pulmonary blood flow raises the pulmonary artery pressure almost proportionately with the increase in blood flow. In pulmonary disease, the pulmonary vascular bed is often affected and the resistance within the pulmonary vessels is increased, so that the pulmonary artery pressure rises. Pulmonary hypertension is considered to be present when the systolic pulmonary blood pressure rises above 30 mm. Hg and the diastolic pressure is above 15 mm. Hg.

Pulmonary hypertension may develop for a number of reasons—an appreciable elevation of the left atrial pressure, an increase in the pulmonary blood flow, obstruction or obliteration of the pulmonary vascular bed, or active pulmonary vasoconstriction. Except for left-to-right cardiac shunts, in which the pulmonary artery pressure is elevated but the vascular resistance is normal, the resistance to blood flow is nearly always increased when pulmonary hypertension develops in respiratory disease.

ELEVATION OF LEFT ATRIAL PRESSURE

If the pulmonary circulatory outflow is impeded (i.e., when the left atrial pressure is elevated) because of an obstruction (such as occurs with *mitral stenosis*) or failure of the left ventricle, due to *aortic valve disease, systemic hypertension, ischemic heart disease* or *cardiomyopathy,* the pressure behind the impediment will rise. Although the raised pressure has certain advantages, in that it maintains a higher level of flow across the obstruction than would otherwise be the case, this is bought at a price. As the pulmonary venous pressure rises, the pulmonary capillary pressure may reach levels in excess of the plasma oncotic pressure (25–30 mm. Hg). As a result, pulmonary interstitial edema may develop, first in the perivascular spaces and later in the alveolar septa. If the transmural pressure becomes very high or if lymphatic drainage is inadequate, alveolar edema may develop. Time is a factor, and levels of pulmonary capillary pressure that may result in severe pulmonary edema in acute situations may be well tolerated in chronic cases. The difference between the two situations is probably related to the development of a more capacious and efficient lymphatic system in the latter case.

When there is pulmonary venous hypertension, the transudation of fluid is maximal in the lower lung regions because the venous pressure is higher there. Lymphatic engorgement is also seen in the lower zones under these circumstances. In addition the pulmonary blood flow is redistributed, with more going to the upper zones, so that the ratio of upper to lower zone blood flow in the erect position may be 1:1 or greater.

INCREASED PULMONARY BLOOD FLOW

If there is a large communication between the right and left ventricles, as in a *ventricular septal defect,* or between the aorta and the pulmonary artery, as in a *patent ductus arteriosus,* the pulmonary blood flow is increased. The left ventricular pressure (in the former situation) or the aortic systolic pressure (in the latter) is transmitted to the pulmonary arterial system so that the pressure in the pulmonary artery is elevated.

OBSTRUCTION OF THE PULMONARY VASCULATURE

The pulmonary vascular resistance rises if the caliber of the pulmonary vessels is reduced or the number of vessels is decreased. Acute obstruction of one pulmonary artery with an inflatable balloon produces variable effects, although it usually causes only a transient rise in the pulmonary artery pressure. This suggests that the vascular bed of the opposite lung, to which the blood has been diverted, is expansile; i.e., previously closed capillaries are opened. This procedure has been used as a prognostic test before a pneumonectomy is performed; if the pressure rises under these circumstances, the surgeon can anticipate that the pulmonary artery pressure and right ventricular pressure will remain elevated following surgery.

In contrast to the experimental acute occlusion of a main pulmonary artery, the pulmonary artery pressure rises if there is acute occlusion of a smaller pulmonary vessel by an embolus. It has been suggested that this rise in pressure is caused by reflex vasoconstriction that is induced by occlusion of small pulmonary arteries but not by obstruction of the main pulmonary arteries. Another hypothesis that has been put forward to explain the pulmonary hypertension is that the vasoconstriction of the pulmonary vessels is caused by the release of *5-hydroxytryptamine,* or *serotonin,* from the blood clot.

OBLITERATION OF THE PULMONARY VASCULATURE

In chronic respiratory diseases such as *fibrosis* or *emphysema,* the pulmonary capillaries may be obliterated, and in *kyphoscoliosis* they may be compressed, so that there is a reduction of the effective capillary bed that is available for perfusion. As a result, the pulmonary vascular resistance may be elevated, and pulmonary hypertension develops.

VASOCONSTRICTION OF THE PULMONARY VASCULATURE

Active pulmonary vasoconstriction is probably a concomitant of many of the other forms of pulmonary hypertension that have been described. Most investigators believe that the pulmonary blood vessels possess tone and, therefore, that the tone can be altered. Hypoxemia and, often, acidemia are common in respiratory insufficiency and probably play a role in pulmonary vasoconstriction and pulmonary hypertension. A number of observers have suggested that the pulmonary vasoconstriction is mediated through the sympathetic fibers. The intense vasoconstriction that occurs after *pulmonary embolism* may be forestalled by a sympathectomy or by the administration of adrenergic-blocking and ganglion-blocking agents. When pulmonary hypertension is present, the infusion of acetylcholine into the pulmonary circulation will often produce a fall in the pulmonary artery pressure, suggesting active dilatation of the pulmonary vessels. The reversal of an elevated pulmonary vascular resistance following surgery for *congenital heart disease* or *mitral valve disease* further suggests that a vasomotor element may be involved. It would seem that, provided intimal changes have not progressed beyond a certain point, removal of the vasoconstrictor stimulus causes regression of the hypertrophy of the vascular smooth muscle.

PRIMARY PULMONARY HYPERTENSION

Primary pulmonary hypertension is a relatively rare condition in which there is neither intrinsic cardiac nor pulmonary disease. The incidence of this condition appears to be slightly greater in females, and the majority of individuals affected are between the ages of 20 and 40. An increase in vascular tone has been implicated, although on pathologic examination the small pulmonary arteries show intimal fibrosis and necrotizing and angiomatoid lesions. In addition there is medial hypertrophy of the small muscular pulmonary arteries and muscularization of the precapillary vessels. The structural changes in the small pulmonary arterial branches result in a progressive increase in pulmonary vascular resistance and pulmonary hypertension. With persistence of the elevated pulmonary vascular resistance, hypertrophy of the right ventricle develops, and ultimately right ventricular failure occurs.

CLINICAL MANIFESTATIONS

The salient symptoms are exertional dyspnea, muscular weakness and fatigue, all of which are probably related to a low cardiac output. Palpitation, exertional substernal and left-sided chest pain and syncopal attacks are present in about one quarter of the cases. The syncope is thought to be due to a drop in left ventricular output as a result of acute elevations of the pulmonary vascular resistance. Hemoptysis occurs occasionally; the mechanism of its production is not clear, although the possibility of *pulmonary emboli* must be considered. The terminal manifestations are characterized by the development of right-sided heart failure, and often there is a sudden demise.

The positive physical signs are usually limited to the heart and those organs that are affected by right ventricular failure. The second pulmonic sound is accentuated and fails to split during inspiration. There is evidence of right ventricular hypertrophy, which is accompanied by distention of the neck veins, hepatomegaly and, later, peripheral edema.

RADIOLOGIC MANIFESTATIONS

A chest roentgenogram demonstrates the right ventricular hypertrophy, a bulging pulmonary artery segment and prominent hilar vessels, with attenuation of the peripheral arterial branches. These findings are associated with normal or diminished intrapulmonary vascular markings.

FUNCTIONAL MANIFESTATIONS

Ventilatory function studies are all within normal limits. Mismatching of ventilation and perfusion is increased so that the $P_{(A-a)}O_2$ is elevated and mild hypoxemia may be present. This is usually associated with hypocapnia and a tendency toward a respiratory alkalemia. Hemodynamic studies performed during cardiac catheterization reveal an elevated pulmonary artery pressure, a normal wedge pressure, and an increased arteriovenous oxygen difference in the presence of a normal systemic blood pressure and a normal or near-normal cardiac output.

PULMONARY EMBOLISM AND INFARCTION

Pulmonary embolism and infarction are major circulatory emergencies. Unfortunately, they are often unsuspected clinically, frequently being discovered only at postmortem examination. However, it is clear that *pulmonary embolism* is one of the most important causes of morbidity and mortality, exceeding pneumonia in some centers.

PATHOGENESIS

Most pulmonary emboli originate as detached portions of venous thrombi located in the deep veins of the lower extremities. Occasionally, the thrombi may be in the right side of the heart, the upper extremities, and, particularly in women, in the veins of the pelvic region. Nonthrombotic materials, such as amniotic fluid, fat, air, bone spicules and fragments of organs, constitute a very small percentage of pulmonary emboli.

Venous thrombosis and pulmonary embolism occur predominantly in bedridden patients, especially in those with cardiac disease and congestive heart failure, or those who have been immobilized following a fracture or multiple injury. The postoperative state is next in importance, especially that following abdominal or pelvic surgery, where there may be injury to the iliac veins. Sitting for long periods in cars, buses or airplanes may also promote stasis and lead to venous thrombosis. Other factors that may predispose individuals to venous thrombosis are *pregnancy, oral contraceptives, varicose veins, carcinoma, obesity, polycythemia vera* or other blood diseases, such as *sickle cell anemia,* particularly if any of these conditions is associated with prolonged bed rest.

The mechanism responsible for the intravascular formation of blood clots is poorly understood. The factors that facilitate the production of intravascular clotting are retardation of the venous circulation, damage to the vessel walls, especially the endothelial surface, and conditions that favor the coagulation of blood. Once a clot fragment loses its anchorage in a peripheral vein or in the right atrium, it is swept rapidly into the pulmonary arteries. Very large thrombi do not progress beyond the larger arteries, but smaller emboli pass into the narrower lobar arteries of the lungs.

Much information about the effects of pulmonary embolism has been learned from animal experimentation. Embolization of the lungs with particulate matter invokes severe pulmonary hypertension, a fall in the systemic pressure, distention of the right cardiac chambers, engorgement of the peripheral veins and, often, death. It is probable that most of these effects are largely mechanical. Nevertheless, when the lungs of the animals are denervated at the height of the embolic reaction, the pulmonary hypertension gradually subsides, the left ventricular output increases and the animals survive. This suggests that embolization produces widespread pulmonary vascular constriction, which is mediated through sympathetic impulses. The vascular constriction might also be due to the local or reflex effects of 5-hydroxytryptamine, or serotonin, which is known to provoke constriction of the pulmonary vasculature, although there is little evidence for this.

PULMONARY INFARCTION

Occasionally an embolus can cause pulmonary infarction. It is less likely to occur when the lungs are healthy and apparently develops only when embolic obstruction of a pulmonary artery is attended simultaneously by some additional factor that retards blood flow through the lungs, such as congestive heart failure, or when the bronchial circulation is compromised. A pulmonary embolus is also more likely to lead to infarction of the lung if alveolar hypoventilation or a pulmonary infection is present.

A pulmonary infarct is usually sterile, and secondary infection is an uncommon feature. Rarely, an abscess may develop in an infarct if the embolus was infected or if necrosis or infection develops secondarily to a bland infarct. Since this type of abscess extends to the pleura, *empyema* may be an added complication.

CLINICAL MANIFESTATIONS

Embolic occlusion of the main pulmonary arteries is usually rapidly fatal. The manifestations of smaller single or multiple embolic episodes are exceedingly varied, and changing symptom patterns are frequent. Although most symptoms and signs of pulmonary embolism are manifest in the respiratory system, the manifestations may suggest a cardiac, neurologic or intra-abdominal disease; in other instances, there may be no symptoms at all. When present, the symptoms may be short-lived, or they may persist for weeks, months or even years.

The diagnosis of pulmonary embolism with or without infarction is based chiefly on the symptoms that result, and only partly on the presence of abnormal physical signs. Pulmonary embolism should be suspected in any elderly bedridden patient who suddenly develops acute dyspnea, chest pain, unexplained vascular collapse or syncope, or who presents with refractory congestive heart failure. In many, pulmonary embolism is promptly followed by signs of circulatory collapse, a rapid and feeble pulse and hypotension, because so little blood passes the blockade in the pulmonary circulation that the left ventricle does not fill adequately and the cardiac output falls. This may result in signs of cerebral ischemia such as restlessness, apprehension, syncope and coma. Occasionally, there is a transient episode of unconsciousness, and in elderly patients, hemiplegia and convulsive phenomena may be the chief signs of pulmonary embolism.

Dyspnea is present in virtually all individuals; it may be mild and hardly noticeable, or it may progress rapidly to gasping respirations that are out of proportion to the amount of lung tissue involved. The difficult breathing has been attributed to stimulation of intrapulmonary receptors. An irritating cough may develop on the second or third day following the infarction. Hemoptysis occurs in only a few cases, although the sputum may be bloody during the early period of an infarction, and dark blood may be expectorated during the healing process.

Pulmonary embolism often presents with sudden chest pain, and in most cases it is either pleuritic in nature or restrosternal and indistinguishable from the pain of myocardial ischemia. Because most infarcts occur in the lower lobes of the lungs, the diaphragm may be involved in the pleuritis and the pain may be referred to the neck and shoulder. On rare occasions there may be severe upper abdominal pain and muscle guarding, which may be due to irritation of the lateral portion of the diaphragm or distention of the liver capsule (if the pulmonary embolism has resulted in acute right-sided heart failure).

Very few cases demonstrate the so-called classic syndrome of pulmonary embolism, i.e., sudden pleuritic chest pain, dyspnea, hemoptysis and fever, with signs of consolidation, a pleural rub and evident venous thrombosis. The physical signs of pulmonary infarction are rarely distinctive, and the physical examination is entirely negative more often than not. Tenderness over the plantar veins of the foot or the muscles of the calves is an early sign of venous thrombosis, and tenderness along the course of the great veins on the inner aspect of the thighs, along with swollen tender inguinal lymph nodes and pitting edema, may develop later. In most cases, however, embolism occurs in the absence of any signs or symptoms of peripheral venous thrombosis.

In most cases the physical signs associated with a pulmonary embolus are due to the development of pulmonary hypertension. An accentuated pulmonic second sound, with narrowing of the normal physiologic splitting, prominent pulsation along the right border of the sternum, and an increased presystolic pulsation or "a" wave of the jugular venous pulse are indicative of pulmonary hypertension and acute dilatation of the right ventricle. An early systolic click may develop, and there is often a short pulmonary ejection murmur. In late cases a murmur of pulmonary incompetence may be heard at the left sternal border. Tachycardia is usually present, and occasionally there may be paroxysmal cardiac arrhythmias, atrial fibrillation or atrial flutter.

Extensive obstruction of the pulmonary vasculature due to multiple pulmonary emboli that may recur over a long period of time may lead to right ventricular hypertrophy and the gradual development of heart failure. When the right ventricle begins to fail, a third heart sound may be heard at the lower sternal edge. Later, tricuspid incompetence may develop, so that a parasystolic murmur that increases during inspiration may be heard. Jugular venous distention is common, and in the late stages, the liver may be enlarged and peripheral edema may develop.

When respiratory signs are present, they are similar to those found with a *pneumonia* or *atelectasis.* Diminished movement, dullness to percussion, diminished breath sounds or bronchial breathing and crackles are often present over the affected area. Localized intercostal tenderness and a pleural friction rub may be present, particularly with an infarction. If a *pleural effusion* develops, both the breath sounds and the vocal fremitus may be diminished.

RADIOLOGIC MANIFESTATIONS

The chest roentgenogram may offer some valuable clues that suggest an acute pulmonary vascular obstruction. For instance, the hilar shadows may be accentuated, and the main pulmonary arteries and the pulmonary artery trunk are dilated. In addition, the diaphragm may be elevated on the side of the embolus, or a platelike atelectasis may be present. Acute gross dilatation of the right atrium and ventricle is rarely seen radiographically, but an elevated systemic venous pressure may be recognized by dilatation of the superior vena cava and azygos vein. Repeated embolic episodes may lead to marked dilatation of the right ventricle and gross dilatation of the pulmonary artery trunk and hilar arteries, along with diminished vascularity in the lung fields.

The radiologic appearance of a pulmonary infarction may suggest minimal or massive collapse of the lung. The opacity frequently has a conical shape, with its apex toward the hilum and its base toward the pleura, or it may be irregular, round or oval. It may present as a hazy clouding or streaking at one base or as a hump filling the costophrenic angle that may change to a well-defined consolidation. The presence of a small pleural effusion may also suggest an underlying embolus.

A lung perfusion scan, supplemented by a ventilation scan, is used most often to investigate the possibility of pulmonary embolism. This entails injection of particles labeled with radioactive iodine or technicium to determine perfusion, whereas radioactive xenon is inhaled to study the distribution of ventilation. Absence of perfusion in a localized area(s) suggests a pulmonary embolus. Clearly, however, if there is a parenchymal infiltration, one cannot say whether the reduced blood flow is due to an infarction or to some other lesion. On the other hand, the absence of a perfusion defect in a well-performed study virtually rules out a pulmonary embolism.

Angiographic examination of the pulmonary vasculature is the most definitive method of diagnosing a pulmonary embolus. This may confirm the dilated major pulmonary artery branches and reveal complete obstruction of segmental or lobar branches of the pulmonary arteries or irregular filling defects. The latter presumably represent adherent, retracted, partially lyzed emboli or thrombi along the walls of the larger arteries. In some cases there may be only retardation of blood flow to one or more lung segments. A follow-up angiogram often reveals complete disappearance of these findings.

Detection of venous thrombosis in the legs has been markedly facilitated by using radiolabeled fibrinogen, which is injected intravenously, and then scanning the extremities. Unfortunately, however, only clots formed in the calves can be detected, and, more importantly, clots in the deep veins of the thigh or pelvis cannot be detected.

FUNCTIONAL MANIFESTATIONS

When a branch of the pulmonary artery is occluded, the alveoli may still be ventilated, and the air leaving these alveoli will have the composition of inspired air; i.e., they constitute part of the physiologic dead space. However, the airways supplying the area of lung whose blood supply has been cut off frequently constrict, and some of the ventilation is then shifted away from nonperfused areas. The mechanism of the bronchoconstriction has not been elucidated, but the low CO_2 concentration in the affected segments, loss of surface-active material in these segments, and release of chemical substances such as histamine or serotonin from the thrombus have been implicated.

The increase in physiologic dead space (i.e., high $\dot{V}/\dot{Q}$ ratios) per se should not cause a fall in arterial Po_2, and yet hypoxemia, generally of moderate degree, is common in patients suffering from a pulmonary embolus. This is presumably because of continued perfusion of poorly ventilated areas of lung (low $\dot{V}/\dot{Q}$ ratios). The P_aCO_2 is usually lower than normal as a result of alveolar hyperventilation. Rarely, carbon dioxide retention due to alveolar hypoventilation develops, because of either a marked rise in the physiologic dead space or an increased work of breathing.

In patients with ***multiple pulmonary emboli,*** the pulmonary vascular bed available for diffusion is reduced. As we have seen earlier, nearly two-thirds of the pulmonary vascular bed must be obliterated before pulmonary hypertension results. However, lesser degrees of mechanical obstruction due to emboli may be associated with considerable functional pulmonary vasoconstriction, so that the pulmonary vascular resistance is usually elevated in patients who have suffered from pulmonary emboli. If this persists, pulmonary hypertension with right ventricular hypertrophy and, eventually, right ventricular failure develop.

PULMONARY ARTERIOVENOUS ANEURYSM

Arteries and veins develop out of a common embryonic capillary plexus, so that opportunities are always present for persistent connections, even after birth. Small arteriovenous communications of the vascular systems of most tissues, including the lungs, normally exist. These communications probably help to adjust to changes in the external and the internal environments. For instance, it is believed that such anastomoses in the skin of the fingers and toes play an important part in heat regulation. The function of arteriovenous anastomoses in the lung is not clear, but it has been suggested that they may act as safety valves to protect the lung capillaries from excessive increases in blood pressure and blood perfusion.

Shunts between large blood vessels or between the chambers of the heart normally exist only during fetal life (see Chapter 6). After birth, about 5 to 7 per cent of the total pulmonary blood flow does not become arterialized to the maximum extent, and so it acts like venous admixture (shunt). The major causes of abnormal vascular shunts are trauma, infection and malignant tumors. In adult life, multiple arteriovenous and other intervascular connections may develop in the lungs in association with chronic infection, such as *bronchiectasis.*

PATHOGENESIS

A *pulmonary arteriovenous aneurysm* is an example of an increase in true venous admixture. This congenital lesion is a pulmonary manifestation of a generalized systemic vascular disorder, *hereditary hemorrhagic telangiectasia,* which is characterized by localized dilatations of small vessels that form telangiectases or angiomata with a tendency to bleed. These tiny ruby lesions are generally seen on the face, the nasopharyngeal and buccal mucous membranes, the lips, and the skin of the body and in the nail beds. The gastrointestinal, respiratory, and genitourinary tracts, and even the brain or spinal cord may be affected. About 60 per cent of patients have a family history of cutaneous telangiectasia. The cause of this inherited lesion remains unknown, but it is believed to be transmitted by a single dominant gene. Both sexes are affected and are able to transmit the disease, but females are more frequently involved. Occasionally, a generation may be skipped.

In most cases, the shunt takes place from a pulmonary artery to a pulmonary vein. One or more branches of the artery usually enter a loculated aneurysmal sac that is drained by a greatly enlarged and often tortuous vein. The aneurysm may also be drained by veins from adjoining lobes, or it may be drained by completely anomalous veins.

It has been suggested that the vascular dilatation may be a manifestation of a generalized weakening of the ground substance in the vessel wall because of a defect of the normal hyaluronidase-inhibiting mechanism. Another suggestion is that the telangiectasis is produced by 5-hydroxytryptamine, which is normally detoxified in the lungs. According to the latter hypothesis, the 5-hydroxytryptamine escapes detoxification by bypassing the lungs via a pulmonary arteriovenous aneurysm. This postulate suggests, therefore, that the multiple telangiectases develop secondarily as a result of a primary pulmonary arteriovenous aneurysm, rather than vice versa.

CLINICAL MANIFESTATIONS

The pulmonary lesion is usually discovered during the third and fourth decades, although occasionally it has been found in children and even in the newborn. The disease may remain stationary for years, but frequently there is a definite tendency toward progression. There appear to be two distinct clinical types: the type that is not associated with any clinical signs, and the type associated with a triad of cyanosis, polycythemia and digital clubbing.

If the shunt is small, there may be no noticeable clinical effects. When the shunt is large, the cardinal symptoms are due to the chronic hypoxemia resulting from shunting of poorly oxygenated blood through the aneurysm. The principal symptoms are dyspnea on exertion, which may be slight at first but later progressively increases in severity, weakness, palpitations, and precordial pain. Neurologic complications are not uncommon; these may consist of headaches, vertigo, convulsions, syncope, paresthesias, diplopia, thick speech, and paresis, as well as cerebrovascular accidents. The neurologic symptoms have been ascribed to a variety of causes, such as cerebral hypoxia and polycythemia, as well as to telangiectasis in the brain with or without associated cerebral thrombosis.

Bleeding is a most important complication, the commonest type being epistaxis from telangiectatic lesions in the nasal mucous membranes. In addition, hemoptysis, hematuria, melena and cerebral hemorrhage may occur because of telangiectatic lesions in the tracheobronchial tree, genitourinary tract, gastrointestinal tract and central nervous system.

Cyanosis, clubbing and occasionally hypertrophic pulmonary osteoarthropathy are present, although cyanosis may not be detectable. When the lesion is large, a murmur is often heard on the chest wall over the site. It is usually continuous and accentuated during systole, and it becomes more intense during deep inspiration, often fading out during expiration.

RADIOLOGIC MANIFESTATIONS

Multiple lesions may be so small as to be barely discernible. A large pulmonary arteriovenous aneurysm is often detected in a routine posteroanterior roentgenogram of the chest. Characteristically, there may be one or more lobulated or spheroid opacities with smooth discrete margins. They may be connected with the hilum by bandlike linear or sinuous opacities. Any segment of either lung may be involved, although there appears to be a predilection for the lower lobes and the right middle lobe. In a few cases, the abnormal shadow may be hidden behind the heart. If multiple tiny lesions are present, no radiologic abnormality may be evident.

Pulsations in the lobulated densities as well as in the hilum may occasionally be seen on fluoroscopic examination. The vascular nature of the lesion may be demonstrated by certain maneuvers, such as the Valsalva and Mueller tests. Although tomography can often give confirmative evidence, angiography is the most definitive and preferable procedure to establish the diagnosis.

FUNCTIONAL MANIFESTATIONS

A pulmonary arteriovenous aneurysm is associated with true venous admixture (i.e., some of the blood from the right ventricle returns to the left side of the heart without becoming fully oxygenated), so that hypoxemia develops. Since the lungs themselves are normal, the hyperventilation induced by the hypoxemia results in hypocapnia. The presence of true venous admixture is confirmed by failure of the P_aO_2 to rise above 500 mm. Hg at sea level when the patient inhales 100 per cent oxygen.

The cardiac output is nearly always normal, although it may be increased if the oxygen tension is very low. Erythropoiesis may be stimulated so that both the red blood cell mass and total blood volume are increased. In some cases, the number of erythrocytes may be normal, and anemia, probably due to the chronic or repeated hemorrhages, may be present.

PULMONARY EDEMA

Pulmonary edema is an excessive accumulation of extravascular water in the lungs. Fluid does not normally accumulate in the lungs, even though the alveolar structure offers little resistance to the passage of fluid from the capillaries. Under ordinary conditions, the osmotic force of 30 mm. Hg exerted by the proteins in the systemic capillaries is neatly balanced by the intracapillary hydrostatic pressure, which is about 25 mm. Hg. In the lungs, however, even in the most dependent lung capillaries, the hydrostatic pressure is only about 10 mm. Hg, and it is even lower in the apices of the lung, indicating a considerable margin of safety for the alveoli. In the healthy lung, there is a continual movement of fluid and, to a lesser extent, protein from the plasma across the endothelium into the interstitial space, whereas the alveolar epithelium is relatively impermeable to fluids other than water. The fluid that moves into the interstitium is removed by the pulmonary lymphatics.

PATHOGENESIS

The continual net flux of fluid and protein from the pulmonary microvasculature into the interstitium is the result of a balance of forces within and around the pulmonary capillaries. This is defined in the following equation for fluid exchange:

$$\dot{Q}f = K(P_{mv} - P_{pmv}) - K\sigma\,(\pi mv - \pi\,pmv)$$

Where Q̇f is the rate of fluid filtration, P the hydrostatic pressure, σ the osmotic pressure in the microvasculature (mv) and perivasculature (pmv) interstitital fluid components, K the filtration coefficient of the microvascular barrier and π the "effective" reflection coefficient of the membrane.

When edema fluid accumulates in the lungs, the factors responsible are essentially the same as those concerned in the formation of edema fluid elsewhere, i.e., any one or a combination of an increased capillary hydrostatic pressure, a diminished colloid osmotic pressure, an increased permeability of the capillary walls, a reduced mechanical pressure in the tissues and interference with the lymph flow. Usually, pulmonary edema is due to either an increased hydrostatic pressure or an increased pulmonary capillary permeability. In high-pressure edema the edema fluid is low in protein, whereas in increased permeability edema it is high in protein.

Increased Hydrostatic Pressure

It is generally thought that the pressure in the interstitial space is about −2 mm. Hg and that the net transmural hydrostatic pressure difference across the pulmonary capillaries is approximately 10 mm. Hg. When the resistance to blood flow out of the lungs is increased, as in *mitral stenosis,* the level of the capillary hydrostatic pressure may rise above that of the colloid osmotic pressure. A pulmonary venous pressure of 20 mm. Hg is considered to be the upper limit of safety, and if the pressure rises above this level, blood pumped into the lung by the right ventricle tends to accumulate behind the obstruction. At high intracapillary pressures, red blood cells and fluid are extravasated because of rupture of capillaries, particularly in the dependent parts of the lungs. If the extravasation occurs at very rapid rates, the ability of the lymphatics to drain the fluid is exceeded, and large amounts may accumulate in the lung.

The precipitation of pulmonary edema by the intravenous infusion of saline, plasma or blood suggests that it may also develop following a sudden increase in the venous return to the lungs, which increases the capillary hydrostatic pressure. The development of acute pulmonary edema when the patient with congestive heart failure is recumbent is an example of this. As long as the patient is in the erect position, the high intracapillary pressure in the areas of the body below the heart protects the lungs, so that edema fluid tends to accumulate primarily in the dependent parts of the body. When the patient lies down at night, however, the edema fluid from the peripheral areas enters the blood stream and increases the venous return to the lungs. As a result, the pulmonary capillary pressure rises, and pulmonary edema may develop. Additional factors that may be involved are an increase in plasma volume and the increased capillary permeability due to hypoxemia that develops during sleep. Acute pulmonary edema is often relieved by factors that reduce venous return, such as venesection, intermittent positive pressure breathing or the application of tourniquets to the extremities.

The mechanism by which pulmonary edema occurs following trauma to the skull, cerebral hemorrhage or an attack of encephalitis is not understood, but it has been proposed that stimulation of the central nervous system induces systemic vasoconstriction through the sympathetic nerves, so that both the resistance to the ejection of blood from the left ventricle and the peripheral venous tone are increased. These act to augment both the pulmonary blood volume and the pulmonary capillary pressure, thereby raising the capillary hydrostatic pressure and producing pulmonary edema.

Diminished Osmotic Pressure

As we have seen, the pulmonary capillary endothelium is permeable to water and, to a lesser extent, to protein. However, because large molecules cannot move across the membrane, there are concentration differences between the capillary and the interstitial space. The osmotic pressure is thought to be about 6 mm. Hg higher in the blood. Coupled with a hydrostatic pressure gradient of about 10 mm. Hg, there is then a net pressure of 4 mm. Hg favoring movement of fluid from the capillaries into the interstitial space. If the osmotic pressure is lowered, the extravascular water content of the lung may rise. A subacute form of pulmonary edema that may be due to reduced colloid osmotic pressure is seen in *uremia, acute nephritis* and *polyarteritis nodosa*. It is possible that the rapid infusion of intravenous fluid could also lead to a reduction in colloid osmotic pressure and so cause acute pulmonary edema.

Increased Capillary Permeability

The permeability of the capillary walls may be altered by chemical, bacterial, thermal or mechanical agents. If the permeability coefficient of the endothelium is altered, liquid can move more readily from the capillary at any particular relationship between hydrostatic and osmotic forces. The greater the change in permeability, the more leak of fluid will occur. In addition, it has been shown that capillary dilatation per se favors the outward movement of fluid. As protein escapes into the tissues, the osmotic gradient across the capillary wall is reduced and further edema is favored. Under these circumstances, the fluid has the characteristics of an exudate; i.e., it has a high protein content. Since the alveolar epithelium is less permeable than the endothelium, the fluid accumulates in the peribronchial and perivascular interstitial spaces. From here it is removed via the pulmonary lymphatics. If the process continues, the liquid will ultimately flood the interstitium and fill the alveoli.

Hypoxemia has been implicated as the most important factor that leads to an increased pulmonary capillary permeability. Although the mechanism of development of high altitude pulmonary edema is not fully understood, hypoxemia undoubtedly plays a role. The frequent association of pulmonary edema and pneumonia at postmortem examination is probably due to pulmonary capillary damage produced by inflammation as well as a local interference with oxygenation. It is likely that the pneumonia not only increases the rate of fluid entry into the alveoli but also decreases the rate of fluid resorption by the lymphatics.

The lungs are irritated by acid gases, such as chlorine and sulfur dioxide, and by certain oxides of nitrogen, such as ammonia and phosgene. The inhalation of water and nitric acid fumes or the ingestion of gasoline may also produce pulmonary irritation. The extent to which such irritants damage the lungs and increase epithelial and vascular permeability depends upon their solubility in water. A highly soluble gas is readily taken out of the inspired air by the first moist tissue it reaches. The upper respiratory tract may, therefore, bear the brunt of its action. On the other hand, a gas with a low solubility creates its greatest damage at the alveolar level. The effects of gas inhalation may vary, therefore, from a slight tracheobronchitis to fatal pulmonary edema.

Reduced Mechanical Pressure

Pulmonary edema can occasionally develop in a patient with severe airway obstruction. During inspiration, the markedly reduced intrapulmonary pressure may exert a suction effect on the capillaries so the serum exudes into the alveoli. In addition, the very negative intrapleural pressure increases the filling of the right side of the heart during inspiration and hinders the flow of blood from the left side of the heart. This may result in a progressive accumulation of blood in the lungs and a consequent increase of the hydrostatic pressure in the capillaries. On the other hand, when both expiratory and inspiratory obstruction is present, pulmonary edema does not appear to develop, presumably because of the balancing effect of the positive intra-alveolar pressure during expiration.

Interference with Lymphatic Flow

Transuded protein and fluid from the pulmonary capillaries can either be removed by the numerous lymphatic collecting channels that are present within the connective tissue surrounding the airways and blood vessels of the lung or move into the alveoli and bronchioli and then be expectorated. Pulmonary edema occurs when the fluid escapes into the lung tissue faster than it can be removed by the lymphatic system. It has been suggested that lymph flow can increase up to ten times above normal when the lungs are healthy. Any factor that decreases the resorption of lymph in the lungs or obstructs the lymphatic channels favors the development of pulmonary edema. Since the lymphatic vessels empty into systemic veins, an elevated systemic venous pressure will have an adverse effect on the resorption of transuded lymph from the lungs.

CLINICAL MANIFESTATIONS

By far the commonest form of pulmonary edema encountered clinically is hydrostatic edema associated with cardiac disease. *Left ventricular failure* and *paroxysmal nocturnal dyspnea* (severe dyspnea and cough that suddenly awaken the patient) frequently occur in patients with *hypertension* and *arteriosclerotic heart disease* or *aortic valvular disease*. *Paroxysmal nocturnal dyspnea* must be differentiated from the nocturnal attack of dyspnea that may develop in cases of chronic bronchitis. That due to *left ventricular failure* improves after the patient sits up or gets up and walks around, whereas the dyspnea due to *chronic bronchitis* characteristically disappears after the expectoration of a plug of sputum.

Acute pulmonary edema may begin with terrifying suddenness, or it may develop gradually, starting as a mild form of *paroxysmal nocturnal dyspnea* with wheezing and then progressing to the full-blown clinical picture, which is characterized by extreme respiratory distress. The breathing is noisy, with audible wheezes or gurgling sounds. The patient must sit up to breathe and has a severe cough; frothy, pink-stained sputum may be so profuse that it pours from the nose as well as from the mouth. The patient is cyanotic and often in a cold sweat; frequently he or she becomes panicky as the sense of impending suffocation grows more vivid. Intense precordial oppression or pain may be present if the edema is due to a *myocardial infarction.*

Moist bubbling crackles may be heard throughout both lungs. Tachycardia is a constant feature, and the blood pressure is usually elevated unless the patient is in shock. Mild forms of edema may subside spontaneously after a few minutes, or the attack may last for hours. It may end fatally during the first attack or during a subsequent episode. The chronic form of pulmonary edema may be insidious, and it often exists with such subtle clinical manifestations that it is easily misdiagnosed by the clinician as *asthma* or *bronchitis.*

Pulmonary edema due to increased vascular permeability is now well recognized as an increasing problem in patients with severe respiratory failure, particularly in association with circulatory shock and acidemia. In these disorders, there is damage to the gas exchange membrane, altered alveolar cell function, alveolar collapse, increased capillary permeability and pulmonary edema. This *adult respiratory distress syndrome* will be discussed in greater detail in the chapter dealing with acute respiratory failure.

RADIOLOGIC MANIFESTATIONS

When pulmonary edema is fully manifest and there is alveolar flooding, one can see a dense, fluffy opacity that spreads outward from the hilar areas into the lungs on the chest roentgenogram. The pulmonary vessels are enlarged and hazy in outline, and the heart shadow is usually increased in size. The peripheral portions of the lungs remain clear, so that the infiltrates have a butterfly shape. Because the alveoli are filled with fluid, the bronchi that traverse the edematous lung are revealed as radiolucent linear arborizations (*air bronchograms*). The central localization of the edema fluid in the lungs has been attributed both to the relatively greater excursion of the peripheral parts of the lung, so that the removal of lymph and fluid is enhanced, and to accessory lymphatic drainage via the pleural lymphatics in these peripheral areas. It is also possible that the x-rays penetrate through less tissue peripherally than centrally. It is important to point out that these radiologic manifestations are evident only when there is alveolar flooding; they are not present in the stage of interstitial fluid accumulation, even though severe functional disturbances may still be present.

FUNCTIONAL MANIFESTATIONS

Even a very marked elevation in mean pulmonary vascular pressure does not greatly affect the distensibility of the lung. When pulmonary edema develops, however, the compliance of the lungs falls considerably and the vital capacity is frequently reduced. As the pulmonary congestion increases, the residual volume falls correspondingly, probably because of bubbles of edema fluid at the mouths of the alveoli. When frank pulmonary edema develops, the resistance to airflow increases by approximately three to four times, presumably because of edema of the airways and free fluid in the tracheobronchial tree.

In moderate degrees of pulmonary congestion and edema, the arterial oxygen tension is usually only slightly lower than normal, but the $P_{(A-a)}O_2$ is markedly widened. In severe edema these alterations are marked, presumably because of continued perfusion of areas of lung in which the alveoli are not ventilated because of edema fluid, resulting in venous-admixture–like perfusion. In the *adult respiratory distress syndrome,* adequate oxygenation may not be achieved even while the patient is inhaling 100 per cent oxygen. The arterial carbon dioxide tension is usually lower than normal, presumably because of the overventilation of well-perfused alveoli that is induced by hypoxemia.

17

PLEURAL DISEASE

The pleural cavity is in reality only a potential space between the visceral pleura, which covers the lungs, and the parietal pleura, which invests the inner surface of the thoracic cage. The pleura is a serous membrane that is lined on its free surface by a single layer of mesothelium, which rests on a subserous, areolar layer that attaches the pleura to the underlying structures. The subserous layer is important, not only because of the considerable elastic tissue that it contains, but also because of its rich network of blood vessels, lymphatics and nerve fibers.

The arterial blood supply of the visceral pleura comes from the bronchial arteries; the venous return is via the pulmonary venous system. The arterial blood supply of the parietal pleura is derived principally from the intercostal and internal mammary arteries, and its venous return takes place through the corresponding veins. The lymphatics of the pleura are closely connected with those of the lungs and the thoracic cage.

The autonomic pulmonary plexus supplies the visceral pleura, whereas the parietal pleura is supplied by the intercostal nerves. There is both a sympathetic and a parasympathetic supply, and their efferent nerve endings lie near the surface of the pleura. Although the visceral layer is apparently completely devoid of pain fibers, the parietal layer is richly endowed with pain fibers, which are derived from the intercostal nerves. Irritation of the parietal pleura produces an exquisitely sharp pain that may be accurately localized to the site of irritation.

Since the outer rim of the parietal layer of the diaphragmatic pleura receives its sensory supply from the lower six thoracic intercostal nerves, irritation of this area results in pain that is referred to the dermatomes of these nerves; i.e., the pain is in the epigastric region or even in the lower abdomen. The central portion of the diaphragmatic parietal pleura receives its sensory supply from the phrenic nerves, which originate from the third, fourth and fifth cervical nerve roots, so that pain originating from the central portion of the diaphragm is referred to the neck and shoulder along the ridge of the trapezius muscle on the same side.

As has been described in Chapter 1, the fall in pleural pressure during inspiration and the inspiratory descent of the diaphragm assists the return of venous blood from the abdomen. Like the blood flow, pulmonary lymph flow is affected by the pleural pressure. During inspiration, lymph is moved from the abdominal cavity into the thoracic portion of the thoracic duct. Because of the valves in the thoracic duct, backward flow is prevented, and the lymph is squeezed into the subclavian vein during expiration.

PLEURAL EFFUSION

The thin layer of lubricating low-protein fluid that separates the pleurae represents a balance between transudation from the pleural capillaries and reabsorption by venules and lymphatics in the visceral and parietal layers. It is felt that fluid is formed at the parietal pleural surface and is absorbed at the surface of the visceral pleura. Just as we saw in the lungs, the movement of fluid into the pleural space is related to the balance between hydrostatic and osmotic forces. An abnormal accumulation of pleural fluid may occur if the hydrostatic pressure is increased; colloid osmotic pressure is decreased; capillary permeability is increased as lymphatic drainage is impaired.

Congestive heart failure, hypoproteinemia or *fluid overload* may lead to a pleural effusion because of the low osmotic pressure in the capillary blood. In these conditions, the fluid is a thin, clear *transudate* and has a protein content of less than 3 per cent and a specific gravity of less than 1.015. Only a few cells, predominantly lymphocytes, are seen microscopically. The fluid does not clot on standing, and no organisms are grown if it is cultured.

In contrast, when the pleural capillary walls are damaged by a disease process, such as *pneumonia* or *tuberculosis,* or when there is interference with lymphatic drainage, as with a *pulmonary neoplasm,* the fluid has the characteristics of an exudate. It is more viscous and less translucent; it may clot on standing, and it has a protein content greater than 3 per cent and a specific gravity higher than 1.015. If it is a bacterial effusion, the offending organism can usually be identified. If it is of recent onset, many polymorphonuclear leukocytes (greater than 1000/ml.) are usually present, but if it has been present for some time, lymphocytes generally predominate. The presence of eosinophilia may indicate *pulmonary infarction, polyarteritis nodosa,* and parasitic and fungal infections and makes the diagnosis of tuberculosis unlikely. If the primary lesion is malignant, tumor cells and red blood cells are frequently demonstrated.

Except for a pleural neoplasm, a pleural effusion is always secondary to some lesion outside the pleura and may be inflammatory, noninflammatory, hemorrhagic, chylous or chyliform.

INFLAMMATORY PLEURAL EFFUSION

An effusion due to inflammation of the pleura is always secondary to an inflammatory process that involves the lung, the mediastinum, the esophagus or the subdiaphragmatic space. In the early stage, there is a "dry" or fibrinous pleurisy (i.e., the inflamed pleural surfaces are covered with fibrin and leukocytes), but there is little increase in pleural fluid. As the lesion progresses, the amount of fluid increases. The fluid is an exudate and possesses the characteristic features that have already been described. In the early stages, the pleural exudate is translucent, has a high fibrinogen content, and is usually described as "serous" or "serofibrinous." In the later stages it may become frankly purulent, and is more opaque and thicker in consistency as the number of polymorphonuclear cells increases.

Empyema

Empyema, an effusion consisting entirely of pus, constitutes the final stage in the progression of an inflammatory exudate. It is an abscess, in that thick, creamy, yellow-green pus is generally confined by adhesions to a localized area of the pleural cavity. It is important to distinguish a purulent exudate from an empyema. In the former, the purulent material is mixed with serous fluid and generally lies free within the pleural space. An *empyema,* or *pyothorax,* is said to be present only when the material consists of pure pus with no serous fluid. The thick, shaggy, fibrinous exudate that is laid down on both the parietal and visceral pleural surfaces as a result of the suppuration tends to localize the collection of pus.

An *empyema* is generally situated in the dependent part of the pleural space, usually in the lateral or posterior aspects. It also very frequently tends to localize in one of the fissures between the lobes of the lung. Aside from an infected traumatic hemothorax or the extremely rare infection of the pleura by a blood-borne septic embolus, all cases of empyema are secondary to a suppurative process in one of the structures adjacent to the pleura, particularly the lungs. Most commonly it develops as a complication of a bacterial pneumonia, chiefly those caused by *Diplococcus pneumoniae, Streptococcus pyogenes* and *Staphylococcus aureus.* Less frequent causes of *empyema* are *septic infarcts, tuberculosis, mycotic infections,* a subdiaphragmatic abscess, or an *amebic abscess* of the liver.

An *empyema* should be suspected if a case of pneumonia is not progressing satisfactorily, particularly if fever and constitutional symptoms persist. In general, the clinical picture is one of sepsis associated with a loculated pleural effusion. A small collection of pus may be absorbed gradually, but it usually persists. If a large empyema remains untreated, septicemia frequently develops. Spontaneous evacuation of the pus may occur either by rupture through the lung into a bronchus *(bronchopleural fistula)* or by extension through the thoracic wall *(empyema necessitans).*

A neglected empyema may have diastrous effects on the thoracic cage and its contents. The extensive inflammatory exudate rapidly becomes organized so that there are thick fibrous adhesions between the two pleural surfaces. The retracted lung and the displaced mediastinum are anchored, and the overlying thoracic cage is retracted and immobile.

NONINFLAMMATORY PLEURAL EFFUSION

A noninflammatory pleural effusion is a clear, pale, straw-colored serous fluid that does not clot on standing; it is a transudate and is referred to as a *hydrothorax.* The pleurae are generally healthy, and the fluid accumulates because of either a diminished osmotic pressure of the blood or retention of sodium. It is, therefore, most commonly found in patients who are suffering from generalized edema secondary to diseases affecting the heart, kidneys or liver. In cardiac decompensation, as well as the nephrotic stage of *chronic nephritis,* the effusions are usually bilateral. For reasons that are not well understood, the *hydrothorax* may be unilateral, involving only the right side; even when it is bilateral, it is frequently predominantly right sided. A unilateral transudate may also result from obstruction of the large intrathoracic veins by a *pulmonary neoplasm* or enlarged mediastinal lymph nodes.

HEMORRHAGIC PLEURAL EFFUSION

When there is frank blood in the pleural space, the condition is referred to as a *hemothorax.* It is commonly caused by trauma to the chest wall and a tear of the intercostal arteries, but it may also occur spontaneously when a subpleural bleb ruptures or a pleural adhesion is torn. The intrapleural bleeding may be slow, continuing over many hours. The blood usually clots very slowly because of the defibrinating effect of the movements of the lung and the heart. If infection should intervene, however, clotting develops very rapidly. In the absence of trauma, if there are more than 10,000 red cells in the fluid, then *malignancy* or a *pulmonary infarction* should be considered. Rarely, the hemothorax may be due to rupture of an intrathoracic blood vessel, such as an *aortic aneurysm.*

Pleural fluid that consists of a mixture of serous fluid and blood so that it is pink or red is *serosanguinous.* This type of effusion is most commonly seen following a *pulmonary infarction.* Other, less frequent causes are a *neoplasm,* either primary (in the pleura) or metastatic (from a primary site elsewhere), *pulmonary tuberculosis,* a *lymphoma* or *hemorrhagic disorders.*

CHYLOUS PLEURAL EFFUSION

The presence of pure chyle in the pleural cavity is known as *chylothorax.* Chyle consists primarily of emulsified fats and is milky white and opalescent. On standing, a creamy supernatant layer develops. Chylous effusions contain chylomucus, and the triglyceride concentration is high. The fat globules stain easily with Sudan III. Clotting does not usually occur, nor does the fluid putrefy. Its specific gravity is greater than 1.012, and it contains a variable quantity of protein. The cellular content is primarily lymphocytic, and it is sterile on culture.

A *chylothorax* results from obstruction of either the thoracic duct and its tributaries or the left subclavian vein. It is most commonly caused by direct neoplastic invasion of the vessels or by the metastatic involvement of the mediastinal lymph nodes, both of which obstruct the thoracic duct and interfere with the normal flow of chyle. Traumatic rupture of the thoracic duct may result from a penetrating or a nonpenetrating wound of the chest wall. Spontaneous rupture may occur in infants on rare occasions. Although chylothorax occurs more commonly on the left side, it may be bilateral. Since the thoracic duct lies outside the pleural cavity, chyle tends to accumulate in the mediastinum before rupturing into the pleural space.

CHYLIFORM PLEURAL EFFUSION

This type of fluid, which is also known as *pseudochyle,* has the superficial appearance of chyle. The fluid has a high cholesterol concentration, but no fat globules can be demonstrated either microscopically or by staining with Sudan III. The milky appearance is due to the fatty degeneration of pus and endothelial cells and occurs in long-standing cases of encysted purulent effusions. This form of effusion is seen occasionally in *tuberculosis,* in *malignancy* and in *rheumatoid disease.*

FIBROTHORAX

A *fibrothorax* is an accumulation of fibrous tissue within the pleural space, usually secondary to a prolonged pleural effusion of any kind, especially a *hemothorax* or an *empyema*. The fibrosed pleurae inevitably reduce the size of the lung so that the diaphragm is usually elevated and the mediastinum is shifted to the affected side.

CLINICAL MANIFESTATIONS

The degree of disability produced by a pleural effusion depends on how rapidly it developed. Very little distress may be experienced, even when a very large effusion is present, if it accumulated slowly. On the other hand, an effusion that developed rapidly may produce extreme respiratory distress.

Breathlessness is a predominant symptom in fibrothorax. A "dry" or fibrinous pleurisy causes chest pain, which varies in severity from a dull, aching discomfort to an excruciatingly severe, sharp, stabbing pain on that part of the chest wall overlying the area of pleural inflammation, which is aggravated by a deep inspiration or by coughing. If the lower part of the pleural space or the peripheral diaphragmatic pleura is involved, the pain may be referred to the lumbar region or the abdominal wall. Irritation of the central portion of the diaphragmatic pleura results in pain along the same side of the neck. Since the pain is caused by movement of the inflamed pleural surfaces over each other, it tends to disappear when the two pleural layers are separated by fluid.

Depending on the underlying cause, the temperature may be either normal or considerably elevated. The fever associated with an *empyema* may be continuous, remittent or intermittent, and it may be accompanied by violent shaking chills as well as "night sweats."

The fluid usually tends to gravitate to the lowest recesses of the pleural space unless it is hindered by adhesions. Since the end-expiratory pressure in the opposite normal pleural space is more negative than that of the affected side, the mediastinum shifts away from the effusion. If the mediastinum is unable to move because of fibrous adhesions, there will be compression of the underlying lung. The mediastinum may also not shift to the unaffected side if there is an underlying *atelectasis,* such as occurs often with a *bronchogenic carcinoma.* Depending on the amount of fluid present, movement is reduced, vocal fremitus is either diminished or absent, and the percussion note varies from dullness to flatness. The breath sounds are usually reduced in intensity or are inaudible, whereas bronchial breath sounds and whispering pectoriloquy may be heard at the upper level of the effusion, particularly if there is compression of lung tissue overlying a patent bronchus.

In a *fibrothorax,* the hemithorax is slightly smaller and there may be retraction and narrowing of the interspaces. Movement is diminished, and the mediastinum is shifted toward the affected side. Vocal fremitus is diminished or absent, and, depending on the degree of fibrothorax present, the percussion note is dull or flat and breath sounds are distant or absent.

CHARACTERISTICS OF PLEURAL FLUID

Although not diagnostic, the characteristics of the pleural fluid help to determine the possible etiology. As indicated earlier, the specific gravity is less than 1.018, and the protein content is less than 2 per cent in a *transudate.* In addition the fluid/serum protein ratio is less than 0.5, the LDH less than 200 I.U. and the fluid/serum LDH ratio less than 0.6. In an exudate, the specific gravity is greater than 1.018, the protein content is greater than 2.5 per cent, the fluid/serum protein ratio greater than 0.5, the LDH greater than 200 I.U. and the fluid/serum LDH ratio greater than 0.6.

A neutrophil count greater than 1000/μl. indicates inflammation, which may be due to a bacterial pneumonia, *pulmonary infarction* or a *subphrenic abscess,* whereas lymphocytes are present in transudates, as well as in *tuberculosis* or other chronic effusions.

The pleural fluid pH is low in *empyema, rheumatoid disease, tuberculosis* and *carcinoma,* whereas the glucose content is low in *tuberculosis* (less than 60 mg./dl.) and in *rheumatoid disease* (less than 30 mg./dl.). In *rheumatoid disease,* rheumatoid factor and *lupus erythematosus,* lupus cells may be present. A pleural fluid amylase level that is elevated and greater than that in the blood suggests an *acute pancreatitis,* but this may also occur with a *pancreatic pseudocyst, esophageal rupture* or *lung carcinoma.*

RADIOLOGIC MANIFESTATIONS

Unless a pleural effusion is very small, it is readily distinguishable by the characteristic shadow it produces (Fig. 100). The fluid casts a dense homogeneous shadow occupying the lowest area of the chest, and its upper border forms a meniscus with a concave downward curve from the chest wall. If the quantity of fluid is small, only the costophrenic angle will be blunted. Fluid occasionally accumulates between the lung and the diaphragm, where it is called **subpulmonic effusion,** and this is easily demonstrated if an x-ray film is taken in the lateral decubitus position.

If the upper level of the fluid is straight and horizontal, then air must be present. This may have been introduced accidentally during an attempted aspiration, or it may be due to a **bronchopleural fistula.**

The mediastinum is generally shifted toward the normal side. If there is no shift, the mediastinum has likely become fixed by adhesions or there is an underlying **atelectasis.**

In a fibrothorax the opacity produced by the thickened pleura may be as dense as that of a pleural effusion. It is distinguished from a pleural effusion by narrower interspaces between the ribs, a shift of the mediastinal structures to the affected side and an elevated and fixed diaphragm.

FUNCTIONAL MANIFESTATIONS

The degree of functional impairment depends on the size of the pleural effusion. As the fluid accumulates and the underlying lung becomes more compressed, the elastic resistance to distention increases, so that the vital capacity will fall and, if measured, the TLC and its compartments will be reduced. Flow resistance is frequently unimpaired, however. If the compressed lung continues to be perfused, there will be venous-admixture–like perfusion and the $P_{(A-a)}O_2$ will be elevated. Hypoxemia may result, but there will be no carbon dioxide retention if the remainder of the alveoli are hyperventilated.

In patients with **fibrothorax** the total lung capacity and vital capacity are frequently markedly reduced, but again there is little increase in airflow resistance. Gas exchange is often affected, and ventilation-perfusion ratios may be considerably altered, so that hypoxemia is present.

Figure 100. Right-sided pleural effusion.

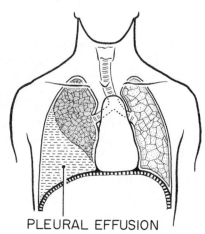

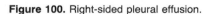

PLEURAL EFFUSION

ABSORPTION OF A PLEURAL EFFUSION

The absorption of a pleural effusion depends on the character and amount of fluid present as well as on the state of the pleurae. A transudate is generally absorbed rapidly once the initial cause of the effusion has been removed. Water, electrolytes and other diffusible substances are absorbed into the capillaries of the subserous areolar layer of the pleurae; protein and other particulate matter are carried away by the lymphatic channels. Absorption of an exudate is considerably hindered by thickening and fibrosis of the pleurae. The fibrin in the fluid must first must become liquefied and the obstructed lymphatics must again become patent before the fluid can be absorbed. If an *empyema* is present, no absorption whatsoever may take place.

PNEUMOTHORAX

The presence of air in the pleural space is referred to as *pneumothorax.* Air can enter the pleural space through either the visceral or parietal pleura as a result of pulmonary disease or a traumatic injury, or it may be deliberately introduced through a needle for therapeutic or diagnostic reasons. Rarely, anaerobic organisms may produce gas within the pleural space if a putrefactive pulmonary abscess ruptures through the visceral pleura.

OPEN PNEUMOTHORAX

In an open pneumothorax, air moves freely in and out of the pleural space during breathing. This may occur in *chest wall trauma* or in a *bronchopleural fistula* resulting from *tuberculosis, bronchogenic carcinoma,* or a *pulmonary infarction.* If it is due to chest wall trauma, the pleural pressure on the affected side will be equal to that of the atmosphere, and unless the mediastinum is bound by fibrous adhesions, it will move to the unaffected side and produce varying degrees of compression of the opposite lung. If the mediastinum shifts from side to side during breathing, some of the air expired from the normal lung may enter and expand the collapsed lung slightly. During the next inspiration, this "rebreathed air" may again be inspired into the normal lung, a condition called *Pendelluft.*

CLOSED PNEUMOTHORAX

In a closed pneumothorax there is no movement of air from the pleural space. This condition may occur spontaneously after rupture of a subpleural bleb or the induction of an artificial pneumothorax.

Spontaneous Pneumothorax

A spontaneous pneumothorax often develops suddenly in a young person who is otherwise healthy, and is usually due to rupture of a subpleural bleb. The blebs may be congenital, but more frequently they are found in association with scars due to some inflammatory disease, such as *tuberculosis*. A pneumothorax also occurs occasionally in other pulmonary diseases, such as *asthma, bronchiectasis, emphysema* and the *pneumoconioses*.

Alveoli may also rupture if they become greatly overdistended as a result of a check-valve obstruction. The air escaping from the ruptured alveoli then tracks along the sheaths of the perivascular structures, the bubbles of air traveling either peripherally (toward the pleural surface) or medially (toward the mediastinum). In either case, a pneumothorax may result because of rupture of either the visceral or mediastinal pleura. This may explain the occasional delay between the time of a precipitating event and the development of pneumothorax.

Traumatic Pneumothorax

A pneumothorax may be produced by a nonpenetrating injury of the chest wall. The sharp edges of fractured ribs may lacerate the parietal and visceral pleura and the underlying lung parenchyma, thereby allowing air to escape into the pleural space. Such injuries frequently cause a hemothorax as well. A traumatic pneumothorax may also be induced by the physician following transthoracic needle biopsy or transbronchial biopsy.

Artificial Pneumothorax

Before the introduction of antituberculous chemotherapeutic agents, the deliberate induction of a pneumothorax was an effective method of treatment of pulmonary tuberculosis. In addition, an artificial pneumothorax is occasionally induced for purely diagnostic purposes. A lesion attached to a rib or the parietal pleura will project into the pneumothorax, whereas an intrapulmonary lesion will not.

TENSION PNEUMOTHORAX

A tear in the visceral pleura may behave like a check-valve and allow air to enter the pleural space during inspiration but prevent it from leaving during expiration. The accumulation of large quantities of air in the pleural space within a short time rapidly increases the pleural pressure above that of the atmosphere. This *tension pneumothorax* is a medical emergency, for, in addition to complete collapse of the affected lung, there is a decided shift of the mediastinum to the opposite side. Venous return to the heart is retarded, so that there is a fall in cardiac output, tachycardia and shock.

CLINICAL MANIFESTATIONS

The severity of the symptoms produced by a pneumothorax depends on the amount of air that has collected in the pleural space and the degree of collapse of the underlying lung. A small pneumothorax may be asymptomatic and produce no abnormal physical findings.

The onset of a spontaneous pneumothorax is usually abrupt and dramatic. The picture of a young man in apparently good physical health who, for no obvious reason, suddenly develops exquisite unilateral chest pain and respiratory distress is very striking. The pain is usually sharp and stabbing in character and is aggravated by breathing and coughing, but occasionally it may be only a dull, aching discomfort. There may be an irritative cough, which is probably due to stimulation of nerve endings in either the pleural space or the walls of the collapsed bronchi.

A patient with a large pneumothorax is frequently in marked respiratory distress, is breathing rapidly and shallowly and may be cyanosed. The skin may be cold and clammy, the pulse rapid and thready, and the blood pressure low. Under these circumstances, one must also consider the possibility of bleeding into the pleural space.

On examination, the affected hemithorax moves poorly or not at all, and the mediastinum is deviated toward the opposite side. Because the ratio of air to solid tissue is increased, the percussion note is hyperresonant. Vocal fremitus is diminished or absent, and the breath sounds are usually faint or inaudible over the affected side. If a bronchopleural fistula is present, the breath sounds may have a bronchial quality. If there is an associated pleural effusion, the percussion note will be dull or flat.

RADIOLOGIC MANIFESTATIONS

Unless it is very small, a pneumothorax presents a characteristic and easily recognizable roentgenographic picture in the upright posteroanterior view. If the collection of air is small, it may not be demonstrable on the inspiratory roentgenogram, but it is often visible if the x-ray film is taken after a maximal expiration. The underlying deflated lung appears somewhat denser than the opposite normal lung, and its periphery is recognized as a thin, fine line running parallel to the upper and lateral margin of the chest cage. The pneumothorax space has a uniform translucency with complete absence of lung markings and is usually predominant in the upper part of the pleural space. If it is complicated by an effusion, the fluid occupies the lowest part of the space, the upper border being straight and horizontal.

FUNCTIONAL MANIFESTATIONS

The degree of functional impairment resulting from a pneumothorax depends upon its size. Although one does not usually measure the lung volume, total lung capacity and residual volume are reduced, and the vital capacity decreases proportionally with the amount of air introduced into the pleural space. For a few hours venous admixture and hypoxemia can be considerable, as perfusion of the collapsed lung persists. Later, the arterial oxygen tension usually rises, apparently because blood is diverted from the collapsed lung to the opposite functioning lung, and only well-oxygenated blood reaches the left side of the heart. If there is paradoxical movement of the chest, air may be shunted back and forth between the normal and the collapsed lung, so that physiologic dead space is increased. In severe cases, alveolar hypoventilation with hypoxemia and hypercapnia may result.

ABSORPTION OF A PNEUMOTHORAX

The air of a pneumothorax is usually absorbed gradually, provided there is no communication between the pleural cavity and the atmosphere. Absorption of the air takes place through the subpleural venous channels, and the speed of absorption depends primarily on the state of health of the pleural surfaces. The process of absorption of air from a pneumothorax is similar to that which takes place when atelectasis develops. The pleural surfaces act as wet membranes, allowing oxygen, carbon dioxide and nitrogen to diffuse through them. Since the partial pressures of the gases in the pneumothorax approximate those of the atmosphere, whereas those in the venous blood are substantially lower, the gases in the pleural space diffuse into the venous blood until the pneumothorax becomes completely absorbed. As the pneumothorax diminishes in size, the lung expands and the total pressure within the space is maintained. Expansion of the lung can be prevented, however, if it has become fibrosed or if the visceral pleura is thickened because of the deposition of fibrin. As with atelectasis, absorption of gas can be accelerated if the air in the pleural space is replaced by oxygen.

CHEST WALL AND
DIAPHRAGMATIC DISEASE

There are wide variations in the general contour of the thoracic cage, but it is usually symmetrical, largely because the thoracic spine is straight under normal circumstances. Since the lungs are enclosed in the semi-rigid bony thoracic cage, any alteration in the contour of the chest or in the function of the respiratory muscles may result in respiratory disturbances even though there is no underlying bronchopulmonary disease.

DEFORMITIES OF THE SPINE

The chest cage may be deformed as a result of spinal abnormalities. Several types of deformity are encountered clinically, the important ones being *scoliosis, kyphosis* and *kyphoscoliosis*.

SCOLIOSIS

The commonest deformity of the thoracic spine is *scoliosis*, which is a lateral curvature of the spine with at least one compensatory curve in the opposite direction, along with some degree of rotation of the vertebrae in their longitudinal axis. This type of deformity is commonly the result of an improper posture. This may occur when an individual repeatedly shifts the body weight onto one leg while standing, so that the body is bent laterally with one shoulder assuming a higher position than the other. Under these circumstances, the tension in the muscles attached to the thoracic spine is unequal, and there is an asymmetrical pull on the transverse spinous processes of the vertebrae. As a result, the vertebral bodies are rotated in the direction of the convexity of the lateral curvature. For reasons that are not fully understood, the majority of lateral curvatures have a convexity to the right. Although this type of deformity can initially be corrected by straightening the spine voluntarily, the deformity can become permanent if the faulty posture is maintained for long periods of time.

In scoliosis, there is a characteristic distortion of the chest cage; the ribs are widely separated on the convex side of the scoliotic spine because of a lateral deviation of the thoracic vertebrae and because rotation of the vertebrae produces angulation of the posterior aspect of these ribs. This results in a bulging of the posterior aspect of the rib cage on the convex side and a flattening of the anterior aspect. On the concave side of the thoracic spine, the ribs are crowded together and their vertebral insertions are rotated. This results in a bulging of the anterior aspect of the chest on this side and a flattening of the posterior aspect.

The scoliosis that follows *poliomyelitis* results from an imbalance of the strength of the trunk muscles and is usually seen within a few years after contracting the disease. In addition to the abnormal rib cage configuration, the ribs tend to lie almost vertically, with very little or no movement of the chest during respiration. The condition is likely to worsen in childhood and may do so quickly during the period when the growth of the vertebral column is most rapid. The rate of deterioration of paralytic scoliosis after the cessation of growth appears to be greater than that for idiopathic scoliosis.

KYPHOSIS

In this type of abnormality, the curvature of the thoracic spine is directed posteriorly. The chest deformity is symmetrical, and the ribs on each side of the chest are widely separated from one another to an equal degree. In elderly individuals a degenerative osteoarthritis often produces a curvature that affects the entire spine. Similarly posterior curvature is often present in the "barrel-chest" deformity, which is associated with chronic airflow limitation.

A less common variety of kyphosis is the angular deformity that is usually associated with a localized protuberance (*gibbus*) that is due to destruction of one or more vertebral bodies by *tuberculous osteomyelitis (Pott's disease)*. The resulting chest deformity consists of a crowding of the ribs that causes the anterior portion of the chest, together with the sternum, to bulge forward in a pigeon-breast manner.

KYPHOSCOLIOSIS

As the name implies, this deformity of the thoracic spine is a combination of kyphosis and scoliosis. Approximately one per cent of the population is affected by this deformity, but it is usually so mild that there are no symptoms.

In the severe form of *kyphoscoliosis*, one side of the chest cage may be so retracted that there is extensive compression of the underlying lung, and the marked protrusion of the opposite side overdistends the underlying lung

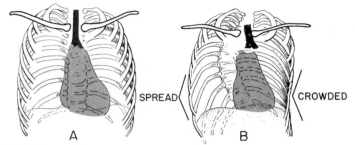

Figure 101. The normal contour of the chest cage **(A)** and that seen in kyphoscoliosis **(B)**.

(Fig. 101). The etiology of the majority of the cases of kyphoscoliosis is unknown, although postural abnormalities have been implicated and there is apparently a hereditary tendency as well. The sequelae of *poliomyelitis* or *Pott's disease* account for most of the remainder.

Functional Manifestations

Minor forms of *kyphosis* and *scoliosis* do not appear to produce significant alterations in pulmonary function. In *kyphosis*, cardiorespiratory disability appears to develop only if the angle of curvature is greater than 20 degrees, and in *scoliosis* only if the curvature is greater than 100 degrees. In *kyphoscoliosis*, on the other hand, even though the kyphosis and the scoliosis are only moderate, the alteration of pulmonary function may be equivalent to that produced by the severe form of either the kyphosis or the scoliosis.

The elastic resistance to distention of both the lungs and the chest wall are increased in *kyphoscoliosis*, so that the vital capacity and the total lung capacity are reduced. The flow resistance is only moderately increased, and the FEV_1/FVC ratio and $\dot{V}_{max}$ at any particular lung volume are usually within normal limits. The minute ventilation is often increased, and the breathing pattern is typically rapid and shallow. Because of compression of the lung, there is often gross mismatching of ventilation and perfusion, so that the $P_{(A-a)}O_2$ is elevated and hypoxemia is present. Because of the rapid shallow breathing and the increased work of breathing, hypercapnia is frequently associated with the hypoxemia.

In the early stages of kyphoscoliosis the pulmonary arterial pressure is usually within the normal range while the individual is at rest, but any requirement for increased pulmonary blood flow (such as during exercise) may be associated with a considerable rise in the mean pulmonary artery pressure. In the later stages of this condition, pulmonary hypertension may be present even at rest. The increased pulmonary vascular resistance is probably due to the additive effects of mechanical compression of the pulmonary vessels and the hypoxemia and acidemia. The work of the right ventricle is increased because of the high pulmonary vascular resistance, so that hypertrophy of the right ventricle, and eventually right-sided heart failure, may develop.

DEFORMITIES OF THE CHEST CAGE

Certain deformities of the anterior aspect of the chest cage are almost certainly hereditary in nature, and they may appear in a family over several generations. These deformities appear to arise because of an impairment of the embryonic development of the septum transversum that later develops into the anterior portion of the diaphragm. Two factors appear to be involved: an abnormal pull on the anterior chest wall by the diaphragm and a disproportionate elongation of the ribs. The type of deformity that develops depends on which factor is predominant.

FUNNEL-CHEST DEPRESSION

Because the cartilages and bony structure of an infant's chest cage are softer and more mobile than those of an adult, a congenital shortening of the diaphragm leads to retraction of the lower anterior chest wall during inspiration. Since the apex of the inspiratory depression is at the xiphisternal junction, this sternal depression becomes fixed as the child develops and its thoracic bony structure becomes more rigid. As a result, the body of the sternum is curved backward, producing a funnel-chest deformity, or *"pectus excavatum."* In a fully developed funnel-chest deformity, the body of the sternum forms a deep depression on the anterior chest wall around the xiphisternal junction. Consequently, the anteroposterior diameter of the chest cage is reduced and the chest cage is longer and narrower than normal.

A funnel-chest deformity, even of moderate severity, is generally asymptomatic, even though there may be some compression of the heart, making it appear enlarged radiologically. In some people, the body of the sternum may be so depressed that the heart is considerably distorted and displaced into the left hemithorax, resulting in compression of the left lung. The distortion of the bronchi may impair drainage, making the patient more susceptible to respiratory infections. In the more severe forms of the deformity, the distortion of the heart and lungs may produce symptoms such as dyspnea, palpitations and cough. In addition, compression of the esophagus may cause dysphagia and other digestive disturbances.

PIGEON-BREAST DEFORMITY

Protruding deformities of the chest wall, which resemble the breast of a pigeon, occur considerably less frequently than do funnel-breast deformities. The protrusion, which is caused by the anterior projection of both the sterum and the costal cartilage, results in a narrowing of the transverse diameter of the chest cage. In some cases, the entire sternum, along with its attached costal cartilages, protrudes forward obliquely and the lowest portion of the sternum becomes the most prominent part of the chest. Another variety of protrusion deformity involves only the costal cartilages, the sternum retaining its normal position. In this type of deformity, only a few successive cartilages on one side may be involved, or the lower costal cartilages bilaterally may be affected.

HARRISON'S GROOVES

Named after the English physician who first described them over a century ago, *Harrison's grooves* are horizontal depressions on the chest wall at sites corresponding to the attachments of the diaphragm. They are often seen in combination with other congenital chest deformities, such as *funnel chest* and *pigeon breast*. The grooves may be unilateral or bilateral, and they may extend laterally along the sixth and seventh costal cartilages and ribs from the xiphoid process to the axilla. It has been suggested that *Harrison's grooves* develop because of a deficiency in development of that portion of the anterior segment of the diaphragm which is attached to the costal cartilages of the sixth and seventh ribs. If this results in an unequal pull on the costal margin, these costal cartilages will be pulled inward by the strong inspiratory contractions of the remainder of the hemidiaphragm. Although most commonly seen in children who have suffered from *rickets*, the condition may also develop in infants suffering from *asthma*, presumably because of the markedly negative intrapleural pressures that they may develop during inspiration.

CHEST TRAUMA

Approximately 25 per cent of the deaths caused by traffic accidents result from chest injuries. Most of these are nonpenetrating, crushing or compression injuries, although occasionally a closed penetrating wound or very rarely, an open penetrating wound may occur.

Crush injuries of the chest are usually nonpenetrating, and they may consist of a single rib fracture, multiple rib fractures, multiple fractures of a single or several ribs, or a fracture of the sternum. Such injuries often result when a person is crushed beneath a heavy object, such as an automobile, or when one receives a direct blow to the chest. They also include a deceleration type of compression injury such as occurs with a head-on collision in which a person is forcefully thrown against the steering wheel, a seat or the front panel of the car. Here, fracture of the ribs is most likely to occur in the midaxillary region. Even if there is no fracture of the ribs or cartilages, there may be such compression of the chest cage in an anteroposterior direction that the sternum is practically brought into contact with the vertebrae. Compression of the chest cage, particularly in elderly people, may result in bilateral fractures of the anterior ends of the ribs, and there may be separation of the costochondral and chondrosternal junctions or even a fracture of the cartilages. If the compressive force is applied in an oblique direction, the ribs may be fractured posteriorly on one side and anteriorly on the other.

When multiple ribs are fractured or several costosternal cartilages are disrupted, a *"flail"* chest may result (Fig. 102). This is a paradoxical movement of the chest wall at the site of the fractures; the affected area is drawn in during inspiration and pushed out during expiration. This is because the atmospheric pressure surrounding the chest pushes the flail area inward when the pleural pressure becomes more negative during inspiration, and it bulges outward when the intrathoracic pressure rises above atmospheric pressure during expiration. As we saw in Figure 101, this may cause shunting of air from one lung to the other during respiration (*"Pendelluft"*), which is equivalent to rebreathing from a dead space. The respiratory rate is usually increased, and it is not uncommon to find considerable hypoxemia and a low P_aCO_2. If bronchial secretions are retained or the patient fatigues, the alveolar ventilation may become inadequate to cope with the carbon dioxide production, and severe hypoxemia and hypercapnia may develop. In severe cases, the cardiac output may fall, and the patient may go into shock.

COMPLICATIONS OF THORACIC INJURY

In addition to the physiologic imbalances created by mismatching of ventilation and perfusion and the development of alveolar hypoventilation, other complications can further aggravate the already disturbed gas exchange. Air is frequently present in the muscle planes and the subcutaneous tissues in nearly all chest injuries. The air may track through the subcutaneous tissues over long distances and may even involve the scalp or the lower extremities. *Mediastinal air* results from the rupture of air vesicles within the lung, the escaped air dissecting its way along the pulmonary vessels into the mediastinum and the neck. It may also be produced by

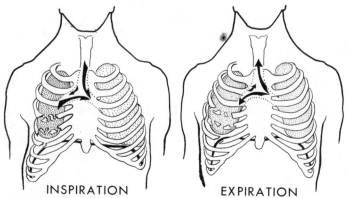

INSPIRATION   EXPIRATION

Figure 102. Paradoxical movement and "Pendelluft" in a flail chest.

rupture of the trachea or an intramediastinal portion of a bronchus. If mediastinal air is present in large quantities, it may compress the great veins, thereby causing serious impairment of the venous return to the heart and a fall in cardiac output. This is usually associated with evidence of respiratory embarrassment, severe substernal pain and occasionally a "crowing" type of respiration due to compression of the trachea. A crunching sound that is synchronous with the heartbeat may be detected by auscultation over the sternum.

If the injury has caused a **hemothorax** or a **pneumothorax**, the alteration in pulmonary function is greatly aggravated, particularly if the air in the pleural space is under tension. In addition, **pulmonary edema** may occur within a few hours after a serious accident. The mechanism of the development of pulmonary edema under such circumstances is not clearly understood.

Extravasation of blood into the pericardial sac as a result of rupture or a wound affecting either a heart chamber or one of the great vessels in the pericardium may also compress the heart and reduce the cardiac output. The blood pressure falls, the pulse pressure becomes smaller, and the cardiac sounds may have a distant quality. Under these circumstances, the jugular venous pressure may rise during inspiration and fall during expiration, presumably because the right atrium cannot enlarge sufficiently to accommodate the increased venous return during inspiration.

DISORDERS OF THE RESPIRATORY MUSCLES

Any disease process that interferes with the normal function of the respiratory muscles may lead to a serious alteration in pulmonary function and the development of respiratory insufficiency. The disturbances in function may vary from mild mismatching of ventilation and perfusion to severe alveolar hyperventilation.

In patients suffering from muscular weakness, progressive polyneuropathy or muscular dystrophy, the thoracic muscles may contract asymmetrically because of variable strength of the intercostal muscles. As a result, different areas of the lung are unequally or asymmetrically inflated, and the inspired gas is distributed abnormally. The resultant mismatching of ventilation and perfusion leads to an increase in the $P_{(A-a)}O_2$ and hypoxemia. Carbon dioxide retention does not occur as long as a sufficient number of perfused alveoli are hyperventilated. On the other hand, if there is excessive muscular weakness, or if an acute respiratory infection should supervene, provision of an adequate alveolar ventilation may become impossible, and severe hypoxemia and carbon dioxide retention can occur. In addition, it has been suggested that the development of respiratory muscle fatigue may play an important role in the development of respiratory failure in patients with chronic respiratory insufficiency.

THE DIAPHRAGM

As we have learned earlier, the primary function of the diaphragm is to enlarge the chest cage vertically during inspiration, but it also plays a part in elevating the lower ribs and the costal margin. Under normal circumstances, the ascent of the diaphragm is purely passive during expiration, and it results because of the expiratory force of the lung elastic recoil and abdominal muscle tone. The mobility of the diaphragm is decreased when it is elevated or depressed as a result of a disease process involving one or both hemidiaphragms.

Paralysis of the Diaphragm

Paralysis of one hemidiaphragm follows interruption of the ipsilateral phrenic nerve, and, provided there are no adhesions, it will rise 3 to 10 cm. higher than the hemidiaphragm on the nonparalyzed side. The nerve supply to the diaphragm may be interfered with, and *diaphragmatic paralysis* develop, as a result of a disease process that affects the nerves directly, as in diphtheria, lead poisoning, alcoholic neuritis or beriberi; or involvement of the nerves by a malignant intrathoracic tumor. Before the advent of chemotherapy and excisional surgery, elevation of the diaphragm was deliberately induced by crushing the phrenic nerve, which was one of the methods used to induce "lung relaxation" during the treatment of pulmonary *tuberculosis*.

When a hemidiaphragm is paralyzed, it is practically motionless during quiet breathing and it may move paradoxically, i.e., upward, if a deep inspiration or a sniff is carried out. This paradoxical movement of a paralyzed diaphragm is produced by several factors. Lowering of the intrapleural pressure during inspiration has a sucking effect on the paralyzed diaphragm, and the rise of intra-adominal pressure, as a result of the inspiratory descent of the normal diaphragm, is transmitted through the abdominal viscera to the undersurface of the paralyzed diaphragm.

Even bilateral paralysis of the phrenic nerves may produce minimal impairment in respiratory function if there is little or no paradoxical movement. If there is considerable paradoxical movement, however, there may be gross maldistribution of inspired air, and if there is increased mismatching of ventilation and perfusion, hypoxemia results.

Eventration of the Diaphragm

The term *"eventration"* is actually a misnomer, for the abdominal viscera do not protrude through an opening in the diaphragm. In this condition, the diaphragm is abnormally elevated, but it still arches smoothly from its costal attachments. In an infant it may develop as a result of a birth injury affecting the brachial plexus. The acquired form of eventration is commonly the end result of paralysis of the phrenic nerve.

Subdiaphragmatic Abscess

The exceedingly rich plexus of lymphatics that traverse the diaphragm forms communications between the pleural and peritoneal spaces, and thus permits the spread of infection from one space to another. Involvement of the subdiaphragmatic space is exceedingly rare in association with pleural or pulmonary suppuration, but a *subdiaphragmatic abscess* often extends into the thorax and causes a *pleural effusion, empyema, pyopneumothorax* or pulmonary suppuration.

A localized collection of purulent exudate or pus in the subdiaphragmatic space may follow any form of intra-abdominal suppuration. It most commonly occurs as a result of *peritonitis* following perforation of a portion of the gastrointestinal tract. The right subdiaphragmatic space is involved five times more frequently than the left .The most common causal organisms are the *Bacillus coli,* the *Staphylococcus* and rarely, gas-forming bacilli. The gas produced by the latter organisms collects within the abscess cavity under the diaphragm and produces a characteristic radiologic appearance that is suggestive of a pneumoperitoneum.

OBESITY

Excessive deposition of fat over the chest wall and abdomen may affect respiratory function, and the alteration in function may be so extensive that respiratory and cardiac failure develop, even if there is no obvious pulmonary or cardiac disease. The increased body mass, with consequent elevation of oxygen consumption and carbon dioxide production, places a stress on the gas transport mechanisms, even at rest. During exercise, the increments in oxygen consumption, ventilation, cardiac output and work of the heart at each level of activity are greater in an obese individual than in one who is not. The increased need for oxygen at rest, and particularly during exercise, must be met in the face of an increased work of breathing, an elevated blood volume, a high pulmonary vascular resistance, and inefficient gas exchange in the lung.

The size of the heart is increased in proportion to the body weight, but the precise mechanisms underlying the development of the cardiac enlargement have not been defined completely. Pulmonary hypertension is frequently present at rest and during exercise in the majority of obese persons, but there is no correlation with the arterial oxygen tension. In fact, exercise may be associated with a rise in arterial Po_2, even when the pulmonary artery pressure increases. Many of the obese individuals with pulmonary hypertension also have systemic hypertension, and the rise in pulmonary artery pressure during exercise is almost regularly accompanied by a rise in pulmonary wedge pressure of the same magnitude, so that the elevated pulmonary artery pressure may be due to the systemic hypertension. However, the increased heart size in obese persons bears no relationship to the presence or absence of systemic hypertension either. On the other hand, obese individuals, especially males, have marked disturbances in gas exchange during sleep, and it is possible that better correlations would be found if values were related to those found during sleep.

Markedly obese individuals may develop a syndrome that consists of cyanosis, twitching, a tendency toward excessive lethargy and drowsiness, and periodic breathing. These features often develop insidiously in a fashion analogous to myxedema, and they may be present for some time before the patient or his relatives realize their significance. It is of interest that Charles Dickens gave a classic description of the syndrome in 1836 in *The Pickwick Papers*. He described "a fat and red-faced boy in a stage of somnolency." This servant-boy, named Joe, was subsequently addressed by his master as "Young Dropsy," "Young Opium-Eater," and "Young Boa Constrictor," terms that were no doubt related to his obesity, somnolence and excessive appetite. Because of the resemblance to this fat boy, obese patients with pulmonary-cardiac failure have been referred to as having the *"pickwickian syndrome."*

In obese individuals the total lung capacity and its subdivisions are frequently reduced, and the respirations are usually rapid and shallow, because the elastic resistance to distention is elevated. In marked obesity there is gross mismatching of ventilation and perfusion, many areas of the lungs being underventilated relative to their perfusion, particularly in the bases, so that hypoxemia results. Often the alveoli at the bases are so compressed that the arterial Po_2 may not arise to expected values even during oxygen breathing.

Although excessive obesity is considered to be the prime factor in the development of the *cardiopulmonary syndrome of obesity*, the exact mechanism by which excessive weight can lead to respiratory failure has not been adequately elucidated. The compliance of the lung-thorax system is considerably reduced, predominantly because of an increase in elastic resistance of the extrapulmonary structures. This elastic resistance increases even further when the patient assumes the supine position, a finding that may possibly explain why obese patients are nursed more easily in the sitting position and why their condition tends to deteriorate if they are kept supine. It is likely that the increased work of breathing, along with the rapid respiratory rate, is responsible for the development of alveolar hypoventilation with hypoxemia and hypercapnia. The oxygen cost of breathing is approximately three times as great in obese persons as it is in healthy persons, and the cost rises precipitously when the ventilation is increased to higher levels.

If the hypoxemia has been present for some time, secondary polycythemia may develop. Hypoxemia and acidemia may increase the pulmonary vascular resistance further so that pulmonary hypertension may be marked. The work of the right ventricle is increased and in some cases, right ventricular hypertrophy and even congestive heart failure may occur. The congestive heart failure is usually characterized by a high cardiac output and "failure" of both ventricles. Venous thrombosis and pulmonary embolism are fairly common in obese patients, and this may account for the clinical picture of chronic cor pulmonale in some patients.

The favorable effect of weight loss supports the theory that excessive obesity is the prime factor in the development of cardiopulmonary failure. Many of the manifestations of the cardiopulmonary syndrome appear to accompany the uncomplicated obese state, and the full-blown syndrome may merely be an accentuation of these manifestations by one or more additional factors. Drowsiness and periodic breathing may be pronounced in obese patients without CO_2 retention or heart failure. However, pronounced CO_2 retention, which is known to be accompanied by drowsiness, may aggravate the previously existing tendency. Similarly, heart failure, which of itself may lead to Cheyne-Stokes respirations, may accentuate the periodic breathing seen in the obese state. Nevertheless, it appears that when the obese state is complicated by mild, and perhaps even clinically insignificant, alterations in function due to lung disease, malfunction of the muscles of respiration, or a central nervous system lesion, then cardiorespiratory failure may develop. It is important to emphasize that the converse is also true, for the superimposition of obesity on pre-existing lung disease may increase the work of breathing sufficiently to lead to alveolar hypoventilation.

RESPIRATORY FAILURE

- PATHOPHYSIOLOGY OF RESPIRATORY FAILURE
- MANAGEMENT OF CHRONIC RESPIRATORY FAILURE
- MANAGEMENT OF ACUTE RESPIRATORY FAILURE

PATHOPHYSIOLOGY OF RESPIRATORY FAILURE

As we have seen, respiratory disease imposes an increased load on the cardiorespiratory system. Patients often compensate for the increased load by increasing the amount of work done by the respiratory muscles or by the heart, and they are often able to maintain normal levels of arterial oxygenation and carbon dioxide elimination. However, if the respiratory muscles are unable to compensate adequately for the increased load, the respiratory system will fail to maintain normal arterial blood gas tensions. This situation is termed *respiratory failure;* i.e., gas exchange is impaired or inadequate, so that the $P_{(A-a)}O_2$ may be altered and hypoxemia with or without hypercapnia may develop.

INADEQUATE OXYGENATION

In discussing oxygenation, it is important to differentiate between hypoxia and hypoxemia. *Hypoxia* is the state in which insufficient oxygen is available to meet the oxidative requirements of the cells of a tissue. Inadequate oxygenation of the tissues may be the consequence of a low oxygen carrying capacity *(anemic hypoxia),* inadequate blood supply *(circulatory hypoxia),* a tissue poison *(histotoxic hypoxia)* or altered cardiopulmonary function, which is associated with a low arterial oxygen tension and content (i.e., *hypoxemia*). Hypoxemia also occurs when one inhales a low inspired oxygen concentration. When it is due to altered function, it may be the result of mismatching of ventilation and perfusion, a diffusion defect, a venous-to-arterial shunt, alveolar hypoventilation or any combination of these abnormalities. In alveolar hypoventilation, carbon dioxide retention is associated with the hypoxemia.

VENTILATION-PERFUSION MISMATCHING

When areas of lung are adequately ventilated but poorly perfused *(dead-space–like ventilation),* hypoxemia does not develop, unless the ventilation of the remaining areas is inadequate to cope˙ with their perfusion. Many patients compensate for an increase in dead-space–like ventilation by increasing the total ventilation; in such patients the P_aCO_2 and carbon dioxide content are frequently low and the arterial pH high.

When areas of lung are poorly ventilated but relatively well perfused, *venous-admixture–like perfusion* is present. The PO_2 in the blood leaving these areas is low and the PCO_2 elevated. Arterial hypoxemia is present, but the PCO_2 in the mixed arterial blood may still be normal or even low if a sufficient number of adequately perfused alveoli are hyperventilated. This compensatory hyperventilation of well-perfused alveoli does not, however, correct the hypoxemia that results from hypoventilation of the other perfused alveoli.

TRUE VENOUS ADMIXTURE

True venous admixture occurs in congenital or acquired venous-to-arterial shunts within either the heart or the lungs. The hypoxemia that results often induces hyperventilation, and since the lungs are usually healthy, the arterial carbon dioxide tension is usually low and the pH high. However, once again, the increased ventilation is not sufficient to correct the hypoxemia. The essential characteristic of the hypoxemia due to this type of disturbance is that the P_aO_2 does not rise above 500 mm. Hg at sea level when 100 per cent oxygen is inhaled. Extensive "shuntlike" or venous-admixture–like perfusion with severe hypoxemia and a low arterial PCO_2 is a feature of the *adult respiratory distress syndrome,* in which there is continued perfusion of edematous or atelectatic alveoli.

DIFFUSION

Hypoxemia due to a pure diffusion defect is probably very rare. However, one may encounter a difficulty in diffusion during exercise if the quality of the alveolocapillary membrane is markedly altered, as in pulmonary fibrosis, or when the capillary bed available for diffusion is considerably reduced, as occurs following a pneumonectomy or as a result of the degenerative processes in emphysema. In most instances, a low diffusing capacity for carbon monoxide is due to mismatching of ventilation and perfusion rather than a diffusion defect. Since carbon dioxide diffuses across the alveolocapillary membrane 20 times more readily than oxygen, it has no difficulty moving into the alveoli. In fact, the arterial carbon dioxide tension is usually low, because the hypoxemic stimulus induces hyperventilation of the alveoli.

INADEQUATE OXYGENATION AND CARBON DIOXIDE ELIMINATION

As has been pointed out earlier, this situation is called *alveolar hypoventilation.* We have seen that the partial pressures of carbon dioxide in the alveoli (P_ACO_2) and in the arterial blood (P_aCO_2) depend on the relationship between the alveolar ventilation ($\dot{V}_A$) and the metabolic production of carbon dioxide ($\dot{V}CO_2$) or oxygen consumption ($\dot{V}O_2$).

$$PCO_2 = \frac{\dot{V}CO_2}{\dot{V}_A} \times 0.863 = \frac{\dot{V}O_2 \times R}{\dot{V}_A} \times 0.863$$

An elevated P_aCO_2 (hypercapnia) develops whenever the alveolar ventilation is inadequate relative to the metabolic production of CO_2 and is always accompanied by hypoxemia unless the patient is inhaling an oxygen-enriched mixture. Thus, *alveolar hypoventilation* develops if the alveolar ventilation falls without a proportionate fall in metabolism or if the oxygen consumption and carbon dioxide production rise without a proportionate increase in alveolar ventilation. As was indicated in Chapter 2, the alveolar ventilation falls if the physiologic dead space increases (tidal volume and respiratory rate remaining constant); the minute ventilation falls, as a result of a cerebral injury, vascular accident (particularly if the cerebrospinal fluid pressure is elevated) or an overdose of depressant drugs; or the respiratory pattern changes (minute ventilation remaining constant), as is seen in diseases of the lungs or chest wall associated with an increase in elastic resistance. Clearly, the work of breathing is particularly important in the genesis of alveolar hypoventilation, for an increased work of breathing may result in the production of more carbon dioxide than can be eliminated by the alveolar ventilation.

PRIMARY VENTILATORY FAILURE

Alveolar hypoventilation with hypoxemia and hypercapnia may develop in the absence of a pulmonary abnormality when the respiratory centers are depressed, as in *drug overdose, anesthesia,* or *cerebrovascular accidents;* in disorders of the spinal cord or respiratory muscles, such as the *Guillain-Barré syndrome, myasthenia gravis* or *muscular dystrophy;* or in disorders of the chest wall, such as *obesity, kyphoscoliosis,* or extensive *trauma.* Unless there is an associated physiologic disturbance, the hypoxemia and hypercapnia of primary ventilatory failure are associated with a normal $P_{(A-a)}O_2$. In such situations, mechanical ventilation and provision of an adequate alveolar ventilation will restore essentially normal blood gas tensions.

RESPIRATORY FAILURE IN NONCARDIOGENIC PULMONARY EDEMA

Severe hypoxemic respiratory failure is encountered with *adult respiratory distress syndrome* (ARDS), a clinical syndrome that may follow any number of sudden catastrophic events that may involve the lungs directly or involve nonthoracic sites with ultimate damage to previously healthy lungs. The syndrome may complicate *trauma,* prolonged *shock* or *hypotension* of any etiology, *burns, fluid overload, bacterial sepsis, aspiration pneumonia, viral pneumonia, fat embolism, drug overdose, inhaled toxins, pancreatitis* or *cardiopulmonary bypass.* Diffuse injury to either side of the alveolocapillary wall develops, and this leads to an increase in pulmonary capillary permeability. The precise pathogenesis has not been elucidated, but humoral agents, toxins, components of the coagulation system, and activation of the complement system have all been implicated.

ARDS manifests itself clinically by marked respiratory distress, diffuse alveolar infiltrates on the chest roentgenogram, reduced lung compliance, decreased functional residual capacity and total lung capacity and severe hypoxemia that is relatively unresponsive to supplemental oxygen; the syndrome is associated with a widened $P_{(A-a)}O_2$ due to mismatching of ventilation and perfusion and physiologic shunting, as well as respiratory alkalosis. Pathologically the lungs are heavy, airless, and on cut section, have the appearance of liver. The collapsed alveoli are usually filled with edema fluid that is rich in protein and cells (i.e., it is a permeability edema). Leukocytes and erythrocytes are present in the interstitium of the lung as well as within the alveoli. Fibrinogen is seen both intravascularly and in the interstitial space, and a hyaline membrane and fibrosis may be present.

RESPIRATORY FAILURE IN INTERSTITIAL LUNG DISEASE

In patients suffering from chronic respiratory failure due to interstitial lung disease, hypoxemia is usually present at rest, and it generally increases during exercise. Hyperventilation with consequent hypocapnia is frequently associated with the hypoxemia. In these patients, mismatching of blood and gas distribution results in hypoxemia, but the alveolar ventilation is usually sufficient to provide an adequate elimination of carbon dioxide at rest. Nevertheless, the added ventilatory demands of heavy exercise or a superimposed bronchial obstruction, infection or pulmonary congestion may precipitate acute respiratory failure with severe hypoxemia and carbon dioxide retention.

RESPIRATORY FAILURE IN CHRONIC OBSTRUCTIVE PULMONARY DISEASE

Chronic alveolar hypoventilation with hypoxemia and hypercapnia is common in patients with chronic airflow limitation, and many patients with *chronic bronchitis, emphysema,* or *cystic fibrosis* become acclimated to the long-term, sometimes severe, alterations in gas exchange. Similarly, in the initial stages of chronic airflow limitation, there are frequently compensatory efforts to overcome any mismatching of ventilation and perfusion by an increase in total ventilation and cardiac work. Later, if the work of breathing is markedly elevated, alveolar hypoventilation with hypoxemia and carbon dioxide retention may develop. The tempo of progression from the first to second stage is highly variable, and indeed, the order in which they appear may vary. Many patients who are maintaining relatively normal blood gas tensions, but at the cost of a marked increase in respiratory work (i.e., *pink puffers*), are much more disabled than others with hypoxemia and hypercapnia who tolerate these marked alterations in blood gas tensions rather than work harder to improve them (i.e., *blue bloaters*). Nevertheless, progressive decompensation is almost invariably associated with an increasing severity of symptoms and is attended by secondary effects of hypoxemia and acidemia and, in some instances, hypercapnia—all of which further compromise respiratory and cardiac function.

When acute respiratory failure develops, the symptoms are those of the precipitating event and those produced by the hypoxemia and hypercapnia. The manifestations of the altered blood gas tensions vary considerably and depend largely on their severity and duration. The symptoms of hypoxemia resemble alcohol intoxication, i.e, incoordination, loss of judgment, restlessness and difficult behavior, whereas those of hypercapnia resemble anesthesia, the patient becoming progressively more somnolent, disoriented and sometimes comatose. Clearly, the central nervous system is particularly vulnerable, and neurologic signs usually predominate. Headache, lassitude, slurred speech, incoordination, restlessness, irritability, tremors and mood fluctuations varying between anxiety, depression and euphoria may be present. Asterixis and papilledema may also occasionally develop. The headache, the papilledema and some of the mental changes may be related to the increase in cerebral blood flow and the elevated cerebrospinal fluid pressure that occur when the arterial carbon dioxide tension rises. The cause of the mental changes is uncertain, although both hypoxia and the narcotic effect of carbon dioxide probably play a role.

Hyperpnea, dyspnea, tachycardia and cyanosis may also be dominant features in some patients. Tachycardia and systolic hypertension are presumably secondary to catecholamine release. Acute hypoxemia and acidemia increase the pulmonary vascular resistance and may precipitate acute right ventricular heart failure. In severely ill patients, where the arterial P_{CO_2} is markedly elevated, generalized cardiovascular collapse with hypotension, profuse sweating and cyanosis may produce a picture resembling other forms of shock.

RESPIRATORY FAILURE IN ASTHMA

Acute asthmatic attacks are characterized by an increase in airflow resistance due to bronchospasm, mucous secretion, inflammation, and edema. In the patient suffering from an acute asthmatic attack, hypoxemia, even when moderately severe, is characteristically associated with a low

P_aCO_2. Hypercapnia does not usually develop until the obstruction becomes especially severe and the FEV_1 falls below about 20 per cent of the predicted value. Nevertheless, a rising P_aCO_2, even into the normal range, in the patient who is having an acute asthmatic attack indicates the development of fatigue and represents a life-threatening emergency.

RESPIRATORY FAILURE IN CHEST WALL OR THORACIC CAGE DISEASES

Diseases affecting the spinal cord, motor nerves, neuromuscular junction and respiratory muscles, such as *polyneuritis, myasthenia gravis* or the *muscular dystrophies,* and conditions affecting the thoracic cage, such as *kyphoscoliosis,* severe *obesity* or *traumatic chest injuries,* often lead to alterations in the distribution of ventilation and perfusion, so that hypoxemia is present. When these alterations are severe, alveolar hypoventilation may supervene. Clearly, if the respiratory muscles fatigue, or if a muscle "relaxant" is administered, even in healthy individuals, the propensity for alveolar hypoventilation is markedly increased.

RESPIRATORY FAILURE IN CENTRAL RESPIRATORY DEPRESSION

Excessive administration of barbiturates, narcotics, opiates, tranquilizers or anesthesia, all of which depress the responsiveness of the respiratory center to carbon dioxide, will cause a fall in minute ventilation and alveolar hypoventilation. A similar situation may occur in patients suffering from a central nervous system infection or increased cerebrospinal fluid pressure as a result of an intracranial tumor, a vascular accident or a head injury. In addition, as has been pointed out earlier, the respiratory system may lose its ability to respond to excessive levels of carbon dioxide in patients with chronic airflow limitation, hypoxemia and carbon dioxide retention.

DIAGNOSIS OF RESPIRATORY FAILURE

Early identification of respiratory failure is extremely important and is facilitated by being aware of the conditions that cause it. The presence of severe air hunger and cyanosis may make the diagnosis of acute respiratory failure easy, but, in the majority of cases, it may not be recognized unless there is a high index of suspicion on the part of the attending physicians, nurses or therapists. The presence or absence of cirrhosis may be misleading, because its recognition is notoriously difficult, and it may not develop until hypoxemia is severe in some cases. In addition, as we have seen, severe hypoxemia may be present without cyanosis, particularly in the presence of anemia.

The onset of restlessness, confusion, tachycardia, and respiratory distress in a patient who is or was in shock, has suffered trauma anywhere in the body, or has a severe infection should lead one to consider the development of severe hypoxemic respiratory failure (i.e., ARDS). Acute hypercapnic respiratory failure should be suspected in any patient who is suffering from bronchopulmonary, chest wall, thoracic cage or central nervous system disease, particularly if the patient is suffering from an acute respiratory infection, *asthma* or acute *heart failure.* Chronic hypercapnic respiratory failure frequently develops insidiously, but it should be suspected when right-sided heart failure and polycythemia are present, since they are frequently associated with chronic hypoxemia and carbon dioxide retention.

The definitive diagnosis of respiratory failure is established by analysis of arterial blood gas tensions and pH. A low P_aO_2 is indicative of *hypoxemia;* a low P_aCO_2 indicates *alveolar hyperventilation;* and a high P_aCO_2 means *alveolar hypoventilation.* In the acutely ill patient, one must also assess the oxygen delivery to the tissues, i.e., the product of the cardiac output per minute and the oxygen content of the blood. Even if the amount of oxygen delivered to the tissues appears to be normal, however, one is not assured that the oxygen utilization is appropriate.

As is shown in Table 16, when the alveolar hypoventilation is acute, hypoxemia (unless oxygen is being administered) and an elevated P_aCO_2 *(respiratory acidosis)* are associated with a plasma bicarbonate and carbon dioxide content that is still in the normal range, but the pH is low *(acidemia).* In chronic alveolar hypoventilation, the hypoxemia (unless oxygen is being administered) and hypercapnia are associated with an elevated bicarbonate and carbon dioxide content and a low serum chloride. The pH is generally just below or at the lower limit of normal because of the elimination of chloride and the retention of base and bicarbonate.

TABLE 16. Arterial Blood Findings in Acute and Chronic Alveolar Hypoventilation

Arterial Blood	Acute	Chronic
P_{O_2}	↓ ↓*	↓ ↓*
P_{CO_2}	↑ ↑	↑ ↑
HCO_3^-	⟷	↑ ↑
CO_2 content	⟷	↑ ↑
pH	↓ ↓	⟷

*Unless on oxygen therapy.

SLEEP DISTURBANCES

Over the past few years, it has become apparent that an increasing number of individuals, with or without obvious cardiopulmonary disease, may suffer from marked disturbances in gas exchange during sleep. Episodes of oxygen desaturation apparently develop even in "healthy" asymptomatic individuals, particularly during REM sleep, and it is possible that the sleep disturbances seen in patients are a normal phenomenon.

Three categories of severe disturbances have been reported during sleep:

1. *Upper airway obstruction,* in which there is no airflow for a period of time even though respiratory efforts are being made.

2. *Central apnea,* in which there is no airflow or breathing efforts.

3. *A mixed disturbance,* in which there is both central apnea and upper airway obstruction during the same episode.

Such sleep disturbances leading to severe hypoxemia are particularly prevalent in the obese male. It is interesting that the syndrome of respiratory disturbances during sleep has rarely been described in females who have not yet reached menopause.

In patients suffering from pulmonary disease, significant hypoxemia may develop during sleep, even though gas exchange may be adequate while awake. It is possible that sleep hypoxemia plays a major role or may even be largely responsible for cardiovascular complications such as *pulmonary hypertension, right ventricular failure* and *cardiac arrhythmias,* as well as *secondary polycythemia,* which may develop in these patients. The implications are clear, and the presence of pulmonary hypertension or polycythemia that is out of proportion to the gas exchange abnormalities elicited during the clinical assessment of a patient should be an indication for the assessment of cardiopulmonary function during sleep.

HEART FAILURE

Heart failure is a frequent manifestation of severe respiratory insufficiency. Although right ventricular failure is far and away the earliest and most frequent event encountered, left ventricular failure may also develop in the later stages of respiratory insufficiency.

RIGHT VENTRICULAR FAILURE

Right ventricular failure develops as a result of a high pulmonary vascular resistance. Although the pathogenetic mechanisms by which the pulmonary vascular resistance is increased may vary from patient to patient, it is believed that hypoxemia and acidemia, which can lead to pulmonary vasoconstriction, are important factors. Other factors that may play a role in increasing the pulmonary vascular resistance are obliteration of pulmonary capillaries, as in *pulmonary fibrosis and emphysema;* compression of the vessels, as in *kyphoscoliosis;* obstruction of the pulmonary vessels, as in *pulmonary embolism;* or an increase in blood volume and viscosity due to secondary polycythemia. The high pulmonary vascular resistance leads to pulmonary hypertension and right ventricular hypertrophy. Eventually right heart failure, the manifestations of which include jugular venous distention, hepatic enlargement and peripheral edema, may develop.

LEFT VENTRICULAR FAILURE

When cardiovascular disease is present, left ventricular failure may develop. The resultant pulmonary congestion leads to mismatching of ventilation and perfusion and increases the work of breathing. In addition, the elevated left atrial pressure increases the pulmonary vascular pressures so that right heart failure may also develop.

SUMMARY

Respiratory failure implies that the respiratory system is unable to provide adequate oxygenation, with or without an adequate elimination of carbon dioxide. Acute hypoxemic failure can develop after a catastrophic event affecting the lungs or nonthoracic sites, and is due to an increased permeability pulmonary edema. Hypercapnic respiratory failure can occur in patients with bronchopulmonary disease, chest wall or thoracic cage disease, or central respiratory depression. The manifestations of respiratory failure may be nonspecific, and definitive recognition of this condition requires analysis of the arterial blood gas tensions and pH.

Although there are specific adjuncts to the therapy for any of the conditions that may be associated with abnormal gas exchange, the management of respiratory failure can be discussed in general terms. For the sake of clarity, the management of acute and chronic failure is dealt with separately in the following two chapters.

20

MANAGEMENT OF CHRONIC RESPIRATORY FAILURE

The management of chronic respiratory insufficiency is discussed before that of acute respiratory failure because it presents a far greater therapeutic challenge to the physician. The results may not be as dramatic or immediate, but the improvement in both function and well-being of the patient with chronic respiratory failure when therapy is intensive can be particularly gratifying. The majority of the following discussion pertains particularly to patients with chronic respiratory failure complicating chronic airflow limitation, i.e., *chronic bronchitis, emphysema, cystic fibrosis,* and severe *asthma,* since patients with these disorders constitute the majority of the patients seen.

GOALS OF MANAGEMENT

The major goals of management of the patient with chronic respiratory insufficiency should be to
1. educate the patient and family about all aspects of the respiratory condition and its management
2. reduce the work of breathing
3. reduce the complications of hypoxemia
4. maximize the patient's ability to perform daily activities
5. prevent acute exacerbations

PATIENT AND FAMILY EDUCATION

Education of patients and their families about the particular respiratory condition and the disturbances in function that have resulted, as well as the goals and all aspects of the treatment, is a major prerequisite for the success of any management program for patients suffering from chronic respiratory insufficiency. The importance of the educational program and the need for repeated and enthusiastic reinforcement by all involved in the patient's care

374

cannot be overemphasized. The beneficial results achieved for a patient depend, in large part, on the extent of the patient's understanding of the condition and the goals of management and the continued optimism and support of the patient by the entire health care team.

If these factors are truly emphasized, the patient will develop confidence in the care providers, an essential ingredient for success. The education of the patient must be complete. It is essential to provide a careful and comprehensive indoctrination about the structural alterations underlying the condition, as well as the status of the functional disturbances, and to ensure that these are fully understood. In addition, the details of the management program must be explained thoroughly, so that the patient and family understand every aspect of the program; cooperation and compliance with the program are thus fostered. One must emphasize all of the factors that may precipitate acute exacerbations of respiratory difficulty and the importance of preventive measures. The mechanism of action of all of the medications that are prescribed, along with their beneficial effects, any potential complications or side effects, and the potential interaction between different medications, must be repeatedly emphasized and clearly understood.

The patient and family must be made to appreciate the chronicity of the pulmonary disorder and, when indicated, the need for aggressive preventive therapy directed at ensuring patent airways at all times. Just as in diabetes, the need for ongoing therapy, no matter how much improvement occurs, is essential. The patient must understand that although therapy may be less intensive at times, it should never be discontinued. This is extremely important, for many patients often reduce or even stop medications because they feel better, only to be readmitted to hospital in an acute exacerbation. Unfortunately, it is also common for many patients to receive excellent attention and care while they are hospitalized, only be discharged from the hospital without proper advice about the need for continuing attention to the minute details of treatment.

The therapeutic approach to chronic respiratory insufficiency is based on the nature of the derangements in respiratory function and the effects of the altered blood gas tensions and acid-base state on other organ systems in the body. Often, maximal improvement in respiratory function occurs only when effective treatment of the secondary phenomena is instituted. Many of the measures used are similar to those used in the management of acute respiratory failure and are directed at a reduction of the work of breathing, reduction of the complications of hypoxemia, increase of alveolar ventilation, improvement in exercise tolerance and the prevention of acute exacerbations.

REDUCTION OF WORK OF BREATHING

The measures used to reduce the work of breathing depend on whether the increase is due to an increased resistance to airflow in the airways or an increased resistance to distention of the lungs or the chest cage.

Relief of Airflow Limitation

The therapy for patients suffering from chronic airflow limitation consists of measures directed at lessening the production and increasing the elimination of secretions and of the use of pharmacologic agents to reverse any bronchospasm.

Reduced Production of Secretions. The removal or avoidance of all possible bronchial irritants or allergens is essential.

ENVIRONMENTAL IRRITANTS OR ALLERGENS. Avoidance of exposure to dusty working conditions, specific occupational irritants or environmental pollution is important, and a change in occupation or residence away from a dusty or smoggy area, although difficult to achieve, may be necessary. Cessation of smoking is imperative (even a single cigarette may cause a measurable increase in airway resistance) and can be particularly effective in lessening symptoms. Similarly, removal of any incriminating allergens, such as household pets, may result in considerable improvement in symptomatology.

UPPER RESPIRATORY TRACT DRAINAGE. It is almost impossible to treat lower airway conditions effectively without concomitant therapy directed at the upper respiratory tract, for both are frequently affected by irritants or allergens. The persistent drainage of secretions from the upper respiratory tract into the tracheobronchial tree (postnasal discharge), particularly during sleep, may be responsible for irritative cough, sputum, chest tightness and wheezing attacks. When a postnasal discharge is present, the patient should be instructed to carry out nasal irrigations by sniffing saline through each nostril on arising and at bedtime. If necessary, a nasal decongestant with minimal rebound may be instilled at bedtime, along with an antihistamine with or without a vasoconstrictive agent.

ESOPHAGEAL REFLUX. Reflux of acid stomach juices, with or without a hiatus hernia, which is fairly common in older individuals and in obese subjects, may be a particularly important factor in the induction of attacks of chest tightness, cough and wheezing. This is particularly true in patients who are receiving theophylline or beta-2-agonists (i.e., patients with chronic airflow limitation), because these agents also relax the esophageal sphincter. Esophageal reflux may induce bronchospasm in two ways: esophageal irritation may induce constriction of the bronchi reflexly, and, in some patients, aspiration of gastric juices into the tracheobronchial tree, particularly during sleep, may cause bronchial irritation and induce mucous secretion and a bronchoreactive state. When symptoms of esophageal reflux are present, the head of the bed should be elevated at least six inches, antacid therapy prescribed, and the patient advised to avoid lifting heavy objects, as well as to avoid alcohol, cigarettes, coffee, colas, and fatty, fried or spicy foods, particularly for several hours before lying down.

INFECTION. Mild chronic respiratory infection is fairly common in patients with chronic airflow limitation. Even though the sputum is clear and mucoid during the day, it is often yellow or green in the mornings, particularly if the inhalation of a nebulized bronchodilator facilitates the expectoration of retained secretions.

Acute pulmonary infections with thick viscid secretions, which may be difficult to expectorate, and inflammatory swelling of the bronchial mucosa increase the amount of airway obstruction and predispose the patient to the development of severe hypoxemia and hypercapnia. Each episode of infection may leave behind a residuum of incompletely resolved inflammation as well as some permanent structural damage. Even a minor cold should be regarded seriously in patients with chronic respiratory insufficiency, for an upper respiratory infection may progress to penumonia or a life-threatening bronchitis and bronchiolitis.

Acute exacerbations are usually due to viral or mycoplasmal infections, but secondary infection by *Hemophilus influenzae* or *Streptococcus pneumoniae* is common. It is therefore important not only to search for evidence of infection and to treat it effectively but also to prevent it. Antibiotics should be given promptly once an infection develops; *tetracycline* (although some *S. pneumoniae* strains are resistant), *ampicillin* and *amoxicillin* are the current antibiotics of choice. When atypical *H. influenzae* strains that are resistant to ampicillin are identified as the pathogen, then *trimethoprim with sulfamethoxazole* or even *chloramphenicol* can be administered, but strict supervision and monitoring are essential in the latter case. The antibiotics should be administered for at least 5 days and preferably until purulence is eliminated and fever and leukocytosis are alleviated.

Some physicians have advocated chronic prophylactic antibiotic therapy because, although acute infections are not prevented, their severity is reduced. However, if proper attention is paid to "bronchial toilet" and retention of secretions is prevented, most acute exacerbations can be prevented, and treatment with antibiotics is recommended only when the sputum is infected.

Increased Elimination of Secretions

THINNING OF SECRETIONS. Although there is no objective evidence to substantiate benefit, one is impressed that hydration of the patient with a daily fluid intake of 30 to 40 ml./kg. body weight does prevent the formation of thick, viscid and crusted secretions, and the ability to raise secretions seems to improve. Also, when the household humidity is maintained above 50 per cent, or bland aerosols and steam are inhaled, patients claim to feel better. The inhalation of detergents, mucolytic agents, and proteolytic enzymes is not recommended, because they have not been shown to be of any greater benefit than aerosolized water or bronchodilator agents. On occasion, the inhalation of these agents may even induce bronchospasm. Similarly, ultrasonic nebulizers that deliver high-density mist have not been shown to be better than simple steaming devices, and they also may have an adverse effect on flow resistance. Expectorants such as saturated solution of potassium iodide and glyceryl guaiacolate do not appear to be of any benefit if adequate hydration is ensured.

POSTURAL DRAINAGE. Postural drainage at frequent intervals often helps to eliminate secretions, particularly if the disease involves a localized area of lung, as in *bronchiectasis.* Benefit in other chronic pulmonary conditions is not as clear-cut, except when the patient has an acute exacerbation.

The posture to be adopted for drainage depends upon the area of lung involved. The upper lobe bronchus is drained best in the upright position. The right middle lobe and the lingular segment of the left upper lobe, which run horizontally and anteriorly, are drained best in the supine position with the head lowermost and the body tilted at an angle of 45 degrees. The superior segments of both lower lobes, which run horizontally and posteriorly, are drained best in the prone position, and the remaining segments of the lower lobes while prone in the Trendelenburg position. While postural drainage is being carried out, the chest should be pummeled with rapid repetitive strokes and vibrated, and then the patient should be encouraged to cough and expectorate secretions. In some patients, manual compression of the lower thorax and the upper abdomen during a slow full expiration may also facilitate the expectoration of secretions.

Relief of Bronchoconstriction

The mainstay in treatment of patients with chronic airflow limitation is agents that lead to reversal of bronchospasm, lessening of bronchial hyperreactivity or both. In the vast majority of patients, these tasks are accomplished by appropriate administration of *theophylline* and *beta-2 agonists.* These agents not only produce bronchodilation but also stimulate mucociliary clearance. In patients with hyperreactive airways *disodium cromoglycate* (cromolyn) may be very beneficial, particularly if there is an antigen implicated or if bronchospasm is induced by exertion. In only a very small number of patients is the addition of chronic corticosteroid therapy for prolonged periods necessary.

Theophylline. Methylxanthines (theophyllines), which are thought to produce bronchodilation because they inhibit phosphodiesterase and elevate cyclic adenosine monophosphate (cAMP), should be prescribed on a daily basis. It is generally considered that theophylline blood levels between 10 and 20 μg./ml. will produce optimal bronchodilation. However, the serum level at which maximum improvement is achieved is extremely variable, and this generalization should be looked upon as only a guide. In some patients, maximum FEV_1 is achieved at serum levels of less than 10 μg./ml.; in others, the highest FEV_1 is not reached until serum levels are greater than 20 μg./ml. Thus, the goal of theophylline therapy should be to achieve the greatest FEV_1 (i.e., the lowest airflow resistance) possible, without inducing side effects, which may vary from nausea and vomiting, cardiac dysrhythmias, headache and nervousness to convulsions. These side effects are more prone to occur at serum levels greater than 20 μg./ml.

Aminophylline may be prescribed in the form of "immediate-release" anhydrous theophylline or sustained-release preparations, the choice depending on the pharmacokinetics of theophylline in a particular patient and the faithfulness with which the oral medications are taken. The amount of oral theophylline prescribed initially depends on the age and size of the patient: 16 mg./kg. of ideal body weight/day or 400 mg/day, whichever is less, has been recommended. After 48 hours, depending on the serum level, the dosage can be increased by about 25 per cent at two- to three-day intervals as long as no intolerance is observed. Conversely, if a dosage is associated with adverse effects, the dosage should be decreased to the previously tolerated level, and the serum concentration at this lower dosage should be measured.

The dosage required to achieve a particular serum level is not the same in all patients, because the metabolism of theophylline varies considerably among individuals. It is particularly affected by the age of the patient: the rate is faster in children and slower in elderly individuals. As seen in Figure 103, a number of other factors affect the rate of metabolism of methylxanthines, and the serum level achieved by a given dosage may vary even in a given patient. Approximately 90 per cent of theophylline is metabolized by the liver, so that a liver disturbance will slow the rate of metabolism of methylxanthines and result in a higher serum level for a given dosage, thereby increasing the likelihood of side effects. Similarly, even when the dosage remains constant, a viral infection, the development of congestive heart failure or the administration of cimetidine or macrolide antibiotics, such as erythromycin or troleandomycin, will raise the serum level (and increase the potential for side effects). Figure 103 illustrates that the converse is also true: cigarette smoking (particularly marijuana smoking), excessive use of alcohol or exposure to environmental pollutants increases the metabolism of theophylline, and in such circumstances, the serum level may be much lower (and bronchospasm greater) than expected for a given dose.

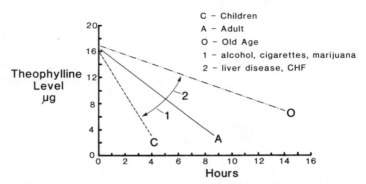

Figure 103. The pharmacodynamics of theophylline. The metabolism of aminophylline is increased in the young child and decreased in old age. The development of liver disease or heart failure, or the administration of drugs such as cimetidine or macrolide antibiotics, raises the blood level for a given dose of aminophylline, whereas alcohol or smoking, particularly of marijuana, results in a marked fall in blood level for a given dose.

Clearly then, the dosage of aminophylline required for a given patient can be affected by any concomitant disease (or medication). In the patient suffering from congestive heart failure or cirrhosis of the liver, the oral dose necessary to achieve a particular serum level, or optimum bronchodilation, will be smaller than that necessary in a healthy individual. Conversely, the oral dose necessary in a smoker will be more than that in a nonsmoker.

It is important that the serum levels be assessed at regular intervals when steady state conditions are present. This is generally not achieved for approximately five half-lives, or about 40 hours, so that measurements made when the patient has not had a stable dosage for at least two days may not be valid for dosage adjustment.

The time of blood sampling depends upon the preparation used: with a solution, the level should be assessed within two hours; with a slow-release preparation, about 4 hours after ingesting the medication. From the above, it is clear that the serum level should also be determined whenever the patient develops increasing symptoms or side effects. A low level (even zero) in a patient who is having increased difficulty may be due to omission of medication, cigarette or marijuana smoking, or excessive alcohol ingestion. Conversely, as we have seen, side effects may develop even with a constant oral dose of theophylline if there are acute alterations of cardiac, hepatic or renal function or when certain medications have been administered.

Beta-2 Agonists. Beta-2 agonists can be administered orally, systemically or by inhalation. The greatest immediate relief of bronchoconstriction is obtained when bronchodilator drugs such as *racemic epinephrine, isoproterenol, isoetharine, terbutaline, metaproterenol,* or *salbutamol* are aerosolized into the tracheobronchial tree. It is our bias to dilute the solution of beta-2 agonist with an equal amount of water or saline.

It is essential that the patient inhale the aerosol properly, for the effectiveness of the aerosolized bronchodilator is very dependent on the manner of administration. Several considerations are important no matter whether a hand bulb or a metered dose type of nebulizer is used (Fig. 104). The nebulizer should deliver a preponderance of small droplets of medication, and these small droplets should be delivered deep into the tracheobronchial tree. The addition of a flex tube or reservoir and a mouthpiece to the nebulizer will foster the delivery of small droplets. Penetration of the bronchodilator deep into the tracheobronchial tree will be facilitated by a very slow deep inspiration and then a breath-hold.

Thus, our recommended method of administration of an aerosolized bronchodilator is the following. After a slow exhalation slightly beyond functional residual capacity, the mouthpiece should be placed between the lips, and the hand bulb (or the metered device, if that is being used) repeatedly squeezed while inhaling very slowly to TLC, as if "sipping hot soup." At the end of the full inspiration, the breath should be held for several seconds to encourage deposition of the drug, and then expiration

Essentials for Effective Inhalation of Bronchodilator

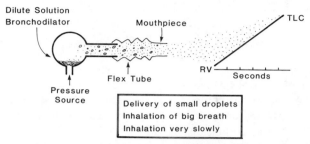

Figure 104. The proper administration of inhaled bronchodilator. Only the smallest droplets should be inhaled as a very slow deep breath is inspired.

should be carried out slowly through pursed lips. The patient should then wait for a minute to determine the effectiveness of the administration, and then attempt to cough up secretions. This will help to ensure that the fine droplets delivered by the ensuing nebulization can exert their effect in the smaller bronchi and bronchioli.

If the patient is unable to coordinate the squeezing of the nebulizer bulb with a slow maximum inspiration, a pressure source (compressed air or oxygen) should be used to nebulize the bronchodilator aerosol. In this case occlusion of a Y tube, which is placed between the pressure source and the nebulizer, allows the patient to control the nebulization during the very slow maximal inspiration. Finally, if a patient is unable to take a big breath or to effectively coordinate the slow inhalation with the aerosolization of bronchodilator, a positive-pressure breathing machine may be necessary to power the nebulization. In both of these cases, the same technique of slow, deep inspirations, a breath-hold and a wait of about one minute between maximum slow inhalations should be encouraged.

For each full treatment, the process of inhalation of the nebulized medication, breath-hold, slow expiration, and wait should be repeated over and over again, until the patient "feels" subjective relief in the lower lateral thoracic areas. Some patients actually feel the penetration of the medication, "air entering," or a feeling of warmth or coolness in the lower lateral chest. Failing recognition of penetration into the lower lateral areas of the chest, the inhalation of medication should be repeated until the pulse rate rises or mild tremor develops.

It must be emphasized that there is no set "dose" (i.e., number of drops or number of inhalations of bronchodilator): the amount of medication and number of inhalations required depend on the severity of the airflow obstruction. In addition, the number of inhalations will vary from patient to patient, or even in a given patient, from day to day. Few inhalations during a treatment will be required if the patient is mildly obstructed, and many inhalations will be necessary if markedly obstructed.

Even though a patient feels relatively free of difficulty, those with chronic airflow limitation should inhale the aerosol bronchodilator in the manner described at least twice daily—every morning on arising and again before retiring. In addition, the patient should inhale the bronchodilator with each episode of chest tightness, cough, wheezing or dyspnea, as well as *before* exposure to agents or events that are known to precipitate symptoms. It is important that patients know their own particular daily pattern of requirement of aerosol bronchodilator, because the need for a greater-than-usual number of "treatments" in a day should be taken as evidence of increasing airway obstruction and as an indication of the need for immediate notification of the attending physician.

Ventilatory function assessment (i.e., the FVC and FEV_1) is an essential component of the follow-up of the patient with airway disease. In the initial evaluation, measurements of ventilatory function before and after a beta-2 agonist provide information about the reversibility of any airflow limitation and the therapeutic effectiveness of the inhaled bronchodilator. When evaluating the potential effectiveness of bronchodilator therapy, one should be guided by the patient's subjective evaluation of relief of symptoms as well as objective improvement in ventilatory function. However, unless clear improvement in flow rates or FVC following bronchodilator indicates the benefit of the agent, a lack of reversibility should not be judged to be present unless the absolute lung volume and isovolume flow rates have been examined. In some cases, the measured values of the FVC and the maximal expiratory flow rates at 75, 50 and 25 per cent of the FVC may underestimate the response to inhaled bronchodilator and suggest a lack of effect of the inhaled bronchodilator. As was seen in Figure 60, the effect of the inhaled bronchodilator on airflow can be assessed only if isovolume flow rates (flow at an equivalent lung volume) are determined.

Atropine and its Derivatives. Aerosolized atropine or methylbromide of *N*-isopropyl nortropine may also improve airflow in some patients. It has been suggested that these agents may be as effective a bronchodilator as beta-2 agents in some patients with chronic airflow limitation. Indeed, the combination of an atropine-like agent and a beta-2 agonist appears to be more effective than either agent alone in some patients. Although adverse side effects may occur with atropine and, to a lesser extent, with the derivative, they deserve a therapeutic trial, particularly in those patients whose FEV_1 remains low despite optimal use of methylxanthines and beta-2 agonists.

Corticosteroids. In the vast majority of patients with chronic airflow limitation, corticosteroids are not indicated. However, in some patients, in whom airflow limitation does not respond significantly despite the appropriate administration of methylxanthines and beta-2 agonists, marked improvement in function may be demonstrated when corticosteroids are added to the therapeutic regimen. Unfortunately, it is not easy to predict which patients will respond favorably; therefore, a brief trial of corticosteroids (40-60 mg./day of prednisone) is justified if symptoms are not controlled and significant improvement in FEV_1 is not achieved with the effective administration of methylxanthines and beta-2 agents.

In addition, corticosteroids are very effective in the management of acute exacerbations of bronchial infection. When it is clear that an acute exacerbation is not being controlled by the standard therapy, very high doses of corticosteroids can be administered for a day or two, and then tapered rapidly until minimal or no drug is taken. As long as there is objective evidence of functional improvement while the patient is receiving this treatment, the corticosteroids should be discontinued if no improvement in FEV_1 is demonstrated.

The adverse effect of corticosteroids include hyperadrenocorticism (with its attendant facial changes), hirsutism, hypertension, fluid retention, skin changes, psychologic alterations, hyperglycemia, peptic ulcer, gastritis, gastrointestinal bleeding and perforation, pancreatitis, glaucoma, cataracts, osteoporosis, aseptic necrosis of bone and myopathy. It is important to point out that these adverse effects are related to both the dosage and the mode of administration. The side effects are greatest when the corticosteroids are administered in divided doses on a daily basis for a period of time, less when a low dose is taken once a day, still less when taken every other day, and least when beclomethasone is inhaled by aerosol.

Reduction of Elastic Resistance

Pulmonary Congestion. Right ventricular failure and fluid retention are important consequences of respiratory failure and the alterations of gas exchange associated with it. The fluid retention and, in some cases, an associated left-sided heart failure, result in pulmonary congestion, which further increases the respiratory work and thus aggravates the respiratory failure. Treatment with diuretics and a restricted salt intake is often sufficient to overcome the fluid retention and heart failure associated with respiratory failure. However, if improvement does not occur after the administration of a diuretic, digitalis may be prescribed, provided that serum electrolyte concentrations are normal. Lessening of the pulmonary congestion lowers the work required to overcome the resistance to lung distention and improves blood and gas distribution, so that arterial blood gas tensions improve. Clearly then, a dual approach to therapy of respiratory failure is required: treatment of the basic disturbances in pulmonary function decreases the tendency to heart failure, and treatment of heart failure improves pulmonary function.

Corticosteroids. In diffuse pulmonary fibrosis, the work of breathing is elevated because the elastic resistance of the lungs is increased. The administration of steroids and, when indicated, removal of a responsible allergen may result in a reduction of the infiltrations and the work of breathing, as well as clinical improvement and an improvement in gas exchange, particularly if the infiltrations are due to sarcoidosis or extrinsic allergic alveolitis.

Weight Loss. As we have seen in Chapter 18, obesity increases the work of breathing, and this may predispose the patient to marked abnormalities in gas exchange. Not only can obesity, per se, lead to respiratory failure, but it can aggravate respiratory failure due to other causes. In individuals with chronic lung disease, the superimposition of obesity may increase the work of breathing markedly, and alveolar hypoventilation (i.e., hypoxemia and hypercapnia) may develop. In such situations, intensive efforts to bring about weight reduction must be instituted. Loss of weight diminishes the work of breathing and leads to a change in respiratory pattern, so that alveolar ventilation is increased. In addition, the matching of ventilation and perfusion is improved, so that arterial blood gas tensions improve.

REDUCTION OF COMPLICATIONS OF HYPOXEMIA

Chronic hypoxemia leads to an elevation of the pulmonary vascular resistance, so that the right ventricular work increases and the right ventricle may fail. In some patients the hypoxemia may be particularly severe during sleep. Indeed, the finding of pulmonary hypertension or polycythemia that is not commensurate with the level of the arterial oxygenation while the patient is awake should arouse suspicion of an associated sleep disturbance.

Low-Flow Oxygen Therapy

The development of portable lightweight oxygen systems has facilitated the use of ambulatory oxygen therapy, thereby allowing a patient to engage in regular daily activities outside of the home. Continuous low-flow oxygen therapy may diminish secondary polycythemia and relieve pulmonary hypertension. On the other hand, it is important that continuous oxygen not be prescribed for patients indiscriminately or unnecessarily.

The indications for continuous oxygen therapy for the ambulant patient are the presence of pulmonary hypertension and cor pulmonale and a resting P_aO_2 of less than 50 mm. Hg at sea level, particularly if it falls during exercise. Nocturnal oxygen is indicated for sleep disturbances that result in hypoxemic episodes. Recently, it has been shown that the survival time in patients with severe chronic airflow limitation is longer when oxygen is administered nearly continuously than when it is given for shorter periods during each day. Significant improvement in neuropsychologic tests and cognitive function, along with lessening of depression, hypochondriasis, hysteria, and "social introversion" have also been demonstrated in such patients while they are receiving oxygen therapy.

INCREASING THE PATIENT'S ABILITY TO CARRY OUT DAILY ACTIVITIES

In many cases, it is necessary to counteract advice given to the patient by others to "take it easy" and to emphasize the need for increased physical activity and fitness. To increase the patient's ability to take part in daily functions, the efforts of all personnel must be maximized and directed at bringing the patient to optimal physiologic and psychologic function. Emphasis should be placed on achieving maximum efficiency of energy utilization, so that the ability of patients to carry out their daily activities is increased.

Breathing Retraining

Breathing retraining is particularly applicable to patients suffering from chronic airflow limitation in which the lungs are frequently hyperinflated, the diaphragms are low and scarcely move, and the accessory respiratory muscles are active during breathing. The patients should be taught a series of exercises to relax the accessory muscles and to carry out "diaphragmatic breathing" exercises simultaneously. Breathing retraining is difficult and time consuming. Indeed, the benefit derived varies directly with the amount of time spent by the physician and physiotherapist in teaching the patient.

Lying in the head-down position enhances the movement of the diaphragm, because it is pushed upward by the abdominal contents. In addition, leaning forward in the upright position helps to relax the accessory respiratory muscles and elevates the diaphragm. Since slow abdominal or diaphragmatic breathing improves the distribution of inspired gas and reduces the work of breathing, patients should be advised to sniff air in slowly (the sniff is a diaphragmatic function) and then expire through pursed lips. The lip pursing raises the pressure in the airways and, along with the slowed expiration, helps to prevent dynamic collapse of the intrapulmonary conducting airways.

Physical Reconditioning

Although excessive physical activity should be avoided during an acute illness, invalidism must be discouraged. Patients with chronic pulmonary disease who continue to be active generally remain in better health and function far more effectively than those who are quiescent. The benefit is due to a more efficient delivery of oxygen to the tissues.

Emphasis should be placed on achieving maximal physical fitness, and patients should be encouraged to gradually increase their exercise tolerance, through daily walking and stair climbing. The program should be tailored to the age and general condition of the patient, but, in general, the graded exercises should begin with the patient walking on the level and then progress by increasing the intensity of the work load on a cycle ergometer or a treadmill or by stair climbing. It is now recognized that such exercise programs allow patients to function at much higher levels of activity with more comfort. The ability of the patient to perform daily tasks can be increased considerably, and mental outlook can be greatly improved. In some patients, the inhalation of supplemental oxygen during exertion will allow them to sustain heavier exercise loads for longer periods. Supplemental oxygen during exercise is usually most effective in those who are markedly limited by their ventilatory capacity or who become progressively hypoxemic during exercise.

It is important to recognize that the level of exercise achievable, although partly related to the status of ventilatory function or gas exchange, is usually unpredictable. Thus, the maximum exercise tolerance cannot be predicted from pulmonary function tests, and one must attempt at all times to achieve maximal exercise capability.

Vocational Guidance

In addition to the intensive efforts of physical and recreational therapists to improve exercise tolerance, meticulous instruction by occupational therapists will teach the patients to perform regular daily activities with maximum efficiency, and in some cases will allow them to return to their regular occupation. If the patient is unable to return to his or her usual employment, it may be possible to alter the work description without fundamentally changing the vocation. If this is also not feasible one should attempt to train the patient in a new vocation. Even if it is not possible for the patient to return to gainful employment, it is important that the physician, in concert with the social worker and all other health professionals, launch a major effort aimed at achieving maximal self-reliance and minimizing dependence on the patient's family and the community.

Psychosocial Management

Although well-integrated patients adjust to chronic disease and cooperate with all modalities of therapy, many display denial and repression, resentment, anger and anxiety. Depression (with associated feelings of hopelessness and worthlessness) is fairly common, and in many instances, the psychologic and emotional problems so affect the patient's response and cooperation that the success of a mangement program may be compromised. The combined efforts of all involved in the patient's care to create an aura of optimism is essential. Indeed, improvement often correlates better with psychologic than with physiologic factors.

PREVENTION OF ACUTE EXACERBATIONS

The course of chronic respiratory disease is punctuated with acute exacerbations requiring repeated hospital admissions. Many acute respiratory insults can be prevented by continued and aggresive therapy directed at ensuring patent airways and at the prevention and treatment of infection. The patient should be instructed regarding the importance of removal of all antigens and irritants, particularly cigarettes. In addition, patients and their families must recognize the need for regular use of oral and nebulized bronchodilators, as well as for adequate hydration and continued exercise. In addition, they and their families should be taught how to recognize signs of deterioration early (Table 17) and how to institute corrective measures or call the attending physician immediately.

Polyvalent influenza vaccine and pneumococcal vaccines should be administered annually, and crowds should be avoided during periods of

TABLE 17. Warning Signals of Impending Respiratory Disability

1. An unusual *increase* in the amount of sputum
2. An unusual *decrease* in the amount of sputum
3. An unusual increase in the consistency and stickiness of the sputum
4. A change in the color of the sputum to either brown, yellow, or green
5. The presence of blood in the sputum
6. An unusual increase in the severity of the breathlessness
7. The development of a feeling of general ill-health
8. The development of swelling of the ankles
9. The need to increase the number of pillows in order to sleep in comfort
10. An unaccountable *increase* or *decrease* in weight
11. Increasing fatigability and lack of energy, with a feeling that more rest is required
12. The development of increasingly frequent morning headaches, dizzy spells, restlessness, loss of libido and insomnia
13. The development during an acute respiratory infection of confusion, disorientation, slurring of the speech and somnolence

known viral epidemics. In general, prophylactic antimicrobial therapy may be useful in patients with bronchiectasis. In patients with chronic airflow obstruction, on the other hand, although prophylactic antibiotics reduce the duration and severity of the exacerbations, they do not appear to lessen the number of acute exacerbations.

Home Care

Repeated hospital admissions or even permanent hospitalization because of the need for frequent medical supervision or mechanical aids to respiration can be prevented if both the patient and the health care providers are meticulous in their attention to details. Unfortunately, such "intensive care" for the nonhospitalized patient may be difficult to provide by even the most highly motivated physician. The management of chronic respiratory insufficiency is time consuming and fraught with frustration; the patient often becomes a burden, and the attending physician tends to "slough" him off. However, regular supervision and guidance must be provided for the patient suffering from severe respiratory insufficiency through frequent visits and counseling by specially trained nurses and, when necessary, physiotherapists or other allied health professionals. This will foster early recognition of deterioration and the immediate institution or intensification of proper therapy. All necessary respiratory care equipment and even humidifiers can be provided in the home when they are indicated, and in some cases a homemaker can assist the family with the housekeeping.

The benefits of intensive home care programs in the management of patients with chronic airflow limitation have been well demonstrated. Cystic fibrosis, which was frequently fatal in early childhood, can now be controlled even through adulthood. Although the morbidity and mortality of patients with moderately severe or severe dysfunction due to chronic bronchitis or emphysema do not appear to have been altered by home care or rehabilitation programs, intensive home therapy and the prevention of acute exacerbations have reduced the requirement for frequent hospital admissions and have allowed the patient to lead a more useful existence. There is symptomatic improvement and a marked increase in exercise tolerance. Indeed, although not yet demonstrated, it is quite possible that the early institution of such continuous and intensive therapy in patients who have only minimal disability will reduce morbidity considerably and may even ultimately reduce mortality.

SUMMARY

Although it has not yet been demonstrated that the natural history of chronic airflow limitation or the rate of deterioration of function is altered by an intensive organized therapeutic program such as is described in this chapter, the fact that the ability of the patient to carry out gainful activity is markedly improved is particularly rewarding. However, the success of the therapeutic regimen depends on the mode of application of the various elements. Measures directed at maintaining optimal lung function and physical performance, effective psychosocial counseling directed at increasing personal motivation, the support of family and friends, and an optimistic attitude on behalf of the attending physician and other health personnel, all play a major role in influencing the response to treatment and improving the "quality of life" in the patient with chronic airflow limitation.

21

MANAGEMENT OF ACUTE RESPIRATORY FAILURE

The development of acute respiratory failure with severe hypoxemia, hypercapnia or both represents a medical emergency that clearly requires immediate therapy. Although only the development of hypercapnia is considered by many to constitute respiratory failure, it is clear that acute hypoxemia without carbon dioxide retention, particularly if progressive, can be especially life threatening and that it requires immediate action.

The management of acute respiratory failure, like that of chronic respiratory insufficiency, is designed to reverse the physiologic disturbances that are present. The aim of therapy should be to restore the patient to health, not merely to achieve "normal arterial gases." Improvement of blood gas tensions and treatment of the underlying respiratory disorder should go hand in hand. The therapy that is instituted consists primarily of measures to improve oxygenation and, when indicated, to reduce the arterial carbon dioxide by lowering the production and increasing the elimination of carbon dioxide.

OXYGENATION

Hypoxemia is the single most lethal consequence of acute respiratory failure. When the cause of the hypoxemia is simply alveolar hypoventilation, the arterial P_{O_2} can be restored to normal levels by provision of an adequate ventilation. However, in most cases, hypoxemia results from increased mismatching of ventilation and perfusion in the lungs, and oxygen enrichment of the inspired air is required.

The aim of oxygen therapy is to increase the amount of oxygen carried in the blood to normal or nearly normal levels. The concentration of oxygen that must be administered in order to raise the arterial oxygen tension to normal levels differs from patient to patient and depends on the type of physiologic disturbance present and the severity of the hypoxemia. In most patients who are suffering from hypoxemic hypoxia, concentrations of 25 to 40 per cent oxygen are more than adequate to return the arterial oxygen tension to normal levels. In cases of circulatory or anemic hypoxia, provision of an adequate oxygen supply to the tissues may necessitate inspired oxygen concentrations that raise the arterial PO_2 well above the normal values, in order to increase the amount carried as dissolved oxygen in the plasma.

OXYGEN THERAPY

There are numerous methods of administering oxygen, and no single method has gained universal favor. The level of oxygenation desired, the reliability and simplicity of the method, and the patient's comfort dictate the optimal method. No matter which mode of administration is chosen, adequate humidification, preferably with jet humidifiers, is essential.

In all patients receiving oxygen therapy, the lowest inspired oxygen concentration that will result in an arterial PO_2 within the normal range should be administered. As has been pointed out by many, high concentrations of oxygen may result in cellular toxicity if administered for more than 48 to 72 hours. In addition to *retrolental fibroplasia*, which may be precipitated by high oxygen concentrations in the newborn infant, lung *congestion, consolidation, atelectasis,* alveolar exudates and the *adult respiratory distress syndrome* have been attributed to the administration of high concentrations of oxygen to adult patients for lengthy periods.

In some patients with chronic hypoxemia and hypercapnia, oxygen administration may result in depression of ventilation and a further rise in arterial PCO_2. However, one can generally correct the hypoxemia without unduly depressing ventilation by the judicious administration of oxygen to such patients using venturi masks, which deliver preset low concentrations of oxygen, or one can deliver oxygen at flow rates of 1 to 2 liters/minute by means of a nasal catheter or cannula. Indeed, a rise in P_aCO_2 when providing adequate oxygenation is not associated with significant deleterious effects and is in no way comparable to the potential danger of severe hypoxemia. A rise in PCO_2 while oxygen is being administered is an indication for intensification of therapy directed at reversing the factors that precipitated the respiratory failure. In some patients, even high concentrations of oxygen may fail to restore the oxygen tension to normal. This is particularly true in patients suffering from the *adult respiratory distress syndrome* or the *infant respiratory distress syndrome,* where there is gross right-to-left shunting.

REDUCTION OF WORK OF BREATHING

Acute exacerbations of respiratory failure are frequently precipitated by an acute *bronchial infection, pneumonia, thromboembolism,* or *pneumothorax.* If one of these is the precipitating cause, it must be treated.

In addition, as indicated in the management of chronic respiratory failure, it is important to reduce the oxygen uptake and carbon dioxide production of the respiratory apparatus by measures directed at reducing the flow resistance or the elastic resistance to distention.

RELIEF OF AIRWAY OBSTRUCTION

Airway obstruction may be increased because of the accumulation of secretions or bronchoconstriction. Thus, therapy must be directed at reducing the production and increasing the elimination of secretions, as well as alleviating bronchoconstriction.

Reduced Production of Secretions

Infection. As we have seen, acute respiratory infection is the most common precipitating cause of respiratory failure in patients with underlying chronic airflow limitation. In most cases, the airway resistance is increased because of thick purulent secretions and inflammatory swelling of the bronchial mucosa. Although most infections are due to viral agents or mycoplasma, a bacterial infection often develops secondarily. The offending bacteria should be identified by smear and culture of the secretions, and their sensitivity to antibiotics should be assessed so that the appropriate antibiotic can be administered. The most common organisms found in such patients are *Streptococcus pneumoniae* and *Hemophilus influenzae,* though there is also a significant incidence of gram-negative infections. Ampicillin represents appropriate initial therapy for the two common organisms, whereas aminoglycosides should be administered if a gram-negative infection is suspected, particularly if the infection develops after admission to a hospital. It must be emphasized that antibiotic treatment should be given only when the secretions are purulent and are associated with clinical evidence of infection. "Chasing" the culture reports with broad-spectrum antibiotics frequently hastens the appearance of resistant strains of bacteria and their associated infections.

Increased Elimination of Secretions

Improved elimination of bronchial secretions is facilitated by efforts to keep them thin and mobile and by physiotherapy. If these measures are not successful, it may be necessary to aspirate the secretions.

Thinning of Secretions. Thinning of bronchial secretions and prevention of crusting are integral requirements for improving the elimination of secretions. The most important measure in this regard is provision of adequate total body hydration. As discussed in Chapter 20, an adequate intake of fluids should be provided. In some cases, warm humidification of the inspired gas will also help liquefy secretions so that they are easier to expectorate, but, as pointed out earlier, nebulized liquefying agents, enzymes and detergents or oral liquefying agents, such as potassium iodide, do not appear to be more effective than water or saline mists or good hydration.

Physiotherapy. The role of physiotherapy in the management of acute respiratory failure cannot be overemphasized. When airway obstruction is associated with the accumulation of secretions, postural drainage is particularly helpful in expediting the elimination of secretions. The foot of the bed should be elevated about 12 inches, and the patient turned from side to side every half hour, while pummeling or clapping the patient's chest with rapid repetitive strokes at frequent intervals. During this procedure, the patient should be encouraged to cough and expectorate secretions.

Endotracheal Suction. If the cough mechanism is inadequate, and secretions are particularly difficult to expectorate, nasotracheal suction and, in some cases, fiberoptic bronchoscopy may be necessary to clear accumulated secretions. To accomplish nasotracheal suctioning, a catheter is inserted into the nose as far as the larynx (usually the distance from the tip of the nose to the ear pinna), with the neck extended, and then is advanced into the trachea during an inspiration. Therapeutic fiberoptic bronchoscopy may be useful, and, in selected patients, total bronchial lavage may be necessary to effectively remove mucous plugs from the bronchi.

Relief of Bronchoconstriction

Relief of bronchospasm, with its attendant lowering of the work of breathing and improvement in alveolar ventilation, is most important. When there is marked airflow obstruction, a loading dose of aminophylline (5 to 6 mg./kg. over 20 to 30 min.) given intravenously usually results in a serum theophylline level of about 12 μg./ml. and improvement in flow resistance. The loading dose should be reduced by 50 per cent if the patient has been taking oral theophylline. Following the loading dose, one should maintain a serum theophylline level of about 12 to 15 μg./ml. by initiating a constant infusion aminophylline drip, the goal being to match the metabolism of the drug with the infusion rate. One must remember that the dose administered will be only an educated guess, so that the blood level of theophylline should be determined as soon as possible. Otherwise, some patients will become toxic and develop seizures or cardiac arrhythmias, whereas others will have subtherapeutic theophylline levels.

In patients with severe bronchial obstruction, particularly those with severe asthma, high doses of systemic corticosteroids, such as methylprednisolone, have been shown to reduce the markedly increased airflow resistance.

In addition, as discussed in the previous chapter, aerosol beta-2 agonists should be administered effectively, i.e., by having the patient take slow, deep breaths of bronchodilator delivered by a nebulizer that delivers small droplets, using either a hand bulb or a pressure source, at frequent intervals. After improvement occurs, the frequency of administration can be reduced.

It has been shown that the hypoxemia may worsen following the administration of aerosol beta-2 agonists or intravenous aminophylline, presumably because of a redistribution of ventilation. However, the transient decrease in arterial P_{O_2} is usually not great, and bronchodilators should not be withheld on this account. Clearly, if there is concern about a drop in P_aO_2, the administration of oxygen together with the bronchodilators is warranted.

RELIEF OF PULMONARY CONGESTION

Left Ventricular Failure

As has been pointed out, left ventricular failure leads to fluid retention and pulmonary congestion. Occasionally patients with acute respiratory failure also have significant congestive heart failure, and this further increases the work of breathing and aggravates the disturbances of gas exchange. Supplemental oxygen is the most potent therapy for patients with pulmonary congestion. When there is evidence of left ventricular failure, the administration of diuretics and a salt-free diet frequently results in improvement in ventilatory function and arterial blood gas tensions, presumably because of a reduction in pulmonary congestion. However, one must be extremely cautious in the use of digitalis, because of the presence of hypoxemia, acidemia, hypercapnia and electrolyte imbalance. In general, it is best to wait until there is a tolerable arterial oxygen tension and all electrolyte abnormalities or acid-base disturbances are corrected before administering digitalis.

IMPROVEMENT OF ALVEOLAR VENTILATION

PATENT AIRWAY

Intensive application of the measures described above and in Chapter 20 will generally result in clinical improvement, so that further modalities are unnecessary. However, in some patients, clearance of secretions may be particularly difficult, or a ventilator may be necessary because of severe hypoxemia or patient fatigue. Clearly, in such cases, it is essential that a patent airway be maintained.

Endotracheal Intubation

Insertion of an endotracheal tube is frequently life saving in patients with laryngeal or tracheal obstruction. Intubation is also indicated in the seriously ill patient with generalized airway obstruction who is comatose, when it is obvious that a safe and effectively patent airway will be difficult to maintain otherwise. This allows oxygenation and provision of assisted or controlled ventilation if it is required and also facilitates suctioning of tracheobronchial secretions. In addition, inflation of the cuff on the endotracheal tube will prevent aspiration of gastrointestinal fluids or upper respiratory secretions.

The choice between nasal or oral intubation is based on clinical grounds and technical considerations. Both have advantages and disadvantages. The nasotracheal tube is more comfortable than the orotracheal tube, but the latter is technically easier to insert. In addition, the orotracheal tube can be shorter and wider, so that it offers less flow resistance and permits better tracheobronchial toilet. Whatever tube is used, it should have the largest possible internal diameter, and its cuff should be highly compliant and capable of holding a large volume at low inflation pressures.

Because of the improved quality of the newer tubes, most endotracheal tubes can be left in place for many days if proper care is taken. Tracheostomy should be considered if an extended period of care is anticipated.

Tracheostomy

When it has been decided that the acute situation will be prolonged, or if, despite intensive nasotracheal suction by the physician and nurse as well as physiotherapy, secretions continue to accumulate and present a problem in management, a tracheostomy may be indicated. However, a tracheostomy is not without complications, and it should not be carried out in haste or without proper precautions. Complications of tracheostomy occur most frequently where the procedure is done hastily in poor surroundings. A tracheostomy, per se, is not an emergency; rather it is the need for a patent airway that is the true emergency, and it is clear that this emergency can be handled by the installation of an endotracheal tube.

Emotional Support. It is important to recognize that emotional problems arise frequently if the patient is intubated or has a tracheostomy, because the patient is unable to talk and communicate with the individuals providing care. Sincere understanding of the patient's problem and careful explanation of all that is being done is extremely important for the patient's emotional status.

Care of the Airway

By far the majority of complications of an endotracheal or tracheostomy tube result from improper care and lack of attention to details. Auscultation over the lateral aspects of both lower lobes and palpation of the upper trachea help determine the level of the lower end of the tube. When the endotracheal tube has been properly positioned, its upper end should be taped securely to the skin and the position then confirmed by a chest x-ray film.

Provision of Humidity. As was pointed out in Chapter 8, approximately 650 ml. of water per day is added to the inspired gas by the upper respiratory tract, particularly the nasal mucosa. When an endotracheal or tracheostomy tube is in place, the inspired air bypasses the upper respiratory tract, so that it is not adequately humidified. Unless evaporation of water from the tracheobronchial tree is prevented, bronchial secretions may become viscid and thick, and crusting may develop. By increasing the moisture content of the inspired air and ensuring adequate hydration of the patient, complications of an artificial airway are minimized. For the spontaneously breathing patient, the inspired air can be humidified by having the patient breathe heated water or saline from a humidifier that is powered by oxygen or compressed air. The humidifier can be connected to the tracheostomy or endotracheal tube by wide-bore tubing connected to a T connector in the tracheostomy or endotracheal tube's opening. If the patient is being ventilated artifically, the inspired gas can be delivered through a heated bypass humidifier of the cascade type.

Prevention of Infection. In addition to bypassing the humidifying properties of the upper respiratory tract, an artificial airway eliminates many of the defenses of the respiratory tract. It is often necessary to suction the tracheobronchial tree, and this may introduce pathogenic bacteria. Clearly then, it is essential to use an aseptic technique and a separate sterile catheter each time the patient requires suctioning. A trap attached to the catheter allows collection of secretions for bacteriologic examination, which should be performed at regular intervals and whenever there is a change in the character of the secretions.

It must be pointed out that all inhalation therapy equipment, particularly humidifiers and nebulizers, may become contaminated with nosocomial organisms, such as ***Pseudomonas aeruginosa,*** and may result in pulmonary infections. This can be avoided by daily sterilization of all tubing and humidifiers or nebulization of weak acetic acid through the humidifiers and nebulizers.

Prevention of Trauma. Since endotracheal suctioning can cause considerable trauma to the trachea and bronchi, the airway should be suctioned only when the accumulation of secretions is detected or, if the patient is on a ventilator, when the ventilator pressure necessary for a given tidal volume rises. The suction catheter should have only a single opening at its tip, because the tracheal mucosa may be sucked into side openings and torn when the catheter moves, especially if a mucous plug blocks the distal opening. A Y tube at the proximal end of the catheter will ensure that suction is not exerted during insertion of the catheter. The catheter should be directed as far down the tracheobronchial tree as possible and then into either the left or right main bronchus by suitable positioning of the head and the tracheostomy tube. The suction catheter should not be left in the tracheobronchial tree for longer than 5 to 10 seconds, particularly in severely hypoxemic patients, and suction should be applied only while the catheter is withdrawn smoothly in a twisting motion.

The mode of inflation of the cuff on the tube is also extremely important in preventing trauma. The cuff, which should be large and easily distensible, should be inflated only enough to approximate the tracheal walls, and no pressure should be exerted on the tracheal mucosa. With proper precautions, pressure necrosis can be avoided and patients can be ventilated indefinitely without tracheal complications.

MECHANICAL VENTILATION

As indicated earlier, the majority of patients suffering from acute respiratory failure can be managed without resorting to the use of a ventilator. Nevertheless, a ventilator is absolutely essential in some patients.

The goals of ventilatory therapy are to provide adequate oxygenation and carbon dioxide elimination, without adverse effects on other organ systems, so as to tide the patient over until the primary injury is rectified and to establish optimal conditions for the early resumption of spontaneous breathing. For the majority of patients, it does not matter whether a pressure-cycled or volume-cycled ventilator is used. With the pressure-cycled ventilator, inspiration terminates after a preselected airway pressure has been reached, so that size of breath delivered will be affected by alterations in flow resistance and the lung and chest wall elastic recoil. With the volume-cycled ventilator, the tidal volume is preset, so that the driving pressure will change with alterations of flow resistance and lung or chest wall compliance. Volume-cycled ventilators are probably more physiologic, since they deliver a fairly constant volume despite changes in resistance or compliance. In addition, the volume-cycled ventilator allows excellent control of the F_IO_2, whereas this may be difficult with a pressure-cycled ventilator.

A ventilator may be used to either assist or control ventilation or to do both (i.e., an assistor controller). When used as an assistor, the ventilator inflates the lungs in response to a drop in airway pressure because of an inspiratory effort by the patient, so that the ventilatory rate is determined by the patient rather than being imposed by the ventilator. Assisted ventilation is particularly useful in patients who require a brief period (hours) of ventilatory support. It is also recommended for longer periods in patients whose respiratory drive mechanism is preserved and who are breathing at a normal or near normal respiratory frequency. It is thought that the need to initiate each breath prevents "disuse" of the muscles of respiration. On the other hand, assisted ventilation in tachypneic patients may lead to hypocapnia and alkalemia, with subsequent impact on cerebral blood flow and cardiac rhythm. Assisted ventilation may also be erratic and unreliable, for the assist mechanism often is either so sensitive that the ventilator autocycles or so insensitive that the ventilator does not respond to the patient's inspiratory effort.

When used as a controller, the ventilator cycles automatically at a preset pattern and is not affected by the patient's inspiratory efforts. This inability to obtain a breath on demand frequently leads to patient apprehension and occasionally may increase the work sufficiently to result in carbon dioxide retention.

When used as an assistor-controller, the ventilator not only controls the respiratory pattern but also assists inspiration whenever a patient attempts to inspire out of phase with the ventilator. In effect, this type of ventilator acts as an assistor as long as the patient's breathing efforts are at a higher rate than the preset respirator rate and as a controller if the respiratory rate drops below the preset value.

Indications for Mechanical Ventilation

The criteria that are commonly used to determine the need for mechanical ventilation in patients suffering from respiratory insufficiency are presented in Table 18, but these parameters must be considered along with an assessment of the clinical situation. Isolated determinations of arterial blood gas tensions, or parameters that reflect the mechanical properties of the respiratory apparatus, are not adequate assessments of the patient's respiratory reserve. A vital capacity that is less than 15 mg./kg. body weight may still be adequate if the patient has an effective cough and is not tiring, and if the arterial blood gas tensions are not increasing progressively. Indeed, progressive deterioration in function and in clinical status is the important determinant that influences the decision about mechanical ventilation.

Controlled mechanical ventilation is indicated in the following situations.

1. When apnea or severe respiratory depression is present, such as may occur following drug overdose, central nervous system dysfunction due to brain trauma or spinal cord injuries, or when there is neuromuscular weakness or paralysis

2. When a patient is unable to maintain adequate spontaneous ventilatory activity while on assisted ventilation

3. When spontaneous ventilatory effort may be deleterious, such as in some cases of flail chest, when splinting of the chest wall is desirable

4. When the application of positive end-expiratory pressure is necessary

5. When a ventilator is operating near its pressure limit or at high respiratory frequencies (greater than 25/min.) and is unable to deliver adequate tidal volumes

Setting the Ventilator

Respiratory Rate and Tidal Volume. When first initiating mechanical ventilation, one generally delivers a large tidal volume (12 to 15 ml./kg.) and a slow respiratory rate (10 to 20 breaths/min.). Smaller breaths may lead to progressive airway or alveolar closure, with a resultant fall in compliance of the lung and, if the unventilated alveoli continue to be perfused, a rise in $P_{(A-a)}O_2$ and fall in P_aO_2. The choice of respiratory rate is arbitrary, but the expiratory time must be sufficiently long to ensure a low mean airway pressure.

TABLE 18. Indications for Ventilatory Support in Adults

Ventilatory Function	Critical Values (Normal Range)
Respiratory rate	>35 (12–20) breaths/min.
Vital capacity	<15 (65–75) ml./kg. body weight*
FEV$_1$	<10 (50–60) ml./kg. body weight
Maximum inspiratory force	<25 (75–100) cm. H$_2$O
Oxygenation†:	
P$_a$O$_2$	<50 (>500 mm. Hg)
Ventilation:	
P$_a$CO$_2$	>55‡ (35–45) mm. Hg
VD/VT	>0.60 (0.25–0.40)

*"Ideal" weight.
†After 10 min. of 100 per cent oxygen.
‡Except in patients with chronic hypercapnia.

To determine whether the respiratory rate and depth chosen provide adequate gas exchange, the arterial blood gas tensions must be assessed. The respiratory rate should be adjusted according to the P_aCO_2, which represents the balance between the metabolic production of carbon dioxide and the alveolar ventilation. From the measured P_aCO_2, any necessary changes in respiratory frequency (f) may be determined:

$$\text{Desired f} = \text{Previous f} \times \frac{\text{Previous } P_aCO_2}{\text{Desired } P_aCO_2}$$

Inspired Oxygen Concentration. Concentrations of inspired oxygen (F_IO_2) of up to 100 per cent may be necessary to ensure adequate oxygenation in some cases. Although high concentrations of oxygen for sustained periods can cause serious lung damage, they should not be withheld for fear of oxygen toxicity if the hypoxemia is severe. Whenever supplemental oxygen is being administered, the P_aO_2 should be followed closely and the F_IO_2 decreased as soon as possible, aiming for a P_aO_2 of 60 to 80 torr and an F_IO_2 of less than 50 per cent.

Pressure and Flow. The pressure required to inflate the lungs will depend on the resistance to airflow in the airways and the compliance of the lungs and chest wall. It will rise whenever the tidal volume and flow are increased, flow resistance rises, or total compliance falls. A pressure-limited ventilator will cut off at the pressure that is preset by the operator. With a volume-limited ventilator, the pressure will vary depending on the impedances to ventilation.

One generally attempts to balance pressure and airflow in such a way as to provide the most rapid flow that can be tolerated comfortably by the patient, allowing sufficient time during expiration for adequate venous return. The pressure limit at which an alarm is triggered on a volume-limited ventilator is set at about 10 to 15 cm. H_2O above the peak pressure developed during mechanical ventilation.

Intermittent Mandatory Ventilation. Intermittent mandatory ventilation (IMV), first described as a useful method of weaning, may be used to assist or control ventilation intermittently. In this system, the patient is allowed to breathe spontaneously, but the ventilator is adjusted to deliver a breath at a preset interval. In current ventilators, which contain demand-valve systems, the ventilator breath is delivered whenever the patient attempts to inspire; i.e., the intermittent mandatory breath is synchronized with the patient's breathing efforts (SIMV). Like all assist-control systems, SIMV serves as a valuable backup system for the patient who does not initiate a breath spontaneously.

Theoretically, IMV has the advantage of allowing one to use very high levels of *positive end-expiratory pressure* (PEEP) or *continuous positive airway pressure* (CPAP). This is because the mean pressure applied by a ventilator over a period of time is low, since a ventilator-initiated inspiration is applied only intermittently. As a result, there will be less impediment to venous return at any given level of end-expiratory pressure. On the other hand, the patient receiving ventilatory support at a low IMV rate who becomes apneic will receive a grossly inadequate alveolar ventilation despite the intermittent mandatory breaths. In addition, spontaneous breathing on an IMV system is associated with an increase in the work of breathing because of the resistance offered by the ventilator tubing.

Positive End-Expiratory Pressure

PEEP is the maintenance of an end-expiratory positive pressure of variable magnitude throughout expiration by the imposition of a threshold resistance (Fig. 105,*A*). **PEEP** is particularly effective in clinical situations characterized by lung units that tend to collapse. As delineated by Ashbaugh et al. in 1969, **PEEP** is indicated in "clinical situations which are characterized by profound hypoxemia, high physiologic shunt, atelectasis, alveolar instability and high cardiac output." The most important indication is the need to raise the P_aO_2 in a patient who is dangerously hypoxemic (P_aO_2 < 50 mm. Hg at an F_IO_2 > 0.5) and who has diffuse, generally uniform, pulmonary infiltrates on the chest roentgenogram. Such a disorder is generally characterized by a lower-than-normal functional residual capacity and a very low lung compliance.

The beneficial effect of **PEEP** derives from the increase in end-expiratory lung volume (FRC), which results from the increase in end-

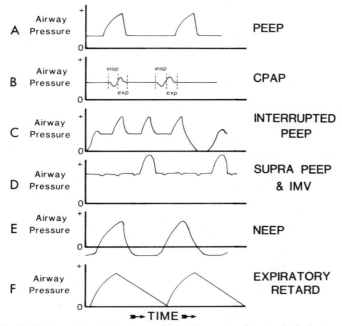

Figure 105. Variations of expiratory pressures that may be applied during mechanical ventilation.

expiratory pressure. This alleviates or helps prevent alveolar collapse, so that the matching of ventilation and perfusion is improved, the gradient for oxygen between the alveolar gas and arterial blood ($P_{(A-a)}O_2$) is reduced and the P_aO_2 rises.

The lowest end-expiratory pressure necessary to achieve a P_aO_2 of 60 to 80 mm. Hg at an F_iO_2 less than 0.5 without interfering with oxygen delivery to the tissues should be applied. One usually first applies 5 cm. H_2O and then assesses gas exchange and the hemodynamic status after about 30 minutes. If the desired goal has not been reached, the pressure can be raised in 5–cm. H_2O increments, provided that no deleterious effects develop.

Continuous Positive Airway Pressure

CPAP (Fig. 105,*B*), first described by Barach, is physiologically similar to PEEP, but CPAP may be applied with or without a ventilator or endotracheal intubation, using either a hood arrangement that encloses the patient's head or a tight-fitting mask. Positive airway pressure is maintained in this system because gas flow is continuous and the patient exhales through an adjustable spring-loaded valve. Although used occasionally in adults, it is used primarily in the management of neonatal hyaline membrane disease.

Interrupted PEEP

Here, the elevation in end-expiratory pressure is interrupted at preset intervals, so that the end-expiratory pressure is allowed to return to zero (ambient pressure) for a period of time (Fig. 105,*C*). Once again, the use of this mode offers a theoretical advantage, because the mean airway pressure over a period of time will be lower and thus there will be less impediment to venous return.

Supra PEEP

This is the application of high levels of positive end-expiratory pressure, usually greater than 15 cm. H_2O (Fig. 105,*D*). It has been suggested that pressures as high as 30 to 40 cm. H_2O, in combination with IMV, will foster rapid reversal of acute respiratory insufficiency if applied early in the management. However, high airway pressures are not without side effects, and they can reduce venous return and cardiac output as well as overdistend and rupture alveoli.

Negative End-Expiratory Pressure (NEEP)

In this situation, a negative pressure is applied during expiration (Fig. 105,*E*). Although this facilitates expiration, it may cause collapse of airways.

Expiratory Retard

Many ventilators include the potential to add an expiratory resistance or to retard exhalation (Fig. 105,*F*). The application of a slight back pressure during expiration, which is similar to the pursed-lip breathing adopted by many patients suffering from chronic obstructive pulmonary disease, is thought to reduce airway collapse and air trapping so that emptying of the lungs is facilitated.

MONITORING THE PATIENT WITH ACUTE RESPIRATORY FAILURE

ASSESSMENT OF CLINICAL STATUS

Frequent examination of the patient by the attending physician and nurse is necessary in order to determine changes in clinical status and to detect secretions, lobar collapse, consolidation or other complications. The attendant at the bedside remains the essential component of patient monitoring. "Laboratory" measurements are only adjuncts that allow the physician and nurse to determine the adequacy of management and recognize trends in the course of the condition and its management.

ASSESSMENT OF GAS EXCHANGE

Arterial Blood Gas Tensions

The partial pressures of oxygen and carbon dioxide in the arterial blood, along with the pH, must be assessed at regular intervals to evaluate the status of gas exchange during the course of management. The P_aO_2 should be maintained between 60 and 80 mm. Hg, and the P_aCO_2 between 35 and 45 mm. Hg. It is important to review the trend in arterial blood gas tensions and acid-base status at all times.

Inspired Oxygen Concentration

Monitoring of the F_IO_2 in all patients receiving supplemental oxygen, and continued efforts to maintain a low inspired concentration, are essential, because oxygen toxicity is a time-dose–related phenomenon. It should be noted that most pressure-cycled ventilators deliver a higher concentration of oxygen than is indicated on the air dilute setting.

Alveolo-Arterial Oxygen Gradient

Knowledge of the F_IO_2 and the arterial blood gas tensions allows estimation of the alveolar oxygen tension (P_AO_2) using a simplified alveolar air equation:

$$P_AO_2 = F_IO_2 - P_aCO_2/R$$

As indicated earlier, R can be assumed to be 0.8 if the patient is breathing room air, and 1.0 if supplemental oxygen is being administered.

As long as the inspired oxygen concentration is kept constant, changes in the alveolo-arterial partial pressure gradient for oxygen ($P_{(A-a)}O_2$) provide the most valuable index of changes in gas exchange over time. The $P_{(A-a)}O_2$ is normally about 10 mm. Hg while the patient is breathing room air, and it increases when gas exchange is altered by shunting, mismatching of ventilation and perfusion or a diffusion defect.

Calculation of $P_{(A-a)}O_2$ while the patient is breathing 100 per cent oxygen is often used to assess the extent of perfusion of unventilated airspaces, i.e., physiologic shunt ($\dot{Q}_s/\dot{Q}_t$). However, in acute lung failure, many alveolar units are minimally ventilated and the inhalation of 100 per cent oxygen may promote absorption atelectasis, thus resulting in even greater shunting of blood. For these reasons, measurement of the $P_{(A-a)}O_2$ and calculation of $\dot{Q}_s/\dot{Q}_t$ are safer and probably more meaningful clinically when determined at an F_IO_2 of 0.50 or less.

Dead-Space/Tidal Volume Ratio

Knowledge of the partial pressure of carbon dioxide in the expired air (P_ECO_2) and the P_aCO_2 allows calculation of the dead-space/tidal volume ratio. From this ratio one can estimate the proportion of the ventilation that is wasted, i.e., lung units that are well ventilated but poorly or not at all perfused:

$$V_D/V_T = (P_aCO_2 - P_ECO_2)/P_aCO_2$$

ASSESSMENT OF ACID-BASE STATUS

Acid-base disturbances are common in respiratory failure, and, if allowed to persist, they may precipitate severe complications. Acidemia, particularly when associated with hypoxemia, can cause marked pulmonary vasoconstriction, precipitate cardiac arrhythmias, and also reduce the response to bronchodilators. Alkalemia may also be associated with a decrease in cardiac output and with disorders of cardiac rhythm, as well as with cerebral irritability and convulsions.

ASSESSMENT OF FLUID BALANCE AND ELECTROLYTES

The balance of fluid intake and output, and the daily weight, should be reviewed regularly, allowing for a catabolic weight loss of 0.5 kg./day. Because of the interplay between changes in hydrogen ion and plasma bicarbonate, along with the extracellular sodium, potassium and chloride, it is also important to determine serial serum and urinary electrolytes and osmolarity. Hypokalemia, if present, leads to a metabolic alkalemia and increases myocardial irritability, whereas the combination of hypoxemia, alkalemia and hypokalemia predisposes the patient to arrhythmias.

In patients suffering from ARDS, fluid retention may occur because one frequently must administer fluid therapy. The type of fluid used is not as important as the amount given, and the goal of such therapy is normalization of the pulmonary vascular pressure. Blood, isotonic salt substances or both should be administered, and the pulmonary vascular pressures should be monitored closely to prevent hypovolemia or excess fluid accumulation in the lungs.

ASSESSMENT OF VENTILATOR FUNCTION

Tidal Volume and Pressure

As we have seen, when a pressure-cycled ventilator is used, gas flow stops whenever the preselected airway pressure has been reached, so the tidal volume delivered will vary with alterations of the mechanical properties of the respiratory system. Here, changes in tidal volume and inspiratory time and thus respiratory rate will reflect changes in flow resistance or the elastic recoil of the lungs and chest wall (Fig. 106,*A*). With a volume-cycled ventilator, flow continues until a preset volume has been delivered, so that the driving pressure will vary with changes in flow resistance or elastic recoil of the respiratory apparatus (Fig. 106,*B*). Thus, a rise in the respiratory rate and fall in tidal volume when a pressure-cycled ventilator is used, and an increase in peak pressure when a volume-cycled ventilator is used, are indicative of the development of airway obstruction (such as mucous plugging, bronchospasm, and displacement of the endotracheal tube) or a fall in lung compliance (such as an atelectasis or a pneumothorax).

Inspired Gas Temperature and Humidity

Adequate humidification of the inspired air must be ensured when an endotracheal or tracheostomy tube is in place. Thus, the temperature of the

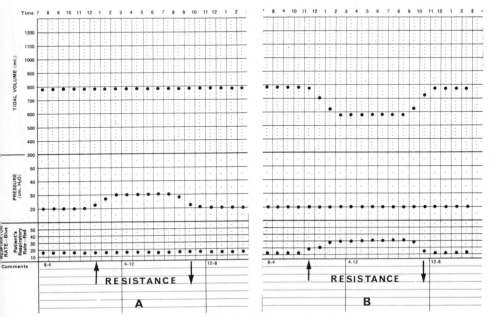

Figure 106. The effect of a change of respiratory resistance on respirator pressure, tidal volume and respiratory rate when a volume-limited ventilator (**A**), and a pressure-limited ventilator (**B**) are being used. Note that when a volume-limited ventilator is in use, an increase in resistance results in a rise in pressure; when a pressure-limited ventilator is in use, an increase in resistance results in a fall in tidal volume and a rise in respiratory rate.

inspired gas, as well as the water level in the ventilator humidifier, must be monitored in order to avoid drying of the airway mucosa and potential obstruction of airways with inspissated secretions.

Total Compliance and Flow Resistance

If inspiration is held at end-inspiration, one can calculate the effective total compliance (C_T) of the lungs and chest wall.

$$C_T = V_T / P_{(insp.\ hold)}$$

The effective compliance is normally greater than 60 ml./cm. H_2O, and a low compliance suggests that the compliance of the lung, chest wall or both is reduced.

At the same time, if the ventilator peak pressure and airflow are known, the resistance to flow (both in the patient and in the ventilator tubing) can be calculated:

$$R = P_{(Peak - Insp.\ hold)} / Flow$$

Best PEEP

When PEEP is being used, one may wish to determine *"best PEEP"* by sequential calculation of the effective compliance at increments of PEEP. This provides a series of compliance values that reach a well-defined maximum, and this is thought to coincide with maximum oxygen transport to the tissues and minimum wasted ventilation. Thus, it is frequently recommended that the level of PEEP be increased until the desired P_aO_2 is reached, provided that the effective compliance increases or remains unchanged.

ASSESSMENT OF HEMODYNAMIC PARAMETERS

In addition to the electrocardiogram and heart rate, which are affected by gas exchange and acid-base status, one should assess the adequacy of the cardiac output and the delivery of oxygen to the tissues.

Cardiac Output

Intermittent assessment of cardiac output (C.O.) is important in order to assess the adequacy of tissue oxygenation. The cardiac output can be measured directly, using either a dye dilution or a thermodilution technique, or it can be calculated from the Fick equation, knowing the oxygen consumption ($\dot{V}O_2$) and the arteriovenous oxygen content difference ($C_{(a-\bar{v})}O_2$):

$$C.O. = \frac{\dot{V}O_2}{C_{(a-\bar{v})}O_2}$$

Since the cardiac output is inversely proportional to $C_{(a-\bar{v})}O_2$, changes in either the cardiac output or $C_{(a-\bar{v})}O_2$ identify hemodynamic alterations and the point beyond which increments in ventilator pressure may have adverse cardiovascular effects.

Mixed Venous Oxygen Tension

The product of cardiac output and arterial oxygen content provides an index of oxygen transport to the tissues, but it does not indicate the amount of oxygen actually required by them. The oxygen tension of the mixed venous blood (P_vO_2), which is the net result of the tissue oxygen supply and demand, is generally used to reflect the adequacy of tissue oxygenation. In general, a P_vO_2 greater than 30 mm. Hg is thought to reflect good tissue oxygenation.

Central Venous Pressure

The central venous pressure normally reflects right ventricular end-diastolic pressure and is at best only an indirect measure of pulmonary artery pressure.

Pulmonary Vascular Pressures

Using the flow-directed balloon-tipped catheter, the pulmonary artery (PAP) and pulmonary capillary wedge (PCWP) pressures can be determined. Over a range of about 5 to 25 mm. Hg, the PCWP closely approximates left atrial pressure (LAP). PCWP correlates poorly with LAP at pressures greater than 25 mm. Hg and when the alveolar pressure is elevated, such as when PEEP is applied.

Systemic Pressure

The systemic blood pressure should also be monitored at regular intervals. The blood pressure may fall either because of a reduction in venous return when very high tidal volumes are being delivered or because of fluid depletion; these causes must be differentiated.

ASSESSMENT OF NUTRITION

General nutritional deficits commonly occur in patients with respiratory failure. Loss of lean body mass and a negative nitrogen balance are part of the physiologic response to injury, but the negative nitrogen balance may decrease muscle strength. Therefore, sufficient calories and essential amino acids must be administered in order to maintain a stable nitrogen balance, weight and metabolism. One should recognize dehydration and hypovolemia (or hypervolemia) early. Potassium depletion may be present because of a poor diet or the administration of diuretics or corticosteroids, and daily supplemental potassium may be necessary to maintain the serum potassium level above 4.0 mEq. In addition, hypophosphatemia may contribute to the perpetuation of respiratory failure.

ASSESSMENT OF OTHER PARAMETERS

Along with the parameters already discussed, a chest roentgenogram should be examined and, in some cases, fluoroscopy may help to assess diaphragmatic–respiratory muscle discoordination. When appropriate, the hematocrit, hemoglobin concentration or both should be measured, because a low hemoglobin will reduce the oxygen-carrying capacity and thus the transport of oxygen to the tissues. Delivery of oxygen to the tissues should be optimized by ensuring a hemoglobin of at least 10 gm./100 ml. of blood and an optimum cardiac output and blood pressure. The white blood cell count and differential; sputum examination and culture, as well as sensitivity to antibiotics; and the stools for occult blood should be assessed, as necessary.

It is also essential to assess muscle function and to ensure maintenance of physical fitness, if at all possible. Activity should be encouraged, and walking on the spot at the bedside or an exercise bicycle should be used well in advance of anticipated weaning, particularly in the patient who has spent a prolonged period being ventilated.

WEANING FROM VENTILATORY SUPPORT

Successful treatment of the underlying pathologic conditions and the factors that precipitated the respiratory failure will usually allow a patient to be weaned from a ventilator. However, this may be difficult if there is an elevated ventilatory requirement due to excessive respiratory stimuli, an increased work of breathing, elevated dead-space–like ventilation or weakness of the respiratory muscles because of disuse, poor nutrition, neuromuscular disease or sedative drugs.

In general, the clinical assessment of the patient and the correction, to the extent possible, of all complications, with repeated evaluation of the ability to cope without ventilatory assistance, remain the most important considerations in weaning. Psychologic preparation of the patient is very important; the degree of need is in direct proportion to the length of time on the ventilator, and counseling must begin long before the patient is disconnected from the ventilator.

Depending on the patient's requirements for ventilation, weaning from PEEP should be carried out before weaning from controlled ventilation, weaning from a ventilator before closing a tracheostomy, and closing a tracheostomy before removing supplemental oxygen.

POSITIVE END–EXPIRATORY PRESSURE

PEEP should be decreased by 5 cm. H_2O, and the patient carefully observed for clinical signs of hypoxemia; the arterial blood gases should be assessed after 10 or 20 minutes. If the clinical and hemodynamic status remains stable and the blood gases do not deteriorate, then the end-expiratory pressure may be lowered further by 5-cm. H_2O increments until only mechanical ventilation is operative. Usually a patient should be monitored for 24 to 36 hours after **PEEP** has been discontinued, before beginning to be weaned entirely from the ventilator.

THE VENTILATOR

The criteria for discontinuation of mechanical ventilation are the converse of those that were considered for its institution. Although different for each patient, the potential ability of the patient to sustain an adequate ventilation without mechanical assistance is classically assessed by determining the strength and endurance of the respiratory muscles, as well as the adequacy of gas exchange.

Patients are generally weaned from a ventilator by having them breathe an oxygen concentration slightly greater than that delivered during mechanical ventilation through a T-piece adaptor connected to a heated nebulizer. The patient's clinical status, vital signs and cardiac rhythm should be monitored at least every 5 to 10 minutes during the patient's first half-hour off the ventilator, and arterial blood gases should be assessed at the end of a half-hour. In patients with limited ventilatory reserve, spontaneous ventilation should be allowed for only 5 to 10 minutes per hour during the early stages of weaning. If this is well tolerated, the time period off the ventilator can be increased by increments of 5 to 15 minutes. In some cases, weaning is facilitated if the time on the ventilator, rather than the time off it, is gradually reduced incrementally.

Intermittent mandatory ventilation has also been advocated for weaning a patient from controlled ventilation. Here the patient is allowed to breathe spontaneously between mandatory inflations produced by a constant-volume ventilator, and weaning is carried out by gradually reducing the number of mandatory breaths per minute. Although there are few objective data to support the contention, it has been suggested that this is physiologically more sound and that it favors a smooth transition from controlled to spontaneous ventilation in that it allows the patient to gradually assume an increasing proportion of the work of breathing. As pointed out earlier, however, it is important to recognize that the work required to breathe through the ventilator tubing may, in itself, impose a considerable additional burden on the patient.

Discontinuation of Weaning

The decision to discontinue weaning attempts and to reinstitute ventilatory support is usually based on a careful clinical evaluation of the extent of the patient's discomfort or anxiety, the development of progressive obtundation, and any deterioration of parameters reflecting respiratory work, gas exchange and cardiac function. In particular, diaphragmatic muscle fatigue and the development of a discoordination between abdominal and chest wall movement are indicative of the need to reinstitute ventilatory support. It has been suggested that electromyography, using surface electrodes, esophageal electrodes or both, and examination of the relationship between high and low frequencies of the EMG may allow recognition of impending diaphragmatic fatigue.

TRACHEOSTOMY TUBE

Once a patient has been weaned from a ventilator for 18 to 24 hours, a fenestrated tube can be inserted in place of the cuffed tracheostomy tube, provided the blood gases and vital signs remain stable. This allows the patient to talk and cough up secretions, and also allows controlled ventilation to be reinstituted, if necessary. If this is well tolerated for a period of time, and if there is no need for further ventilatory support, the fenestrated tube can be removed and the tracheostomy site covered with a dry sterile dressing.

SUPPLEMENTAL OXYGEN

Patients should be weaned from supplemental oxygen as soon as is safely possible. The P_aO_2 should be maintained at about 60 mm. Hg, because further alveolar hypoventilation and CO_2 retention may occur if too much oxygen is given inadvertently. In patients suffering from ARDS, intrapulmonary shunting and ventilation-perfusion abnormalities may persist following termination of controlled ventilation, so that this may require supplemental oxygen. Improvement usually occurs after a few days, in which case the inspired oxygen can be reduced accordingly. In all patients, the arterial blood gas tensions should be measured 20 minutes after the F_IO_2 has been reduced to that of room air, in order to ensure that the patient can tolerate a prolonged period without supplemental oxygen.

THE INTENSIVE CARE UNIT

From the previous discussion, it is clear that the management of acute respiratory failure requires close attention to minute details and regular monitoring of vital parameters. However, the continuous availability of both personnel who are sufficiently trained to understand basic mechanisms of disturbed function and the sophisticated equipment used to treat or monitor the critically ill patient is virtually impossible on a general medical or surgical ward of a hospital. In addition, a coordinated effort and continuity of care are particularly difficult on general wards because of frequent staff changes and the staff's divided responsibilities in caring for other patients on the ward. For these reasons, it is recommended that all critically ill patients be cared for in a special area staffed by highly trained personnel.

PERSONNEL

The health care personnel must be able to recognize and manage not only acute respiratory failure, but also acute circulatory, acid-base, fluid and electrolyte disturbances. They are under constant pressure and must continually assess each patient or undertake measures aimed at maintaining or improving respiratory, cardiovascular, renal and cerebral function as well as acid-base, fluid, electrolyte and nutritional status. Attention to very minute details is necessary, changes in patient status must be recognized immediately, and emergencies must be handled quickly and effectively. In many cases, completely new directions in therapy must be undertaken.

This kind of attention and care must be provided throughout the day and night and cannot be a part-time occupation on the part of the attending personnel. Although it is usually recognized that only a full-time trained nursing staff can provide the technical competence required for the care of the very ill patient, this concept is much less readily accepted for house staff and medical staff. Like the nurse, a doctor who is not constantly involved in such care cannot maintain the technical competence and expertise necessary. The busy practicing physician or surgeon and the house staff also have divided responsibilities that may keep them occupied with patients in the office, on other wards or, in the case of the surgeon, in the operating room. Thus, they are not always immediately available when they are needed, and their suggestions or directions for treatment frequently come after a crisis situation has already been handled and therapy instituted.

FACILITIES

The intensive care facility should be air-conditioned, with frequent air changes and easy control of temperature and humidity. There must be ample outlets for oxygen, compressed air, suction and electricity at each bed station. Since ventilators and monitoring equipment are often necessary during the course of management, there must be sufficient space around each bed to permit easy use of such equipment. A portable x-ray unit is essential, and, if it is feasible, equipment for electroencephalography, radioisotope lung scans and cardiac output should also be available; facilities for electronic monitoring of essential parameters must be present at each bed station to help the nurse manage the patient.

A laboratory with capability for measurement of blood gas tensions and pH, blood volume, serum electrolytes and osmolarity, as well as blood smears, sputum and urine must be immediately accessible. There should also be a conference room, storage space for bulky equipment such as respirators, cooling apparatus, circo-electric beds, and pacemakers, as well as a waiting room for relatives.

Because of the broad approach that is necessary for the management of the critically ill patient, it is also clear that there is little to recommend a special unit dedicated solely to the management of acute respiratory failure. By the same token, separate medical and surgical units involve unnecessary duplication of equipment and trained personnel, for the disturbances in function are similar in both types of patients and many management requirements are the same.

ORGANIZATION

The details of the organization of a unit designed to care for critically ill patients are necessarily different in various centers, but there are certain general principles that are applicable in most units. To ensure continuous advances and innovations in the investigation of the critically ill patient and to stay in the forefront of their care, an attitude of inquiry and repeated evaluation of all procedures being used is necessary. This can proceed effectively only if those involved in the evaluation and clinical research are in control of the patient management.

In addition, the full-time personnel in the unit, under a director, are best equipped to evaluate potential admissions and discharges and to initiate a discharge if necessary. If control of admissions and discharges is not exercised by the staff of the unit, inappropriate deployment of resources may result.

To ensure the ready availability of the resources of the entire health team for each critically ill patient, the care of the patient should be coordinated by an experienced nurse at the bedside. In addition, full-time residents or, if these are not available, full-time physicians should coordinate a team of specialists in various fields as well as the attending physician and be responsible for the investigation and total care of all patients admitted to the unit. The nurse at the bedside should be responsible for applying the therapeutic measures decided upon by the attending team as well as for coordinating the activities of physiotherapists, respiratory therapists, occupational therapists and social workers, who play a vital role in both the management and rehabilitation of the patients. In this way, conflict or duplication is avoided, and there is a coherent treatment and investigation plan for the nurses and other members of the care team to follow. It is also important that an adequate number of nurses' assistants, such as aides and orderlies, as well as clerical workers be available to ensure optimum care and record keeping.

Organization of an "intensive care" unit in the manner described, with a full-time staff, facilitates virtually continuous teaching at the bedside. Through orderly rounds, all personnel can gain an insight into the capabilities and limitations of equipment or monitoring apparatus. Patients can be discussed by all members of the health team, and procedures and their rationale, as well as the therapeutic plan, can be explained to the health team. In this way, a true "esprit de corps" is developed, and all feel that they are truly taking an active role in the planning process and in the management of the critically ill patients.

SUGGESTED READING

Section I. Basic Considerations

Agostoni, E.: Mechanics of the pleural space. Physiol. Rev. 1972; *52*:57–128.

Allman, P. C., and Dittner, D. S. (eds.): Respiration and Circulation. Bethesda, MD., American Society for Experimental Biology, 1971.

Angus, J. E., and Thurlbeck, W. M.: Number of alveoli in the human lung. J. Appl. Physiol. 1972; *32*:483–485.

Anthonisen, N. R., Danson, J., Robertson, P. C., and Ross, W. R. D.: Airway closure as a function of age. Respir. Physiol. 1969; *8*:58–65.

Astrand, P. O., and Rodahl, D.: Textbook of Work Physiology. New York, McGraw-Hill, 1970.

Barton, A. D., and Laurenco, R. V.: Bronchial secretions and mucociliary clearance. Arch. Intern. Med. 1973; *131*:140–144.

Bates, D. V., Macklem, P. T., and Christie, R. V.: Respiratory Function in Disease. Philadelphia, W. B. Saunders Co., 1971.

Bellingham, A. J., Detter, J. C., and Lenfant, C.: Regulatory mechanisms of hemoglobin oxygen affinity in acidosis and alkalosis. J. Clin. Invest. 1971; *50*:700–706.

Brain, J. D., Proctor, D. F., and Reid, L. M. (eds.): Respiratory Defense Mechanisms, Part I and Part II. New York, Marcel Dekker, 1977.

Briscoe, T. J.: Carotid body: structure and function. Physiol. Rev. 1971; *51*:437–495.

Brodovsky, D. M., Macdonell, J. A., and Cherniack, R. M.: The respiratory response to carbon dioxide in health and emphysema. J. Clin. Invest. 1960; *39*:724–729.

Byrne-Quinn, E., Weil, J. V., Sodal, I. E., Filley, G. F., and Grover, R. F.: Ventilatory control in the athlete. J. Appl. Physiol. 1971; *30*:91–98.

Campbell, E. J. M., Agostoni, E., and Davis, J. N.: The Respiratory Muscles: Mechanics and Neural Control, 2nd ed. London, Lloyd-Luke (Medical Books) Ltd., 1970.

Campbell, E. J. M., Westlake, E. K., and Cherniack, R. M.: The oxygen consumption and efficiency of the respiratory muscles of young male subjects. Clin. Sci. 1959; *18*:55–64.

Campbell, E. J. M., Westlake, E. K., and Cherniack, R. M.: Simple methods of estimating the oxygen consumption and efficiency of the breathing muscles. J. Appl. Physiol. 1957; *11*:303–308.

Cherniack, R. M.: Pulmonary function testing. Semin. Respir. Med. 1983; *4*:171–266.

Cherniack, R. M.: Pulmonary Function Testing. Philadelphia, W. B. Saunders Co., 1977.

Cherniack, R. M.: The oxygen consumption and efficiency of the respiratory muscles in health and emphysema. J. Clin. Invest. 1959; *38*:494–499.

Cherniack, R. M.: The physical properties of the lung in chronic obstructive pulmonary emphysema. J. Clin. Invest. 1956; *35*:394–404.

Cherniack, R. M., and Snidal, D. P.: The effect of obstruction to breathing on the ventilatory response to CO_2. J. Clin. Invest. 1956; *35*:1286–1290.

Chernick, V.: Respiratory problems in children. Semin. Respir. Med. 1979; *1*:99–186.

Clements, J. A.: Surface phenomena in relation to pulmonary function. Physiologist 1962; *5*:11–28.

411

Cumming, G.: Gas mixing efficiency in the human lung. Respir. Physiol. 1967; 2:213–224.

Davies, G., and Reid, L.: Growth of the alveoli and pulmonary arteries in childhood. Thorax 1970; 25:669–681.

Derenne, J. P., Macklem, P. T., and Roussos, C.: The respiratory muscles: mechanics, control and pathophysiology. State of the art. Am. Rev. Respir. Dis. 1978; 118:119–133, 373–390, 581–601.

Ekblom, B., Astrand, P. O., Saltin, B., Stenberg, J., and Wallstrom, B.: Effect of training on circulatory response to exercise. J. Appl. Physiol. 1968; 24:518–528.

Farrell, P. M., and Avery, M. E.: Hyaline membrane disease. State of the art. Am. Rev. Respir. Dis. 1975; 111:657–688.

Filley, G. F.: Acid-Base and Blood Gas Regulation. Philadelphia, Lea and Febiger, 1971.

Finch, C. A., and Lenfant, C.: Oxygen transport in man. N. Engl. J. Med. 1972; 286:407–415.

Fishman, A. P.: Respiratory gases in the regulation of the pulmonary circulation. Physiol. Rev. 1961; 41:214–280.

Forster, R. E.: Exchange of gases between alveolar air and pulmonary capillary blood: pulmonary diffusing capacity. Physiol. Rev. 1957; 37:391–405.

Gell, P. G. K., Coombs, P. S., and Lackman, P. J. (eds.): Clinical Aspects of Immunology. Oxford, Blackwell Press, 1975.

Grassino, A., Goldman, M. D., Mead, J., et al.: Mechanics of the human diaphragm during voluntary contractions: Status. J. Appl. Physiol. 1978; 44:829–839.

Green, G. M.: Alveobronchiolar transport mechanisms. Arch. Intern. Med. 1973; 131:109–114.

Green, G. M.: Lung defense mechanisms. Med. Clin. North Am. 1973; 57:547–562.

Green, G. M., Jakob, G. J., Low, R. B., and Davis, G. S.: Defense mechanisms of the respiratory membrane. Am. Rev. Respir. Dis. 1977; 115:479–514.

Gross, D., Grassino, A., Ross, W. R. D., et al.: Electromyogram pattern of diaphragmatic fatigue. J. Appl. Physiol. 1979; 46:1–7.

Gross, K. W., Klaus, M., Tooley, W. H., and Weisser, K.: The response of the new-born to inflation of the lungs. J. Physiol. (Lond) 1960; 151:551–565.

Guyton, A. C., Granger, H. J., and Taylor, A. E.: Interstitial fluid pressure. Physiol. Rev. 1971; 51:527–563.

Guz, A.: Clinical aspects of the nervous control of breathing. Acta Physiol. Pol., 1971; 22: (Suppl. 2):445–458.

Hills, A. G.: Acid-Base Balance: Chemistry, Physiology, Pathophysiology. Baltimore, Williams & Wilkins Co., 1973.

Hirschman, C. V., McCullough, R. E., and Weill, J. V.: Normal values for hypoxic and hypercapnia ventilatory drives in man. J. Appl. Physiol. 1975; 38:1095–1098.

Hocking, W. G., and Golde, D. W.: The pulmonary alveolar macrophage. N. Engl. J. Med. 1979; 301:580–587, 639–645.

Howell, J. B. L., and Campbell, E. J. M. (eds.): Breathlessness. Philadelphia, F. A. Davis Co., 1966.

Huber, G. L.: Respiratory tract defenses. Semin. Respir. Med. 1980; 1:187–280.

Hyatt, R. E., Okeson, G. C., and Rodarte, J. R.: Influence of expiratory flow limitation on the pattern of lung emptying in normal man. J. Appl. Physiol. 1973; 35:411–419.

Ishizaka, K., and Ishizaka, T.: IgE and reagin hypersensitivity. Ann. N.Y. Acad. Sci. 1971; 190:443–456.

Johnson, R. L., and Miller, J. M.: Distribution of ventilation, blood flow and gas transfer coefficients in the lung. J. Appl. Physiol. 1968; 25:1–15.

Jones, N. L.: Exercise testing in pulmonary evaluation: Clinical applications. N. Engl. J. Med. 1975; 293:339–342.

Jones, N. L.: Exercise testing in pulmonary evaluation. N. Engl. J. Med. 1975; 293:541–544, 647–650.

Jones, N. L., and Campbell, E. J. M.: Clinical Exercise Testing, 2nd ed. Philadelphia, W. B. Saunders Co., 1982.

Junod, A. F.: Metabolism, production and release of hormones and mediators in the lung. State of the art. Am. Rev. Respir. Dis. 1975; 112:93–108.

Kaltreider, H. B.: Expression of immune mechanisms in the lung. State of the art. Am. Rev. Respir. Dis. 1976; 113:345–379.

Kendig, E. L., and Chernick, V.: Disorders of the Respiratory Tract in Children, 4th ed. Philadelphia, W. B. Saunders Co., 1983.

Lenfant, C., and Sullivan, K.: Adaptation to high altitude. N. Engl. J. Med. 1971; *284*:1298–1309.

Leusen, I.: Regulation of cerebrospinal fluid composition with reference to breathing. Physiol. Rev. 1972; *52*:1–56.

Levison, H., and Cherniack, R. M.: Ventilatory cost of exercise in chronic obstructive pulmonary disease. J. Appl. Physiol. 1968; *25*:21–27.

Lob, L., Goldman, M., and Newsom-Davis, J.: The assessment of diaphragm function. Medicine 1977; *56*:165–169.

Lugliani, R., Whipp, B. J., Searl, C., and Wasseman, K.: Effect of bilateral carotid-body resection on ventilatory control at rest and during exercise in man. N. Engl. J. Med. 1971; *285*:1105–1114.

Macklem, P. T.: Tests of lung mechanics. N. Engl. J. Med. 1975; *293*:339–342.

Macklem, P. T.: Relationship between lung mechanics and ventilation distribution. Physiologist 1973; *16*:580–588.

Macklem, P. T.: Obstruction in small airways: a challenge to medicine. Am. J. Med. 1972; *52*:721–724.

Macklem, P. T., Woolcock, A. J., Hogg, J. C., Nadel, J. A., and Wilson, N. J.: Partitioning of pulmonary resistance in the dog. J. Appl. Physiol. 1969; *26*:798–805.

Matsuba, K., and Thurlbeck, W. M.: The number and dimensions of small airways in non-emphysematous lungs. Am. Rev. Respir. Dis. 1971; *104*:516–524.

Mead, J.: Mechanical properties of lungs. Physiol. Rev. 1961; *41*:281–330.

Middleton, E., Jr., Reed, C. E., and Ellis, E. F. (eds.): Allergy: Principles and Practice. St. Louis, C. V. Mosby Co., 1978.

Milic-Emili, J.: Clinical methods for assessing the ventilatory response to carbon dioxide and hypoxia. N. Engl. J. Med. 1975, *293*:864–865.

Milic-Emili, J., and Grunstein, M. M.: Drive and timing components of ventilation. Chest 1976; *70*:131S–133S.

Mitchell, R. A., and Berger, A. J.: Neural regulation of respiration. State of the art. Am. Rev. Respir. Dis. 1975; *111*:206–224.

Naimark, A., and Cherniack, R. M.: Compliance of the respiratory system and its components in health and obesity. J. Appl. Physiol. 1960; *15*:377–382.

Otis, A. B.: The work of breathing. Physiol. Rev. 1954; *34*:449–458.

Otis, A. B., Fenn, W. D., and Rahn, H.: Mechanics of breathing in man. J. Appl. Physiol. 1950; *2*:592–607.

Pengelly, L. D., Rebuck, A. S., and Campbell, E. J. M. (eds.): Loaded Breathing. Edinburgh, Churchill Livingstone, 1974.

Polgar, G., and Promadhat, V.: Pulmonary Function Testing in Children: Techniques and Standards. Philadelphia, W. B. Saunders Co., 1971.

Porter, R. (ed.): Breathing: Hering Breuer Centenary Symposium. London, J. A. Churchill, 1970.

Pride, N. B., Permutt, S., Riley, R. L., and Bomberger-Barnea, B.: Determinants of maximal expiratory flow from the lungs. J. Appl. Physiol. 1967, *23*:646–662.

Proctor, D. F.: The upper airways: nasal physiology and defense of the lungs. Am. Rev. Respir. Dis. 1977; *115*:97–129, 315–342.

Proctor, D. F., Andersen, I., and Lundquist, G.: Clearance of inhaled particles from the human nose. Arch. Intern. Med. 1973; *131*:132–139.

Rochester, D. F., and Campbell, E. J. M.: International symposium on the diaphragm. Am. Rev. Respir. Dis. 1979; *199*:1–177.

Rowell, L. B.: Human cardiovascular adjustments to exercise and thermal stress. Physiol. Rev. 1974; *54*:75–159.

Saltin, G., and Astrand, P.O.: Maximal oxygen uptake in athletes. J. Appl. Physiol. 1967; *23*:353–358.

Scarpelli, E. M.: The Surfactant System of the Lung. Philadelphia, Lea and Febiger, 1968.

Soren, S. C.: The chemical control of ventilation. Acta Physiol. Scand. 1971; *361* (Suppl.):1–72.

Staub, N. C.: Pulmonary edema. Physiol. Rev. 1974; *54*:678–811.

Stossel, T. P.: Phagocytosis. N. Engl. J. Med. 1974; *290*:717–723, 774–780, 833–839.

Szentwanyi, A.: The beta adrenergic theory of the atopic abnormality in bronchial asthma. J. Allergy 1968; *42*:203.

Szidon, J. P., Pietra, G. G., and Fishman, A. P.: The alveolar-capillary membrane and pulmonary edema. N. Engl. J. Med. 1972; *286*:1200–1204.

Thurlbeck, W. M.: Chronic Airflow Obstruction in Lung Disease. Philadelphia, W. B. Saunders Co., 1976.

Thurlbeck, W. M.: Postnatal growth and development of the lung. State of the art. Am. Rev. Respir. Dis. 1975; *111*:803–844.

Tomasi, T. B., Jr.: Secretory immunoglobulins. N. Engl. J. Med. 1972; *287*:500–506.

Wagner, P. D., Laravuso, R. B., Uhi, R. R., and West, J. B.: Continuous distributions of ventilation-perfusion ratios in normal subjects breathing air and 100% O_2. J. Clin. Invest. 1974; *54*:54–68.

Wanner, A.: Clinical aspects of mucociliary transport. State of the art. Am. Rev. Respir. Dis. 1977; *116*:73–125.

Wasserman, K., and Whipp, B. J.: Exercise physiology in health and disease. State of the art. Am. Rev. Respir. Dis. 1975; *112*:219–250.

Wasserman, K., Whipp, B. J., and Castagna, J.: Cardiodynamic hyperpnea: hyperpnea secondary to cardiac output increase. J. Appl. Physiol. 1974; *36*:457–464.

Weibel, E. R.: How does lung structure affect gas exchange? Chest 1983; *83*:651–675.

Weibel, E. R.: Morphological basis of alveolar-capillary gas exchange. Physiol. Rev. 1974; *53*:419–495.

Weibel, E. R.: Morphometry of the Human Lung. New York, Academic Press, 1963.

Weil, J. V., Byrne-Quinn, E., Sodal, I. E., Friesen, W. D., Underhill, B., Filley, G. F., and Grover, R. F.: Hypoxic ventilatory drive in normal man. J. Clin. Invest. 1970; *49*:1061–1072.

Weiser, R. S., Myrvik, Q. N., and Pearsall, N. N.: Fundamentals of Immunology for Students of Medicine and Related Sciences. Philadelphia, Lea and Febiger, 1969.

West, J. B.: Respiratory Physiology: The Essentials. Baltimore, Williams & Wilkins Co., 1974.

West, J. B., Dollery, C. T., and Naimark, A.: Distribution of blood flow in isolated lung; relation to vascular and alveolar pressures. J. Appl. Physiol. 1964; *19*:713–724.

Whipp, B. J., and Wasserman, K.: Alveolar-arterial gas tension differences during graded exercise. J. Appl. Physiol. 1969; *27*:361–365.

Whitelaw, W. A., Derenne, J. P., and Milic-Emili, J.: Occlusion pressure as a measure of respiratory center output in conscious man. Respir. Physiol. 1975; *23*:181–199.

Widdicombe, J. G., and Sterling, G. M.: The autonomic nervous system and breathing. Arch. Intern. Med. 1970; *126*:311–329.

Williams, M. H. (ed.): Disturbance of respiratory control. Clin. Chest Med. 1980; *1*:1.

Woolcock, A. J., Vincent, N. J., and Macklem, P. T.: Frequency dependence of compliance as a test for obstruction in the small airways. J. Clin. Invest. 1969; *48*:1097–1106.

Section II.   Manifestations of Respiratory Disease

Bates, D. V., Macklem, P. T., and Christie, R. V.: Respiratory Function in Disease. Philadelphia, W. B. Saunders Co., 1971.

Campbell, E. J. M., Agostoni, E., and Davis, J. N.: The Respiratory Muscles: Mechanics and Neural Control, 2nd ed. London, Lloyd-Luke (Medical Books) Ltd., 1970.

Cherniack, L.: Chest movements in respiratory diseases. Can. Med. Assoc. J. 1950; *62*:266.

Coury, C.: Hippocratic fingers and hypertrophic osteoarthropathy: A study of 350 cases. Br. J. Dis. Chest 1960; *54*:202–209.

Delp, M. H., and Manning, R. T.: Major's Physical Diagnosis: An Introduction to the Clinical Process, 9th ed. Philadelphia, W. B. Saunders Co., 1981.

Fraser, R. G., and Paré, J. A. P.: Diagnosis of Diseases of the Chest, 2nd ed., vol. 2. Philadelphia, W. B. Saunders Co., 1978.

Guz, A.: Respiratory sensations in man. Br. Med. Bull. 1977; *33*:175–177.

Howell, J. B. L., and Campbell, E. J. M. (eds.): Breathlessness. Philadelphia, F. A. Davis Co., 1966.

Kendig, E. L., and Chernick, V.: Disorders of the Respiratory Tract in Children, 4th ed. Philadelphia, W. B. Saunders Co., 1983.

Murray, J. F.: The Normal Lung: The Basis for Diagnosis and Treatment of Pulmonary Diseases. Philadelphia, W. B. Saunders Co., 1976.

Lillington, G. A., and Jamples, R. W.: A Diagnostic Approach to Chest Diseases. Baltimore, Williams & Wilkins Co., 1977.

Pengelly, L. D., Rebuck, A. S., and Campbell, E. J. M. (eds.): Loaded Breathing. Edinburgh, Churchill Livingstone, 1974.

Porter, R. (ed.): Breathing: Hering Breuer Centenary Symposium. London, J. A. Churchill, 1970.

Section III.   Assessment of Respiratory Disease

Anderson, H. A.: Transbronchoscopic lung biopsy for diffuse pulmonary diseases. Results in 999 patients. Chest 1978; *73*:734S–740S.

Anderson, H. A., Fontana, R. S., and Harrison, E. G., Jr.: Transbronchoscopic lung biopsy in diffuse pulmonary disease. Dis. Chest 1965; *48*:187–192.

Ashkutosh, K., and Keighley, J. F. H.: Diagnostic value of serum angiotensin converting enzyme in lung disease. Thorax 1976; *31*:552–557.

Chai, H., Farr, R. S., Froehlich, L. A., et al.: Standardization of bronchial inhalation challenge procedures. J. Allergy Clin. Immunol. 1975; *56*:323–327.

Cherniack, L.: Chest movements in respiratory diseases. Can. Med. Assoc. J. 1950; *62*:266.

Cockcroft, D. W., Killian, D. N., Mellon, J. J. A., and Hargreave, F. E.: Bronchial reactivity to inhaled histamine. A method and clinical survey. Clin. Allergy 1977; *7*:235–243.

Dutra, F. R., and Geraci, C. L.: Needle biopsy of the lung. JAMA 1954; *155*:21–24.

Felson, B.: Chest Roentgenology. Philadelphia, W. B. Saunders Co., 1973.

Fraser, R. G., and Paré, J. A. P.: Diagnosis of Diseases of the Chest, 2nd ed., vol. 1. Philadelphia, W. B. Saunders Co., 1977.

Godwin, J. D., Speckman, J. M., Fram, E. K., et al.: Distinguishing benign from malignant pulmonary nodules by computed tomography. Radiology 1982; *144*:349–351.

Hargreave, F. E., Pepys, J., Longbottom, J. L., and Wraith, D. G.: Bird breeder's (fancier's) lung. Lancet 1966; *1*:445–449.

Hayes, M., and Taplin, G. V.: Lung imaging with radioaerosols for the assessment of airways disease. Semin. Nucl. Med. 1980; *10*:243–251.

Hyson, E. A., and Ravin, C. E.: Radiographic features of mediastinal anatomy. Chest 1979; *75*:609–613.

Juhl, J. H.: The Essentials of Roentgen Interpretation, 4th ed., New York, Harper & Row, 1981.

Kendig, E. L., and Chernick, V.: Disorders of the Respiratory Tract in Children, 4th ed. Philadelphia, W. B. Saunders Co., 1983.

Lillington, G. A., and Jamples, R. W.: A Diagnostic Approach to Chest Disease: Differential Diagnoses Based on Roentgenographic Patterns, 2nd ed. Baltimore, Williams & Wilkins Co., 1977.

Line, B. R., Fulmer, J. D., Reynolds, H. Y., et al.: Gallium-67 citrate scanning in the staging of idiopathic pulmonary fibrosis: correlation with physiological and morphological features and bronchoalveolar lavage. Am. Rev. Respir. Dis. 1978; *118*:355–365.

Line, B. R., Hunninghake, G. W., Keogh, B. A., et al.: Gallium-67 scanning to stage the alveolitis of sarcoidosis: correlation with clinical studies, pulmonary function studies and bronchoalveolar lavage. Am. Rev. Respir. Dis. 1981; *123*:440–446.

Middleton, E., Jr., Reed, C. E., and Ellis, E. F. (eds.); Allergy: Principles and Practice, St. Louis, C. V. Mosby Co., 1978.

Neumann, R. D., Sostman, H. D., and Gottschalk, A.: Current status of ventilation-perfusion imaging. Semin. Nucl. Med. 1980; *10*:198–217.

Parker, C. D., Belbo, R. E., and Reed, C. E.: Methacholine as a test for bronchial asthma. Arch. Intern. Med. 1965; *155*:452.

Pepys, J., and Hutchcroft, B. J.: Bronchial provocation tests in etiology, diagnosis and analysis of asthma. State of the art. Am. Rev. Respir. Dis. 1975; *112*:829–860.

Phelps, M. E.: Emission computed tomography. Semin. Nucl. Med. 1977; *7*:337.

Potts, D. W., Levin, D. C., and Sahn, S. A.: Pleural fluid pH in parapneumonic effusions. Chest 1976; *70*:328–331.

Sackner, M. A.: Bronchofiberscopy. State of the art. Am. Rev. Respir. Dis. 1975; *111*:62–88.

Sagel, S. S.: Special Procedures in Chest Radiology. Philadelphia, W. B. Saunders Co., 1976.

Sahn, S. A.: Evaluation of pleural effusions and pleural biopsy. *In* Petty, T.L. (ed.): Pulmonary Diagnostic Techniques. Philadelphia, Lea and Febiger, 1975, pp. 105–131.

Sanderson, D. R.: Diagnostic techniques. Semin. Respir. Med. 1981; *3*:1–58.

Schaner, E. G., Change, A. E., Doppman, J. L., et al.: Comparison of computed and conventional whole lung tomography in detecting pulmonary nodules: a prospective radiologic-pathologic study. Am. J. Radiol. 1978; *131*:51–54.

Schwarz, M. I.: The idiopathic interstitial pneumonias. Semin. Respir. Med. 1979; *1*:47–54.

Wagner, H. N., Jr.: The use of radioisotope techniques for the evaluation of patients with pulmonary disease. State of the art. Am. Rev. Respir. Dis. 1976; *133*:203–218.

Weiser, R. S., Myrvik, Q. N., and Pearsall, N. N.: Fundamentals of Immunology for Students of Medicine and Related Sciences. Philadelphia, Lea and Febiger, 1969.

Wolinsky, E.: Nontuberculous mycobacteria and associated diseases. State of the art. Am. Rev. Respir. Dis. 1979; *119*:107–160.

Zornoza, J., Snow, J., Jr., Lukeman, J. M., et al.: Aspiration biopsy of discrete pulmonary lesions using a new thin needle. Radiology 1977; *123*:519–520.

Section IV. The Patterns of Respiratory Disease

Anderson, C. M., and Goodchild, M. C.: Cystic Fibrosis: Manual of Diagnosis and Management. Oxford, Blackwell, 1976.

Austin, K. F., and Orange, R. P.: Bronchial asthma: the possible role of the chemical mediators of immediate hypersensitivity in the pathogenesis of subacute chronic disease. Am. Rev. Respir. Dis. 1975; *112*:423–436.

Bartlett, J. G., and Finegold, S. M.: Anaerobic infections of the lung and pleural space. State of the art. Am. Rev. Respir. Dis. 1974; *110*:56–77.

Bates, D. C., Macklem, P. T., and Christie, R. V.: Respiratory Function in Disease. Philadelphia, W. B. Saunders Co., 1971.

Bates, D. V.: Chronic bronchitis and emphysema. N. Engl. J. Med. 1968; *278*:546–551, 600–604.

Brigham, K. L.: Pulmonary edema. Semin. Respir. Med. 1983; *4*:267–300.

Burwell, C. S., Robin, E. D., Whaley, R. D., and Bickelmann, A. G.: Extreme obesity associated with alveolar hypoventilation: a Pickwickian syndrome. Am. J. Med. 1956; *21*:811–818.

Cherniack, R. M.: Respiratory effects of obesity. Can. Med. Assoc. J. 1959; *80*:613–616.

Cherniack, R. M.: The oxygen consumption and efficiency of the respiratory muscles in health and emphysema. J. Clin. Invest. 1959; *38*:494–499.

Cherniack, R. M.: The physical properties of the lung in chronic obstructive pulmonary emphysema. J. Clin. Invest. 1956; *35*:394–404.

Cherniack, R. M., Cuddy, T. E., and Armstrong, J. B.: The significance of pulmonary elastic and viscous resistance in orthopnea. Circulation 1957; *15*:859–864.

Chernick, V.: Respiratory problems in children. Semin. Respir. Med. 1979; *1*:99–186.

Crystal, R. G., Fulmer, J. D., Roberts, W. C., et al.: Idiopathic pulmonary fibrosis: clinical, histologic, radiographic, physiologic, scintigraphic, cytologic and biochemical aspects. Ann. Intern. Med. 1976; *85*:769–788.

Davidson, P. T.: Mycobacterial diseases of the lungs. Semin. Respir. Med. 1981; *2*:233–239.

di Sant'Agnese, P. A., and Davis, P. B.: Cystic fibrosis in adults. Am. J. Med. 1979; *66*:121–132.

di Sant'Agnese, P. A., and Davis, P. B.: Research in cystic fibrosis. N. Engl. J. Med. 1976; *295*:481–485, 534–541, 597–602.

Drutz, D. J., and Catanzaro, A.: Coccidioidomycosis. State of the art. Am. Rev. Respir. Dis. 1978; *117*:559–585, 727–771.

Farrell, P. M., and Avery, M. E.: Hyaline membrane disease. State of the art. Am. Rev. Respir. Dis. 1975; *111*:657–688.

Fink, J. N.: Hypersensitivity pneumonitis. *In* Middleton, E. Jr., Reed, C. E., and Ellis, E. F. (eds.): Allergy: Principles and Practice, St. Louis, C. V. Mosby Co., 1978.

Fishman, A. P.: Chronic cor pulmonale. State of the art. Am. Rev. Respir. Dis. 1977; *114*:775–794.

Fishman, A. P., and Renkin, E. M.: Pulmonary edema. Bethesda, American Physiological Society, 1979.

Fletcher, C., Peto, R., Trinker, C., and Speizer, F. E.: The Natural History of Chronic Bronchitis and Emphysema. New York, Oxford University Press, 1976.

Fraser, R. G., and Paré, J. A. P.: Diagnosis of Diseases of the Chest, 2nd ed., vol 1. Philadelphia, W. B. Saunders Co., 1977.

Gadek, J., Hunninghake, G. W., Zimmerman, R., et al.: Pathogenetic studies in idiopathic pulmonary fibrosis. Chest 1979; *75*:264–265.

Goodwin, R. A., Jr., and Des Prez, R. M.: Histoplasmosis. State of the art. Am. Rev. Respir. Dis., 1978; *117*:929–956.

Hamman, L., and Rich, A. R.: Acute diffuse interstitial fibrosis of the lungs. Bull. Johns Hopkins Hosp. 1944; *74*:177–212.

Hamman, L., and Rich, A. R.: Fulminating diffuse interstitial fibrosis of the lungs. Trans. Am. Clin. Climatol. Assoc. 1935; *51*:154–163.

Hance, A. J., and Crystal, R. G.: The connective tissue of lung. State of the art. Am. Rev. Respir. Dis. 1975; *112*:657–712.

Hoidal, J. R., and Niewohner, D. E.: Pathogenesis of emphysema. Chest 1983; *83*:679–685.

Hogg, J. C., Macklem, P. T., and Thurlbeck, W. M.: Site and nature of airway obstruction in chronic obstructive lung disease. N. Engl. J. Med. 1968; *278*:1355–1360.

Hunninghake, G. W., and Fauci, A. S.: Pulmonary involvement in collagen vascular diseases. State of the art. Am. Rev. Respir. Dis. 1979; *119*:471–504.

Janoff, A., White, R., Carp, H., Havel, S., Dearing, R., and Lee, D.: Lung injury induced by leukocytic proteases. Am. J. Pathol. 1979; *97*:111–129.

Kaufman, B. J., Ferguson, M. H., and Cherniack, R. M.: Hypoventilation in obesity. J. Clin. Invest. 1959; *38*:500–507.

Kendig, E. L., and Chernick, V.: Disorders of the Respiratory Tract in Children, 4th ed. Philadelphia, W. B. Saunders Co., 1983.

Kueppers, F., and Black, L. F.: Alpha₁-antitrypsin and its deficiency. State of the art. Am. Rev. Respir. Dis. 1974; *110*:176–194.

Lichtenstein, L. M., and Austen, K. F.: Asthma: Physiology, Immunopharmacology and Treatment. New York, Academic Press, 1977.

Lieberman, J.: Clinical syndromes associated with deficient lung fibrinolytic activity. N. Engl. J. Med. 1959; *260*:619–626.

Light, R. W., MacGregor, M. I., Luchsinger, P. C., et al.: Pleural effusions: the diagnostic separation of transudates and exudates. Ann. Intern. Med. 1972; *77*:507–513.

Lillington, G. A., and Jamples, R. W.: A Diagnostic Approach to Chest Diseases. Baltimore, Williams & Wilkins Co., 1977.

Lindskog, G. E., and Halaxz, N. A.: Spontaneous pneumothorax: A consideration of pathogenesis and management with review of 72 hospitalized cases. Arch. Surg. 1957; *75*:693–698.

Lockhart, C. H., and Battaglia, J. D.: Croup (laryngotracheal bronchitis) and epiglottitis. Pediatr. Ann. 1977; *6*:262–269.

Loughlin, G. M., and Taussig, L. M.: Pulmonary function in children with a history of laryngotracheobronchitis. J. Pediatr. 1979; *94*:365–369.

Loughlin, G. M., and Taussig, L. M.: Upper airway obstruction. Semin. Respir. Med. 1979; *1*:131–146.

McCombs, R. P.: Diseases due to immunologic reactions in the lungs. N. Engl. J. Med. 1973; *286*:1186–1194, 1245–1252.

McFadden, E. R., Jr., Ingram, R. H., Jr., Hynes, R. L., and Wellman, J. J.: Predominant site of flow limitation and mechanisms of post-exertional asthma. J. Appl. Physiol. 1977; *42*:746–752.

Middleton, E., Jr., Reed, C. E., and Ellis, E. F. (eds.): Allergy: Principles and Practice, St. Louis, C. V. Mosby Co., 1978.

Mitchell, D. N., and Scadding, J. G.: Sarcoidosis. State of the art. Am. Rev. Respir. Dis. 1974; *110*:774–802.

Morgan, W. K. C., and Seaton, A.: Occupational Lung Diseases. Philadelphia, W. B. Saunders Co., 1975.

Moser, K. M.: Pulmonary embolism. State of the art. Am. Rev. Respir. Dis. 1977; *115*:829–852.

Nadler, H., Rao, G., and Taussig, L. M.: Cystic fibrosis. *In* Stanbury, J. B., Wyngaarden, J. B., and Fredrickson, D. S. (eds.): The Metabolic Basis of Inherited Disease. New York, McGraw-Hill, 1978.

Naimark, A., and Cherniack, R. M.: The compliance of the respiratory system and its components in health and obesity. J. Appl. Physiol. 1960; *15*:377–382.

Norris, R. M., Jones, J. G., and Bishop, J. M.: Respiratory gas exchange in patients with spontaneous pneumothorax. Thorax 1968; *23*:427–433.

Pagtakhan, R. D., and Chernick, V.: Bronchiolitis. *In* Moss, A. J. (ed.): Pediatrics Update: Reviews for Physicians. Elsevier North Holland, Inc., New York, 1980.

Pagtakhan, R. D., Wohl, M. E., and Chernick, V.: Bronchiolitis. Semin. Respir. Med. 1979; *1*:99–105.

Pepys, J.: Hypersensitivity Diseases of the Lungs due to Fungi and Organic Dusts. Basel, Switzerland, S. Karger, 1969.

Pepys, J., and Davies, R. J.: Occupational asthma. *In* Middleton, E., Jr., Reed, C. E., and Ellis, E. F. (eds.): Allergy: Principles and Practice. St. Louis, C. V. Mosby Co., 1978.

Pepys, J., and Hutchcroft, B. J.: Bronchial provocation tests in etiologic diagnosis and analysis of asthma. State of the art. Am. Rev. Respir. Dis. 1975; *112*:829–860.

Petty, T. L.: Chronic respiratory insufficiency. Semin. Respir. Med. 1979; *1*:1–98.

Pierce, A. K., and Sanford, J. P.: Aerobic gram-negative bacillary pneumonias. State of the art. Am. Rev. Respir. Dis. 1974; *110*:647–658.

Potts, D. W. Levin, D. C., and Sahn, S. A.: Pleural fluid pH in parapneumonic effusions. Chest 1976; *70*:328–331.

Rankin, J., Haeschke, W. H., Callies, Q. C., and Dickier, A.: Farmer's lung. Physiopathologic features of the acute interstitial granulomatous pneumonitis of agricultural workers. Ann. Intern. Med. 1962; *57*:606–626.

Reid, L.: The Pathology of Emphysema. Chicago, Year Book Medical Publishers, 1967.

Reid, L.: Measurement of the bronchial mucous gland layer: a diagnostic yardstick in chronic bronchitis. Thorax 1960; *15*:132–141.

Roberts, R. C., and Moore, V. L.: Immunopathogenesis of hypersensitivity pneumonitis. State of the art. Am. Rev. Respir. Dis. 1977; *116*:1075–1090.

Robin, E. D., Cross, C. E., and Zellis, R.: Pulmonary edema. N. Engl. J. Med. 1973; *288*:239–246, 292–304.

Ruckley, C. V., and McCormick, R. J. M.: The management of spontaneous pneumothorax. Thorax 1966; *21*:139–144.

Sahn, S. A.: Evaluation of pleural effusions and pleural biopsy. *In* Petty, T. L., (ed.): Pulmonary Diagnostic Techniques. Philadelphia, Lea and Febiger, 1975, pp. 105–131.

Scadding, J. G., and Hinson, K. F. W.: Diffuse fibrosing alveolitis (diffuse interstitial fibrosis of the lungs). Correlation of histology at biopsy with prognosis. Thorax 1967; *22*:291–304.

Schatz, M., Patterson, R., and Fink, J.: Immunologic lung disease. N. Engl. J. Med. 1979; *300*:1310–1320.

Schwarz, M. I.: The idiopathic interstitial pneumonias. Semin. Respir. Med. 1979; *1*:47–54.

Staub, N. C.: Lung water and solute exchange. New York, Marcel Dekker, 1978.

Staub, N. C.: Pathogenesis of pulmonary edema. State of the art. Am. Rev. Respir. Dis. 1974; *109*:358–372.

Staub, N. C.: Pulmonary edema. Physiol. Rev. 1974; *54*:678–811.

Straus, R. H., McFadden, E. R., Jr., Ingram, R. H., Jr., and Jaeger, J. J.: Enhancement of exercise-induced asthma by cold air. N. Engl. J. Med. 1977; *297*:743.

Szentwany, A.: The beta adrenergic theory of the atopic abnormality in bronchial asthma. J. Allergy 1968; *42*:203.

Thurlbeck, W. M.: Chronic Airflow Obstruction in Lung Disease. Philadelphia, W. B. Saunders Co., 1976.

Thurlbeck, W. M., Henderson, J. A. M., Fraser, R. G., and Bates, D. V.: Chronic obstructive lung diseases: a comparison between clinical, roentgenologic, functional, and morphologic criteria in chronic bronchitis, emphysema, asthma, and bronchiectasis. Medicine 1970; *49*:81–145.

Turner-Warwick, M.: Immunological aspects of systemic diseases of the lungs. Proc. R. Soc. Med. 1974; *67*:541–547.

Weiser, R. S., Myrvik, Q. N., and Pearsall, N. N.: Fundamentals of Immunology for Students of Medicine and Related Sciences. Philadelphia, Lea and Febiger, 1969.

Weiss, E. B., and Segal, M. S.: Bronchial Asthma: Mechanisms and Therapeutics. Boston, Little, Brown & Co., 1976.

Williams, M. H.: Asthma and airway reactivity. Semin. Respir. Med. 1980; *1*:4.

Wohl, M. E. B., and Chernick, V.: Bronchiolitis. State of the art. Am. Rev. Respir. Dis. 1978; *118*:759–781.

Wood, R. E., Boat, T. F., and Doershuk, C. F.: Cystic fibrosis. State of the art. Am. Rev. Respir. Dis. 1976; *113*:833–878.

Yam, L. T.: Diagnostic significance of lymphocytes in pleural effusions. Ann. Intern. Med. 1967; *66*:972–982.

Ziskind, M., Jones, R. N., and Weill, H.: Silicosis. State of the art. Am. Rev. Respr. Dis. 1976; *113*:643–666.

Section V.   Respiratory Failure

Bachofen, M., Bachofen, H., and Weibel, E. R.: Lung edema in the adult respiratory distress syndrome. *In* Fishman, A. P., and Fenkim, E. M. (eds.): Pulmonary Edema. Bethesda, Md., American Physiological Society, 1979.

Bergofsky, E. H.: Respiratory failure in disorders of the thoracic cage. 1979; *119*:643–670.

Block, A. J.: Oxygen administration in the home. Am. Rev. Respir. Dis. 1977; *115*:897–899.

Block, A. J., Boysen, P. G., Wynne, J. W., et al.: Sleep apnea, hypopnea and oxygen desaturation in normal subjects. N. Engl. J. Med. 1979; *300*:513–517.

Campbell, E. J. M.: The J. Burns Amberson Lecture. The management of acute respiratory failure in chronic bronchitis and emphysema. Am. Rev. Respir. Dis. 1967; *96*:626–639.

Cherniack, R. M.: The management of acute respiratory failure. Chest 1970; *58*(Suppl. 2):427–436.

Cherniack, R. M.: The management of respiratory failure in chronic obstructive lung disease. Ann. N.Y. Acad. Sci. 1965; *121*:942–958.

Cherniack, R. M., and Goldberg, I.: The effect of nebulized bronchodilator delivered with and without IPPB on ventilatory function in chronic obstructive emphysema. Am. Rev. Respir. Dis. 1965; *91*:13–20.

Cherniack, R. M., and Hakimpour, K.: The rational use of oxygen in respiratory insufficiency. JAMA 1967; *199*:178–182.

Cherniack, R. M., Handford, R. G., and Svanhill, E.: Home care of chronic respiratory disease. JAMA 1969; *208*:821–824.

Cherniack, R. M., and Svanhill, E.: Long-term use of intermittent positive-pressure breathing (IPPB) in chronic obstructive pulmonary disease. Am. Rev. Respir. Dis. 1976; *113*:721–728.

Chester, E. H., Belman, M. J., Bahler, R. C., Baum, G. L., Schey, G., and Bach, P.: Multidisciplinary treatment of chronic pulmonary insufficiency. 3. The effect of physical training on cardiopulmonary performance in patients with chronic obstructive pulmonary disease. Chest 1977; *72*:695–702.

Dudley, D. L., and Welke, E.: How to Survive Being Alive. New York, Doubleday, Inc., 1977.

Farrell, P., and Avery, M. E.: Hyaline membrane disease. State of the art. Am. Rev. Respir. Dis. 1975; *111*:657–688.

Fernandez, E., and Cherniack, R. M.: The use and abuse of ventilators. *In* Isselbacher, K. J., Adams, R. D., Braunwald, E., Martin, J. B., Petersdorf, R. G., and Wilson, J. D. (eds.): Principles of Internal Medicine (Update II). New York, McGraw-Hill, 1982, pp. 165–184.

Flenley, D. C.: Respiratory failure. Scott. Med. J. 1970; *15*:61–72.

Grant, I., Heaton, R. K., McSweeny, A. J., Adams, K. M., and Timms, R. M.: Neuropsychologic findings in hypoxemic chronic obstructive pulmonary disease. Arch. Intern. Med. 1982; *142*:1470–1476.

Guilleminault, C., Eldridge, F. L., and Dement, W. C.: Insomnia with sleep apnea. A new syndrome. Science 1973; *181*:856–858.

Guilleminault, C., Telkion, A., and Dement, W. C.: The sleep apnea syndromes. Ann. Rev. Med. 1976; *27*:465–484.

Harris, P.: Principles of management of cor pulmonale. Chest 1970; *58*(Suppl. 2):437–440.

Hudson, L. D.: Adult respiratory distress syndrome. Semin. Respir. Med. 1981; *2*:99–174.

James, O. F.: Critical care medicine. Semin. Respir. Med. 1982; *3*:219–312.

Leith, D. E., and Bradley, M.: Ventilatory muscle strength and endurance training. J. Appl. Physiol. 1976; *41*:508–516.

Lertzman, M. M., and Cherniack, R. M.: Rehabilitation of patients with chronic obstructive pulmonary disease. State of the art. Am. Rev. Respir. Dis. 1976; *114*:1145–1166.

McSweeny, A. J., Grant, J., Heaton, R. K., Adams, K. M., and Timms, R. M.: Life quality of patients with chronic obstructive pulmonary disease. Arch. Intern. Med. 1982; *142*:473–478.

Medical Research Council Working Party: Long-term domiciliary oxygen therapy in chronic hypoxic cor pulmonale complicating chronic bronchitis and emphysema. Lancet 1981; *1*:681.

Mendella, L. A., Manfreda, J., Warren, C. P. W., and Anthonisen, N. R.: Steroid response in stable chronic obstructive pulmonary disease. Ann. Intern. Med. 1982; *96*:17–21.

Miller, W. F.: Rehabilitation of patients with chronic obstructive lung disease. Med. Clin. North Am. 1967; *51*:349–361.

Nicotra, M. B., Rivera, M., and Awe, R. J.: Antibiotic therapy of acute exacerbations of chronic bronchitis. A controlled study using tetracycline. Ann. Intern. Med. 1982; *97*:18–21.

Nocturnal Oxygen Therapy Trial Group. Continuous or nocturnal oxygen therapy in hypoxemic chronic obstructive lung disease: a clinical trial. Ann. Intern. Med. 1980; *93*:391–398.

Pardy, R. L., Rivington, R. N., Despas, P. J., and Macklem, P. T.: The effect of inspiratory muscle training on exercise performance in chronic air flow limitation. Am. Rev. Respir. Dis. 1981; *123*:426–433.

Petty, T. L.: Intensive and Rehabilitation Care. Philadelphia, Lea and Febiger, 1982.

Petty, T. L.: Chronic respiratory insufficiency. Semin. Respir. Med. 1979, *1*:1–98.

Petty, T. L.: Chronic Obstructive Pulmonary Disease. New York, Marcel Dekker, 1978.

Petty, T. L.: Ambulatory care for emphysema and chronic bronchitis. Chest 1970; *58*(Suppl. 2):441–448.

Petty, T. L., Ashbaugh, D. G.: The adult respiratory distress syndrome (clinical features, factors influencing prognosis and principles of management). Chest 1971; *60*:233–239.

Phillipson, E. A.: Regulation of breathing during sleep. State of the art. Am. Rev. Respir. Dis. 1977; *115*:217S–224S.

Remmers, J. E., DeGroot, W. S., Sauerland, E. K., et al.: Pathogenesis of upper airway occlusion during sleep. J. Appl. Physiol. 1978, *44*:931–938.

Riley, I. D., Tarr, P. J., Andrew, M., et al.: Immunization with a polyvalent pneumococcal vaccine: Reduction of adult respiratory morbidity in a New Guinea Highland community. Lancet 1977; *1*:1338–1341.

Rowlett, D. B., and Dudley, D. L.: Psychosocial and psychophysiologic issues in COPD. Psychosomatics 1978; *19*:273.

Schaffer, A. J., and Avery, M. E.: Diseases of the Newborn, 4th ed. Philadelphia, W. B. Saunders Co., 1977.

Wolfsdorf, J., Swift, D. L., and Avery, M. E.: Mist therapy reconsidered: an evaluation of the respiratory deposition of labelled water aerosols produced by jet and ultrasonic nebulizers. Pediatrics 1969; *43*:799–808.

Wynne, J. W., Block, A. J., Hemenway, J., et al.: Disordered breathing and oxygen desaturation during sleep in patients with chronic obstructive lung disease (COLD). Am. J. Med. 1979; *66*:573–579.

INDEX